New Perspectives on Cardiovascular Disease: Women's Treatment and Management

New Perspectives on Cardiovascular Disease: Women's Treatment and Management

Editors

Silvia Maffei
Antonella Meloni

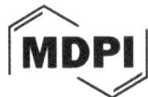

Basel • Beijing • Wuhan • Barcelona • Belgrade • Novi Sad • Cluj • Manchester

Editors

Silvia Maffei
Fondazione Toscana Gabriele
Monasterio, Cardiovascular
Endocrinology and
Metabolism Medicine
and Surgery
Pisa
Italy

Antonella Meloni
Department of Radiology
Fondazione G. Monasterio
CNR-Regione Toscana
Pisa
Italy

Editorial Office
MDPI
St. Alban-Anlage 66
4052 Basel, Switzerland

This is a reprint of articles from the Special Issue published online in the open access journal *Journal of Clinical Medicine* (ISSN 2077-0383) (available at: https://www.mdpi.com/journal/jcm/special_issues/women_cardiovascular).

For citation purposes, cite each article independently as indicated on the article page online and as indicated below:

Lastname, A.A.; Lastname, B.B. Article Title. *Journal Name* **Year**, *Volume Number*, Page Range.

ISBN 978-3-7258-0735-2 (Hbk)
ISBN 978-3-7258-0736-9 (PDF)
doi.org/10.3390/books978-3-7258-0736-9

© 2024 by the authors. Articles in this book are Open Access and distributed under the Creative Commons Attribution (CC BY) license. The book as a whole is distributed by MDPI under the terms and conditions of the Creative Commons Attribution-NonCommercial-NoDerivs (CC BY-NC-ND) license.

Contents

Jack Charles Barton, Anna Wozniak, Chloe Scott, Abhisekh Chatterjee,
Greg Nathan Titterton, Amber Elyse Corrigan, et al.
Between-Sex Differences in Risk Factors for Cardiovascular Disease among Patients with
Myocardial Infarction—A Systematic Review
Reprinted from: *J. Clin. Med.* **2023**, *12*, 5163, doi:10.3390/jcm12155163 . . . . **1**

Anna Vittoria Mattioli, Valentina Selleri, Giada Zanini, Milena Nasi, Marcello Pinti,
Claudio Stefanelli, et al.
Physical Activity and Diet in Older Women: A Narrative Review
Reprinted from: *J. Clin. Med.* **2023**, *12*, 81, doi:10.3390/jcm12010081 . . . . **14**

Valentina Bucciarelli, Anna Vittoria Mattioli, Susanna Sciomer, Federica Moscucci,
Giulia Renda and Sabina Gallina
The Impact of Physical Activity and Inactivity on Cardiovascular Risk across Women's Lifespan:
An Updated Review
Reprinted from: *J. Clin. Med.* **2023**, *12*, 4347, doi:10.3390/jcm12134347 . . . . **27**

Luca Fazzini, Mattia Casati, Alessandro Martis, Ferdinando Perra, Paolo Rubiolo,
Martino Deidda, et al.
Gender Effect on Clinical Profiles, Pharmacological Treatments and Prognosis in Patients
Hospitalized for Heart Failure
Reprinted from: *J. Clin. Med.* **2024**, *13*, 881, doi:10.3390/jcm13030881 . . . . **46**

Silvia Maffei, Antonella Meloni, Martino Deidda, Susanna Sciomer, Lucia Cugusi, Christian
Cadeddu, et aL.
Cardiovascular Risk Perception and Knowledge among Italian Women: Lessons from IGENDA
Protocol
Reprinted from: *J. Clin. Med.* **2022**, *11*, 1695, doi:10.3390/jcm11061695 . . . . **59**

Christine Friedrich, Mohamed Salem, Thomas Puehler, Bernd Panholzer, Lea Herbers, Julia
Reimers, et al.
Sex-Specific Risk Factors for Short- and Long-Term Outcomes after Surgery in Patients with
Infective Endocarditis
Reprinted from: *J. Clin. Med.* **2022**, *11*, 1875, doi:10.3390/jcm11071875 . . . . **70**

Jose M. De Miguel-Yanes, Rodrigo Jimenez-Garcia, Javier De Miguel-Diez,
Valentin Hernández-Barrera, David Carabantes-Alarcon, Jose J. Zamorano-Leon, et al.
Differences in Sex and the Incidence and In-Hospital Mortality among People Admitted for
Infective Endocarditis in Spain, 2016–2020
Reprinted from: *J. Clin. Med.* **2022**, *11*, 6847, doi:10.3390/jcm11226847 . . . . **84**

Beatrice Dal Pino, Francesca Gorini, Melania Gaggini, Patrizia Landi, Alessandro Pingitore
and Cristina Vassalle
Lipoprotein(a), Cardiovascular Events and Sex Differences: A Single Cardiological Unit
Experience
Reprinted from: *J. Clin. Med.* **2023**, *12*, 764, doi:10.3390/jcm12030764 . . . . **96**

Raffaella Ronco, Federico Rea, Amelia Filippelli, Aldo Pietro Maggioni and Giovanni Corrao
Sex-Related Differences in Outpatient Healthcare of Acute Coronary Syndrome: Evidence from
an Italian Real-World Investigation
Reprinted from: *J. Clin. Med.* **2023**, *12*, 2972, doi:10.3390/jcm12082972 . . . . **105**

Federica Moscucci, Susanna Sciomer, Silvia Maffei, Antonella Meloni, Ilaria Lospinuso, Myriam Carnovale, et al.
Sex Differences in Repolarization Markers: Telemonitoring for Chronic Heart Failure Patients
Reprinted from: *J. Clin. Med.* **2023**, *12*, 4714, doi:10.3390/jcm12144714 . . . . **117**

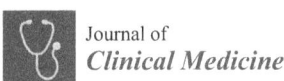

Systematic Review

Between-Sex Differences in Risk Factors for Cardiovascular Disease among Patients with Myocardial Infarction—A Systematic Review

Jack Charles Barton [1,*], Anna Wozniak [1], Chloe Scott [1], Abhisekh Chatterjee [2], Greg Nathan Titterton [3], Amber Elyse Corrigan [4], Ashvin Kuri [3], Viraj Shah [2], Ian Soh [5] and Juan Carlos Kaski [6]

[1] Critical Care and Perioperative Medicine Research Group, William Harvey Research Institute, Queen Mary University of London, London E1 4NS, UK; anna.wozniak3@nhs.net (A.W.); chloe.scott19@nhs.net (C.S.)
[2] Department of Medicine, Faculty of Medicine, Imperial College London, London SW7 2AZ, UK; abhisekh.chatterjee20@imperial.ac.uk (A.C.); viraj.shah19@imperial.ac.uk (V.S.)
[3] Barts and the London School of Medicine and Dentistry, Queen Mary University of London, London E1 4NS, UK; g.n.titterton20@smd.qmul.ac.uk (G.N.T.); a.a.kuri@smd17.qmul.ac.uk (A.K.)
[4] Department of Medicine, Kings College London, London SE5 9RS, UK; amber.corrigan1@nhs.net
[5] St. George's University of London, London SW17 0RE, UK; ian.soh23@gmail.com
[6] Molecular and Clinical Sciences Research Institute, St. George's University of London, London SW17 0RE, UK; jkaski@sgul.ac.uk
* Correspondence: jack.barton@nhs.net

Abstract: Between-sex differences in the presentation, risk factors, management, and outcomes of acute myocardial infarction (MI) are well documented. However, as such differences are highly sensitive to cultural and social changes, there is a need to continuously re-evaluate the evidence. The present contemporary systematic review assesses the baseline characteristics of men and women presenting to secondary, tertiary, and quaternary centres with acute myocardial infarction (MI). Over 1.4 million participants from 18 studies, including primary prospective, cross sectional and retrospective observational studies, as well as secondary analysis of registry data are included in the study. The study showed that women were more likely than men to have a previous diagnosis of diabetes, hypertension, cerebrovascular disease, and heart failure. They also had lower odds of presenting with previous ischaemic heart disease and angina, dyslipidaemia, or a smoking history. Further work is necessary to understand the reasons for these differences, and the role that gender-specific risk factors may have in this context. Moreover, how these between-gender differences are implicated in management and outcomes also requires further work.

Keywords: risk factors; myocardial infarction; sex; gender; women

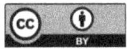

1. Introduction

Sex- and gender-bias is ubiquitous within medicine [1–3]. Cardiovascular medicine, and the management of myocardial infarction (MI) in particular, has long been considered a 'disease for men'. Yet, whilst there is a higher incidence of MI in men, women tend to experience greater mortality when adjusting for age and other known confounders [4,5]. Women who survive also tend to report lower quality of life post-MI irrespective of age of presentation [6,7].

Even for the most well-evidenced therapies such as percutaneous coronary intervention (PCI), data overwhelmingly suggests that women are offered PCI less frequently, whilst experiencing lower success rates and increased complication rates [5,8–10]. Such differences span the entire spectrum of MI care, from acute treatment to chronic management, with women also experiencing lower rates of enrolment in cardiac rehabilitation programmes [11]. Adverse outcomes are exacerbated by ethnicity and socioeconomic status, making subsets of the population particularly vulnerable [12].

Psychosocial factors and systemic bias are also key contributors to worse outcomes in women [5,13]. Some data even suggests that adjusting for said bias all but removes the gender-outcome gap [12]. Clinical guidelines are also susceptible, given that the majority of the evidence base from which they are derived reports data collected disproportionately from men [14].

Genetic and phenotypical differences between genders explain a proportion of the differences in observed outcomes. For example, there are known gender differences in the pathophysiology of MI. Women tend to experience a greater degree of plaque erosion and embolisation, and also experience more diffuse atherosclerotic disease [15]. They are also more likely to develop microvascular and endothelial dysfunction, making their pathology less amenable to conventional therapies [15]. It follows, then, that the risk factors associated with MI in women may not be the same as those associated with MI in men. Even for shared risk factors, prevalence and associated risk are likely to vary. The same can be said for presenting clinical features [16]. In turn, these factors are likely to contribute to delayed, or incorrect diagnosis in women.

Considering the disproportionate risk faced by women, and the gender differences in the pathophysiology and presentation of MI in women, it is not enough to merely be cognisant of one's own individual and systemic bias. We must instead evaluate the unique and dynamically changing factors which drive gender-based differences in presentation and outcomes, and integrate these findings into the evidence base underlying clinical guidelines and decision making in clinical practice. For example, whilst previous systematic reviews in this area have identified fixed risk factors in women, such as the post-menopausal loss of oestrogenic protection [17], others have identified dynamic factors that are influenced by changes to the cultural and political landscape including but not limited to physical inactivity, dietary choices, cigarette smoking, and contraceptive choices [17–19]. Sex-specific risk factors (which will not be addressed exhaustively in the present review) are also likely to play a major role, but are not generally included in risk assessment algorithms in clinical practice [5,15]. Greater understanding of these risk factors will inform better clinical and policy decisions that are applicable to both men and women. It could be argued that work in this field to date has contributed to the significant improvement already observed in bridging the gendered MI gap [20].

A first step in updating the literature is to consider the presence of shared, known cardiovascular risk factors between genders, and identify current knowledge gaps in the field that require further investigation. We have performed a systematic review of the last ten years of literature in order to achieve this.

2. Materials and Methods

The protocol for this systematic review was registered on PROSPERO (PROSPERO ID: CRD42022373892). It was conducted in accordance with the PRISMA statement [21].

2.1. Selection Criteria

Studies were considered if they reported risk factors by gender in those who had experienced MI either as baseline characteristics, primary, or secondary outcome. Prospective observational and retrospective observational studies of either primary or secondary data, including data originating from registries, were considered. For inclusion, the paper must have been published between January 2012 and September 2022, must have been written in English (or translated), and must have been available via institutional access.

Study population/participant inclusion criteria: any adult $\geq$ 16 y/o presenting to a secondary/tertiary care facility with myocardial infarction as defined by clinical evidence of acute myocardial ischaemia with a rise of cardiac high-sensitivity cardiac troponin T (>14 ng/L OR at least one value >99th percentile) or troponin I (>0.04 ng/mL at least one value >99th percentile), within 6 h of the onset of symptoms and at least one of the following: symptoms of myocardial ischaemia (cardiac chest pain); new or increased and persistent ST-segment elevation in at least two contiguous leads of ≥ 1 mm in all leads, other than V2-3 where elevation is ≥ 2.5 mm in men <40 y/o, ≥ 2 mm in men > 40 y/o, ≥ 1.5 mm in women; new horizontal or downsloping ST depression ≥ 0.5 mm in two contiguous leads and/or T wave inversion >1 m in two contiguous leads with prominent R wave or R/S ratio > 1; pathological Q waves; new or recent onset left bundle branch block; dynamic troponin T or I rise (>20% variation); regional wall motion abnormality evidenced on cardiac imaging performed within the Emergency Department [22,23]. Alternatively, studies were included if they fulfilled all other criteria and patients were deemed to have acute coronary syndrome by the senior clinician in charge of their care if the criteria for myocardial infarction was not otherwise explicitly described within the methodology, or if appropriate local or regional definition of MI was applied.

2.2. Literature Search

Two researchers (JB, GNT) performed an initial database search of MEDLINE, EMBASE, and CENTRAL, which was conducted between 16 and 25 November 2022. Search terms for each database can be found in Supplementary Materials.

2.3. Study Selection and Data Extraction

All titles were screened by seven researchers (JB, AW, GNT, NW, CS, VS, IS), split into teams of two/three screening one database per team. If article titles were deemed to meet inclusion criteria by the two screening researchers, they were uploaded to Mendeley (Mendeley.com accessed on 20 November 2022; Mendeley Ltd., London, UK). References were then downloaded as an RIS rile and uploaded to Rayyan (rayyan.ai 4 December 2022; Rayyan Systems Inc., Cambridge, MA, USA). Duplicates were then removed.

Each article was then screened by a minimum of two researchers (all except JB, AK and JCK) to assess suitability. Where there was non-consensus between the two screening researchers, a third reviewer (JB) was sought from the research team. If the abstract was deemed to meet inclusion criteria a full paper review was then conducted, again by two researchers with a third opinion sought (primary author—JB) if there was non-consensus after initial screening.

Data extraction was undertaken at the point at which the second, or third assessor if non-consensus, deemed the study to meet inclusion criteria after full text review and was undertaken by a group of three researchers (JB, AK, AC). Information extracted included article title and DOI, citation and reference information, year of publication, study type, country/countries of data collection, number of centres, start and end date of data collection, recruitment method, participant characteristics and demographic details, prevalence of reported risk factors, inpatient mortality by sex, and additional information deemed relevant by the researcher.

2.4. Quality Assessment/Risk of Bias

Risk of bias assessment was undertaken if the second, or third assessor if non-consensus, deemed the study to meet inclusion criteria after full text review. One researcher not involved with initial data screening (AK) performed risk of bias assessment using the Newcastle–Ottawa Scale [24]. Each study was assessed as either high, medium, or low quality after assessment of the following domains: selection; comparability; outcome. Second opinion was sought with the lead author (JB) as deemed necessary. Outcomes of the risk of bias assessment are presented in Supplementary File S1.

2.5. Statistical Analysis

Meta-analysis was not performed due to high heterogeneity between studies. Heterogeneity was attributed to a combination of primary and secondary data sources, as well as prospective and retrospective observational studies in heterogenous populations.

Fisher's exact test and pooled odds ratios were calculated using contingency tables for all included risk factors. Alpha level was set at <5%.

3. Results

3.1. Search Results

The PRISMA flow diagram is presented in Figure 1. A total of 117 unique studies underwent full text review, 99 were excluded (see Figure 1).

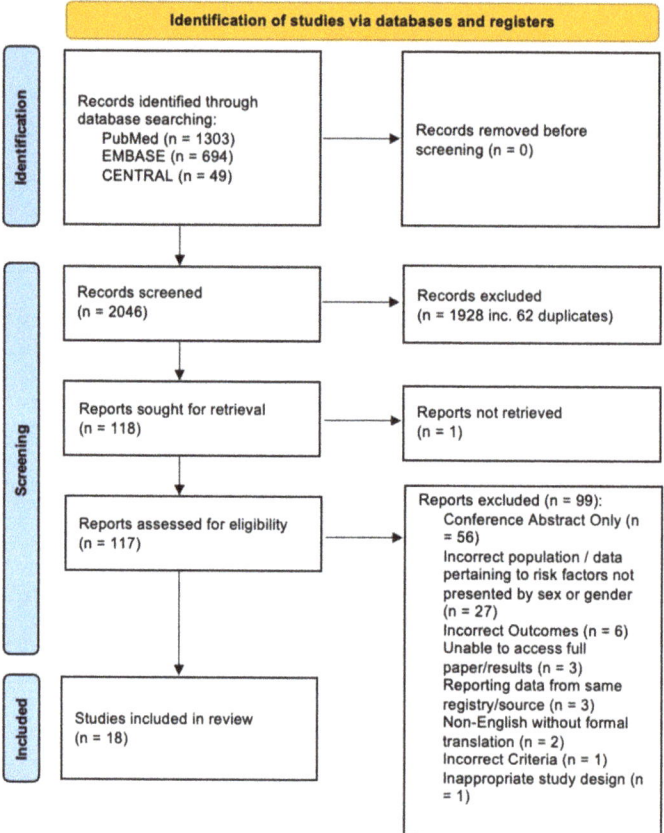

Figure 1. PRISMA flow diagram of the search and screening process.

3.2. Study Characteristics

Of the eighteen included studies, eleven were based in Europe (two in the United Kingdom [25,26], one in Germany [27], one in Iceland [28], one in Portugal [29], two in Sweden [30,31], one in Switzerland [32], one in Italy [33], one in the Netherlands [34], one in France [35]), two in the United States of America [16,36], two in India [37,38], one in Iran [39], one in Vietnam [40], and one in Australia [41]. Thirteen of the included studies were retrospective cohort studies [16,26–36,40], two were prospective cohort studies [25,41], two were cross-sectional studies [37,39], and one was a retrospective analysis of a prospective interventional trial [38]. In total, 580,524 women (median = 1021; IQR = 5431) and 898,800 men (median = 3220.5; IQR = 15,215.8) were included across the studies. See Table 1 for study characteristics.

Table 1. Characteristics of included studies. Myocardial infarction (MI); percutaneous coronary intervention (PCI); ST-elevation myocardial infarction (STEMI).

First Author, Year of Publication	Country	Study Design	Population	Recruitment Method	Women (%)	Men (%)	Mean/Median Age (SD/IQR) Women	Mean/Median Age (SD/IQR) Men
Ahmadi et al. (2015) [39]	Iran	Cross sectional	Patients admitted with acute MI	Registry data	5717 (27.55)	15,033 (72.45)	65.4 (12.6)	59.6 (13.3)
Asleh et al. (2021) [36]	United States of America	Retrospective cohort	Patients admitted with acute MI	Retrospective electronic chart review	764 (39)	1195 (61)	73.8 (14.1)	64.2 (14)
Bajaj et al. (2016) [37]	India	Cross-sectional	Patients admitted with acute MI	Prospective recruitment of patients presenting with acute MI	50 (50)	50 (50)	62 (SD not reported)	56.5 (SD not reported)
Baumann et al. (2016) [27]	Germany	Retrospective cohort	Patients undergoing emergency PCI for acute MI	Registry data	216 (26.9)	587 (73.1)	66.8 (14.1)	60.9 (12.8)
Canto et al. (2012) [16]	United States of America	Retrospective cohort	Patients admitted with acute MI	Registry data	481,581 (42.11)	661,932 (57.89)	73.9 (12.4)	66.5 (13.2)
Dreyer et al. (2013) [41]	Australia	Prospective cohort	Patients attending PCI centre with STEMI.	Registry data	234 (25.66)	678 (74.34)	67 (14)	60 (13)
Gardarsdottir et al. (2022) [28]	Iceland	Retrospective cohort	Patients who underwent acute coronary angiography for acute MI	Retrospective analysis of prospective interventional trial dataset	625 (24.1)	1969 (75.9)	With STEMI: 68.5 (13.3) With NSTEMI: 71.0 (11.4)	With STEMI: 61.9 (12.1) With NSTEMI: 67.1 (11.6)
Khraishah et al. (2021) [38]	India	Retrospective analysis of prospective interventional trial	Patients admitted with acute MI	Prospective recruitment of all patients undergoing primary PCI at centre	5191 (24.29)	16,183 (75.71)	65 (12)	58 (12)
Krishnamurthy et al. (2019) [25]	United Kingdom	Prospective cohort	Patients undergoing primary PCI for STEMI	Retrospective electronic chart review	826 (27.09)	2223 (72.91)	69 (20)	60 (19)
Leurent et al. (2014) [35]	France	Retrospective cohort	Patients admitted with STEMI within 24 h.	Registry data	1174 (23.48)	3826 (76.52)	68.8 (14)	60.8 (12)
Nguyen et al. (2014) [40]	Vietnam	Retrospective cohort	Patients admitted with acute MI	Registry data	101 (33.44)	201 (66.56)	70 (10)	64 (12)
Ortalani et al. (2013) [33]	Italy	Retrospective cohort	Patients undergoing PCI for acute MI.	Registry data	5093 (27.75)	13,258 (72.25)	72.3 (11.2)	64.6 (12.1)
Radovanovic et al. (2012) [32]	Switzerland	Retrospective cohort	Patients presenting with STEMI.	Registry data	5786 (26.76)	15,834 (73.24)	71.5 (12.6)	62.9 (13)
Rashid et al. (2020) [26]	England and Wales	Retrospective cohort	Patients admitted with a diagnosis of NSTEMI	Registry data	40,811 (29.7%)	96,455 (70.3%)	Low Risk: 65 (55–74); Intermediate Risk: 69 (60–76); High Risk: 72 (62–79)	Low Risk: 60 (52–68); Intermediate Risk: 64 (56–72); High Risk: 66 (56–75)

Table 1. Cont.

First Author, Year of Publication	Country	Study Design	Population	Recruitment Method	Women (%)	Men (%)	Mean/Median Age (SD/IQR) Women	Mean/Median Age (SD/IQR) Men
Redfors et al. (2015) [31]	Sweden	Retrospective cohort	All patients treated for acute MI	Registry data	17,068 (35.47)	31,050 (64.53)	75 (12)	68 (12)
Roque et al. (2020) [29]	Portugal	Retrospective cohort	Patients admitted with acute MI	Registry data	14,177 (28.87)	34,936 (71.13)	72(12)	67(13)
Strömbäck et al. (2017) [30]	Sweden	Retrospective cohort	Patients admitted with acute MI	Registry data	242 (23.8)	775 (76.2)	61.3 (8.3)	55.8 (8.4)
Velders et al. (2013) [34]	Netherlands	Retrospective cohort	Patients who underwent primary PCI for STEMI	Prospective recruitment of all patients undergoing PCI for STEMI	868 (24.92)	2615 (75.08)	67.6 (13.1)	61.8 (11.9)

3.3. Quality Assessment

All studies were deemed to be of high quality, with the exception of Roque et al. [29] which was deemed to be of medium quality. See the Supplementary Materials for the full risk of bias assessment.

3.4. Risk Factors

Data pertaining to the odds of reported risk factors and baseline characteristics of women and men with myocardial infarction are presented in Table 2. Pooled odds ratios are displayed in Figure 2.

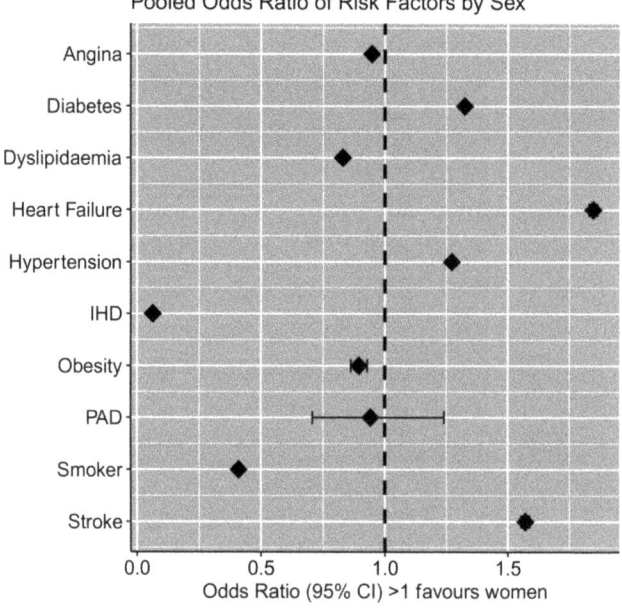

Figure 2. Pooled odds ratios for reported cardiovascular risk factors. Ischaemic heart disease (IHD); peripheral arterial disease (PAD). Note: ischaemic heart disease and angina reported independently as per results.

Table 2. Reported prevalence of baseline characteristics and risk factors of included studies. Myocardial infarction (MI); ST-elevation myocardial infarction (STEMI).

Citation	Obesity			Diabetes			Hypertension			Stroke			Dyslipidaemia/ Hypercholesterolaemia			Angina			Heart Failure			IHD/Previous Myocardial Infarction			Peripheral Artery Disease			Current/Ex Smoker		
	W	M	p	W	M	p	W	M	p	W	M	p	W	M	p	W	M	p	W	M	p	W	M	p	W	M	p	W	M	p
Ahmadi et al. (2015) [39]				33.4	18	<0.001	53.7	28.6	<0.001				25.3	15	<0.001													20.1	28.5	<0.001
Asleh et al. (2021) [36]				25.8	23.2	<0.001	79.9	62.4	<0.001				66.1	63.4	0.234													16.7	25	<0.001
Bajaj et al. (2016) [37]				52	24	0.004	46	28	0.062																			0	44	<0.001
Baumann et al. (2016) [27]				24.1	24.3	0.952	68.1	54.8	<0.001				24.1	32.5	0.021							13	18.2	0.08				35.6	55.5	<0.001
Canto et al. (2012) [16]				33.2	27		60.9	52.7		12.5	9.3		27.6	31.9		15	14.8		23.7	14.7		24	27.6					18	29	
Dreyer et al. (2013) [41]				32	27	0.24	60	45	<0.001				52	48	0.37							26	21	0.19						
Gardarsdottir et al. (2022) [28]				13	12	0.5	55	47	0.01													11	17	0.02				36	40	0.3
Khraishah et al. (2021) [38]				53.6	41.4	<0.001	61.2	42.4	<0.001																1	1	1	3.2	39.8	<0.001
Krishnamurthy et al. (2019) [25]				14.4	12.5	0.51	47.1	35.1	<0.01				30.6	30.5	0.95							10	13.5	0.02	2.1	2.8	0.43	59.6	70.4	<0.01
Leurent et al. (2014) [35]				13	11	0.06	54	36	<0.001													4	8	<0.001				26	41	<0.001
Nguyen et al. (2014) [40]				22.8	13.9		66.3	55.7					9.9	2	0.003	2	5	0.17	0	0.5	NA							1	48.3	<0.001
Ortalani et al. (2013) [33]				29.2	21.5		76.1	62		1.2	1.1		53.9	52.5					6.1	3.7		24.7	28.1					19.8	34.3	
Radovanovic et al. (2012) [32]	18.8	18.8	<0.001	22.4	17.3	<0.001	50.8	65	<0.001				49.8	53.8	<0.001							30.1	31.5	0.08						
Rashid et al. (2020) [26]				25.7	24.2		58.5	51.7					39.7	40.2		27.0	28.3		26.4	24.7					4.4	5.2		49.7	65.0	
Redfors et al. (2015) [31]				21	18	<0.001	48	38	<0.001				13	14	0.013							17	20	<0.001				21	24	<0.001
Roque et al. (2020) [29]	23.8	20.4	<0.001	26	35.9	<0.001	60.4	75.9	<0.001	8.2	6.8	<0.001							8	5	<0.001							8.5	32.6	<0.001
Strömbäck et al. (2017) [30]				33.5	20.1	<0.001	57.9	40.8	<0.001																			44.2	37.4	0.01
Velders et al. (2013) [34]				14.2	10.2	<0.001	45.9	32.5	<0.001	6.9	6.1	0.418	21.8	23.6	0.282							7.1	12.1	<0.001				40.6	47.8	0.001

All of the included studies [16,25–41] reported prevalence of diabetes and hypertension. Women had higher odds of having both a pre-existing diagnosis of diabetes (OR 1.33; CI 1.32–1.34; $p < 0.001$) and/or a diagnosis of hypertension (OR 1.27; CI 1.26–1.28; $p < 0.001$).

A total of 16 studies reported current/ex-smoking status [16,25–31,33–40]. Women had lower odds of having a smoking history (OR 0.41; CI 0.41–0.41; $p < 0.001$).

A total of 12 studies reported prevalence of dyslipidaemia or hypercholesterolaemia [16,25–27,31–34,36,39–41]. Women had significantly lower odds of presenting with these diagnoses (OR 0.83; CI 0.82–0.84).

When "ischaemic heart disease", "previous PCI", or "previous coronary artery bypass graft" was reported by the authors [25–27,30–34,36,40] women were reported to experience significantly lower odds (OR 0.06; CI 0.063–0.065; $p < 0.001$). When authors reported anginal history without preceding MI, PCI, coronary artery bypass graft, or when authors reported anginal history independent of ischaemic heart disease [26,36,39], women experienced marginally lower odds (OR 0.95; CI 0.94–0.96; $p < 0.001$).

Women had higher odds of having a previous diagnosis of heart failure (OR 1.85; CI 1.83–1.86; $p < 0.001$), although this was only reported by five of the included studies [26,28,32,36,39].

Three of the included studies reported prevalence of peripheral arterial disease [25,26,37], with non-significant difference observed between groups (OR 0.94; CI 0.71–1.24; $p = 0.73$).

History of stroke/cerebrovascular disease was reported in four of the included studies [28,32,33,36]. Women experienced greater odds (OR 1.57; CI 1.55–1.59; $p < 0.001$).

4. Discussion

The present manuscript discusses the findings of a large systematic review of 18 studies, including over 1.4 million patients. We have described the variation in prevalence of common, shared cardiac risk factors in men and women presenting with MI. Our data show that women are more likely to have pre-existing diabetes, heart failure, hypertension, and stroke prior to presenting with MI in comparison to men. By contrast, they experience lower odds of dyslipidaemia, angina and ischaemic heart disease, and smoking history. The relationships observed likely represent an amalgamation of a complex, dynamic interaction between biological, social, and cultural factors [42,43]. These factors undoubtedly impact the effectiveness of public health interventions.

Our findings largely support and update those reported by other high quality prospective observational studies [44–47]. Previous reviews have also demonstrated variation in the hazards associated with disproportionate risks, particularly those relating to diabetes, smoking, and hypertension [18,42,45]. Diabetes, for example, is known to increase the risk of MI in females by four-fold, in comparison to only two-and-a-half-fold in men [48]. By increasing the scope of our initial search and inclusion criteria, we have included studies that would not allow us to evaluate the hazards associated with the risks reported. We were thus also unable to examine the interaction between risk factors, how these interactions may be moderated by gender and sex, and what potential implications this has on patient outcomes. Continuous analysis of such data, particularly that pertaining to high quality prospective studies as well as case–control data which report data on matched controls, is necessary to prevent disproportionate bias in the future.

The included studies also failed to report variables which would have provided a more meaningful insight into the sex- and gender-differences of the most clinically relevant risk factors. Many reported diabetes mellitus in its entirety without distinguishing between types 1 and 2, or the other many subtypes of the condition. The methods of data collection employed also necessitated the use of previous allocated diagnoses, meaning that variables, particularly those relating to continuous data, could not be reported. For example, in a large retrospective cohort study of over 11,000 MI events, Rapsomaniki et al. [49] recently demonstrated the importance of distinguishing between diastolic and systolic blood pressure when evaluating one's risk of MI. Subtle differences in likely pathophysiology may also explain some of the discordance between our findings and those of other studies which were not included. For example, Smilowitz et al. [50] reported similar rates of dyslipidaemia in men and women, with women experiencing marginally higher prevalence than men. Importantly, the authors reported lower rates of dyslipidaemia in non-obstructive coronary artery disease, a condition which is more prevalent in women and one that many of the studies included in our review failed to consider. Furthermore, Huxley et al. [18] highlighted the importance of considering the hazards associated with less prevalent risk factors in women, such as cigarette smoking. However, their findings are incongruous with other large prospective observational trials [43], suggesting that there is a need to further interrogate the risk factors in question and how they interact with themselves in addition to other confounders and colliders.

A total of 11 of the included studies reported death rate by gender [16,26–29,33–35,38–40]. However, we did not examine this data given that the included papers did not explore the well-established interaction between age, comorbidity, and treatment modality [51–54], the latter of which is particularly important, given that women experience greater complication rates [55,56] and, whilst having benefitted from advancements in technology such as drug eluding stents, remain at greater risk of suboptimal outcomes. This is in part due to suboptimal postprocedural TIMI flow grade [57]. The papers also failed to address the well-reported discrepancy between genders of non-obstructive coronary artery disease, a condition experienced far more commonly in women [58,59].

It is not unlikely that a proportion of the reported data represent discrepancy in prevalence, severity, and management of MI as well as other comorbidities and confounders [42]. This, in turn, reflects both fixed biological variables [59] as well as variables relating to the well-evidenced gender bias present within healthcare [60]. Thus, our data and that of others before us represent an important opportunity for healthcare providers. Firstly, healthcare providers may be able to better risk stratify those with clinical features of MI at the point of presentation. Pre-hospital physicians and paramedics, emergency department doctors, cardiologists, inpatient physicians, triage nurses, and all of the members of the multi-disciplinary team assessing patients must recognise the increased prevalence of diabetes, heart failure, hypertension, and stroke in women presenting with MI. They must also remain cognisant of the fact that this population are less likely to receive gold-standard treatment in a timely manner, and thus may experience worse outcomes when compared to their gender- and sex-matched counterparts. Thus, active conscious effort must be made to counter the disadvantages that women may face. It also highlights a need to consider the effect of our policies and interventions on gender and sex, and how adaptations to these may disproportionately affect women. There is clear variation in the risk factors present in women and men, and males and females, presenting with MI, only some of which can be explained by biological variation. Thus, there must be an active effort to consider these factors when targeting primary prevention and evaluating our care pathways. Further research is needed to understand how these factors interact with public health interventions, and how we can better account for them in the future. Finally, and perhaps most importantly, our paper further emphasises the need for researchers to consider the implications of gender and sex [61]. In doing so, we must understand how these are implicated by research methodology, and how we can reduce bias within our study design. In this instance, due to a need to examine the data of others, we have unavoidably conflated gender and sex for this article. This is inappropriate and represents an area of academic medicine where improvement is urgently needed. Researchers in the future should aim to make clear the difference between biological sex and gender in their data and report their findings as such, where possible. Doing so will result in more meaningful and applicable data to guide clinicians and policy makers in the future.

Our data are not without limitations. In addition to the aforementioned, we have not adjusted the odds of investigated risk factors to account for variation in known and unknown confounders, including but not limited to age, which were noted to be lower in men across all included studies. This decision was made to meet our intention to provide clinically meaningful data to front door clinicians. We have not examined the relationship between these risk factors and patient outcomes, as justified above. We have also only chosen to focus on those presenting with MI, rather than considering the relative incidence between those who do and those who do not suffer from cardiovascular disease. We have not included sex-specific risk factors in this review but are aware of the importance of those risk factors may have in specific populations. Again, this was an unavailable consequence of our search strategy meeting the primary aim of expanding our inclusion criteria to include papers reporting relevant outcome data from men and women presenting with MI, as opposed to considering large population-based studies prone to bias and often reporting data pertaining to a wider range of cardiovascular diseases.

Further research is necessary to re-evaluate and update the prevalence of risk factors for cardiovascular disease in the general population. Ideally, research would consist of high-quality meta-analyses of prospective cohort studies in addition to more frequently cited retrospective observational data, which is growing in age. There is also a need for continuous re-evaluation of all of the hazards associated with the presence of risk factors in those presenting with MI, and how these are affected by gender and sex. This will contribute to the growing body of literature which has done so for risk factors most prone to cultural variation, such as cigarette smoking [18]. In doing so, one must consider the biopsychosocial variables that are likely to moderate gender- and sex-related risk, including but not limited to disproportionate risks pertaining to socioeconomic status and health literacy [62,63]. A greater understanding of such relationships will better inform our interventions, policies, and decision making in the future.

5. Conclusions

There is a disparity in the distribution of shared cardiovascular risk factors between men and women presenting with MI. We must continually re-evaluate the prevalence of these risk factors to better guide our diagnostic reasoning and clinical decision making. Furthermore, there is a need for researchers to consider the implications of sex and gender on their study design, and to report data both by sex and gender, as opposed to conflating the two. Further research is needed to re-evaluate the prevalence of shared and independent risk factors for cardiovascular disease, and the subsequent development of MI, in the general population. There is also a need for continuous re-evaluation of the hazards associated with the presence of risk factors, and how these are affected by gender and sex. In doing so, one must consider the biopsychosocial variables that are likely to moderate gender- and sex-related risk.

Supplementary Materials: The following supporting information can be downloaded at: https://www.mdpi.com/article/10.3390/jcm12155163/s1, Table S1: Risk of bias assessment; File S1: Search terms.

Author Contributions: Conceptualization, J.C.B.; methodology, J.C.B., G.N.T., A.W., C.S., A.E.C., V.S., I.S. and J.C.K.; formal analysis, J.C.B. and A.C.; data curation, J.C.B., G.N.T., A.W., C.S., A.E.C., V.S. and I.S.; visualization, J.C.B.; writing, J.C.B., A.E.C., A.W. and A.K.; supervision, J.C.K.; project administration, J.C.B. All authors have read and agreed to the published version of the manuscript.

Funding: This research received no external funding.

Institutional Review Board Statement: Ethical review and approval were waived for this study due to the fact that it is a secondary analysis of previously published data.

Informed Consent Statement: Not applicable.

Data Availability Statement: All reported data will be made available on request by contacting the corresponding author.

Conflicts of Interest: The authors declare no conflict of interest.

References

1. Clayton, J.A. Studying both sexes: A guiding principle for biomedicine. *FASEB J. Off. Publ. Fed. Am. Soc. Exp. Biol.* **2015**, *30*, 519–524. [CrossRef] [PubMed]
2. Beery, A.K.; Zucker, I. Sex bias in neuroscience and biomedical research. *Neurosci. Biobehav. Rev.* **2011**, *35*, 565–572. [CrossRef] [PubMed]
3. Heinrich, J.; Gahart, M.T.; Rowe, E.J.; Bradley, L. Drug Safety: Most Drugs Withdrawn in Recent Years Had Greater Health. Risks for Women. U.S. Government Accountability Office; 2001. Available online: https://www.gao.gov/products/gao-01-286r (accessed on 17 April 2023).
4. Camacho, X.; Nedkoff, L.; Wright, F.L.; Nghiem, N.; Buajitti, E.; Goldacre, R.; Rosella, L.C.; Seminog, O.; Tan, E.J.; Hayes, A.; et al. Relative contribution of trends in myocardial infarction event rates and case fatality to declines in mortality: An international comparative study of 1·95 million events in 80·4 million people in four countries. *Lancet Public Heal* **2022**, *7*, e229–e239. [CrossRef] [PubMed]
5. Mehta, L.S.; Beckie, T.M.; DeVon, H.A.; Grines, C.L.; Krumholz, H.M.; Johnson, M.N.; Lindley, K.J.; Vaccarino, V.; Wang, T.Y.; Watson, K.E.; et al. Acute Myocardial Infarction in Women: A Scientific Statement from the American Heart Association. *Circulation* **2016**, *133*, 916–947. [CrossRef]
6. Westin, R.C.L. Differences in Quality of Life in Men and Women with Ischemic Heart Disease: A Prospective Controlled Study. *Scand. Cardiovasc. J.* **1999**, *33*, 160–165. [CrossRef]
7. Shumaker, S.A.; Brooks, M.; Schron, E.B.; Hale, C.; Kellen, J.C.; Inkster, M.; Wimbush, F.B.; Wiklund, I.; Morris, M. Gender differences in health-related quality of life among postmyocardial infarction patients: Brief report. CAST Investigators. Cardiac Arrhythmia Suppression Trials. *Women's Heal* **1997**, *3*, 53–60.
8. Guo, Y.; Yin, F.; Fan, C.; Wang, Z. Gender difference in clinical outcomes of the patients with coronary artery disease after percutaneous coronary intervention: A systematic review and meta-analysis. *Medicine* **2018**, *97*, e11644. [CrossRef]
9. Potts, J.; Sirker, A.; Martinez, S.C.; Gulati, M.; Alasnag, M.; Rashid, M.; Kwok, C.S.; Ensor, J.; Burke, D.L.; Riley, R.D.; et al. Persistent sex disparities in clinical outcomes with percutaneous coronary intervention: Insights from 6.6 million PCI procedures in the United States. *PLoS ONE* **2018**, *13*, e0203325. [CrossRef]
10. Nicolas, J.; Claessen, B.E.; Cao, D.; Chiarito, M.; Sartori, S.; Qiu, H.; Goel, R.; Nardin, M.; Roumeliotis, A.; Vogel, B.; et al. A sex paradox in clinical outcomes following complex percutaneous coronary intervention. *Int. J. Cardiol.* **2020**, *329*, 67–73. [CrossRef]
11. Samayoa, L.; Grace, S.L.; Gravely, S.; Scott, L.B.; Marzolini, S.; Colella, T.J. Sex Differences in Cardiac Rehabilitation Enrollment: A Meta-analysis. *Can. J. Cardiol.* **2014**, *30*, 793–800. [CrossRef]
12. Iribarren, C.; Tolstykh, I.; Somkin, C.P.; Ackerson, L.M.; Brown, T.T.; Scheffler, R.; Syme, L.; Kawachi, I. Sex and Racial/Ethnic Disparities in Outcomes after Acute Myocardial Infarction: A cohort study among members of a large integrated health care delivery system in northern California. *Arch. Intern. Med.* **2005**, *165*, 2105–2113. [CrossRef]
13. Greenwood, B.N.; Carnahan, S.; Huang, L. Patient–physician gender concordance and increased mortality among female heart attack patients. *Proc. Natl. Acad. Sci. USA* **2018**, *115*, 8569–8574. [CrossRef]

14. Regitz-Zagrosek, V.; Seeland, U. Sex and Gender Differences in Clinical Medicine. In *Handbook of Experimental Pharmacology*; Springer: Berlin/Heidelberg, Germany, 2012; p. 214. [CrossRef]
15. Geraghty, L.; Figtree, G.A.; Schutte, A.E.; Patel, S.; Woodward, M.; Arnott, C. Cardiovascular Disease in Women: From Pathophysiology to Novel and Emerging Risk Factors. *Hear. Lung Circ.* **2020**, *30*, 9–17. [CrossRef]
16. Canto, J.G.; Rogers, W.J.; Goldberg, R.J.; Peterson, E.D.; Wenger, N.K.; Vaccarino, V.; Kiefe, C.I.; Frederick, P.D.; Sopko, G.; Zheng, Z.-J.; et al. Association of Age and Sex with Myocardial Infarction Symptom Presentation and In-Hospital Mortality. *JAMA* **2012**, *307*, 813–822. [CrossRef]
17. Stangl, V.; Baumann, G.; Stangl, K. Coronary atherogenic risk factors in women. *Eur. Hear. J.* **2002**, *23*, 1738–1752. [CrossRef]
18. Huxley, R.R.; Woodward, M. Cigarette smoking as a risk factor for coronary heart disease in women compared with men: A systematic review and meta-analysis of prospective cohort studies. *Lancet* **2011**, *378*, 1297–1305. [CrossRef]
19. Rosendaal, F.; Helmerhorst, F.; Vandenbroucke, J.P. Female Hormones and Thrombosis. *Arter. Thromb. Vasc. Biol.* **2002**, *22*, 201–210. [CrossRef]
20. Mosca, L.; Barrett-Connor, E.; Wenger, N.K. Sex/Gender Differences in Cardiovascular Disease Prevention: What a difference a decade makes. *Circulation* **2011**, *124*, 2145–2154. [CrossRef]
21. Page, M.J.; McKenzie, J.E.; Bossuyt, P.M.; Boutron, I.; Hoffmann, T.C.; Mulrow, C.D.; Shamseer, L.; Tetzlaff, J.M.; Akl, E.A.; Brennan, S.E.; et al. The PRISMA 2020 statement: An updated guideline for reporting systematic reviews. *BMJ* **2021**, *372*, 71. [CrossRef]
22. Thygesen, K.; Alpert, J.S.; Jaffe, A.S.; Chaitman, B.R.; Bax, J.J.; Morrow, D.A.; White, H.D.; ESC Scientific Document Group. Fourth universal definition of myocardial infarction (2018). *Eur. Heart J.* **2018**, *40*, 237–269. [CrossRef]
23. Domieniek-Karłowicz, J.; Kupczyńska, K.; Michalski, B.; Kapłon-Cieślicka, A.; Darocha, S.; Dobrowolski, P.; Wybraniec, M.; Wańha, W.; Jaguszewski, M. Fourth universal definition of myocardial infarction. Selected messages from the European Society of Cardiology document and lessons learned from the new guidelines on ST-segment elevation myocardial infarction and non-ST-segment elevation-acute coronary syndrome. *Cardiol. J.* **2021**, *28*, 195–201. [CrossRef] [PubMed]
24. Wells, G.A.; Shea, B.; O'Connell, D.; Pereson, J.; Welch, V.; Losos, M.; Tugwell, P. The Newcastle–Ottawa Scale (NOS) for Assessing the Quality of Nonrandomised Studies in Meta-Analyses. The Ottawa Hospital Research Institute. Available online: http://www.ohri.ca/programs/clinical_epidemiology/oxford.asp (accessed on 20 May 2023).
25. Krishnamurthy, A.; Keeble, C.; Burton-Wood, N.; Somers, K.; Anderson, M.; Harland, C.; Baxter, P.D.; McLenachan, J.M.; Blaxill, J.M.; Blackman, D.J.; et al. Clinical outcomes following primary percutaneous coronary intervention for ST-elevation myocardial infarction according to sex and race. *Eur. Hear. J. Acute Cardiovasc. Care* **2017**, *8*, 264–272. [CrossRef] [PubMed]
26. Baumann, S.; Huseynov, A.; Koepp, J.; Jabbour, C.; Behnes, M.; Becher, T.; Renker, M.; Lang, S.; Borggrefe, M.; Lehmann, R.; et al. Comparison of Serum Uric Acid, Bilirubin, and C-Reactive Protein as Prognostic Biomarkers of In-Hospital MACE Between Women and Men with ST-Segment Elevation Myocardial Infarction. *Angiology* **2015**, *67*, 272–280. [CrossRef] [PubMed]
27. Rashid, M.; Curzen, N.; Kinnaird, T.; Lawson, C.A.; Myint, P.K.; Kontopantelis, E.; Mohamed, M.O.; Shoaib, A.; Gale, C.P.; Timmis, A.; et al. Baseline risk, timing of invasive strategy and guideline compliance in NSTEMI: Nationwide analysis from MINAP. *Int. J. Cardiol.* **2019**, *301*, 7–13. [CrossRef]
28. Gardarsdottir, H.R.; Sigurdsson, M.I.; Andersen, K.; Gudmundsdottir, I.J. Long-term survival of Icelandic women following acute myocardial infarction. *Scand. Cardiovasc. J.* **2022**, *56*, 114–120. [CrossRef]
29. Roque, D.; Ferreira, J.; Monteiro, S.; Costa, M.; Gil, V. Understanding a woman's heart: Lessons from 14,177 women with acute coronary syndrome. *Rev. Port. Cardiol.* **2020**, *39*, 57–72. [CrossRef]
30. Strömbäck, U.; Vikman, I.; Lundblad, D.; Lundqvist, R.; Engström, Å. The second myocardial infarction: Higher risk factor burden and earlier second myocardial infarction in women compared with men. The Northern Sweden MONICA study. *Eur. J. Cardiovasc. Nurs.* **2016**, *16*, 418–424. [CrossRef]
31. Redfors, B.; Angerås, O.; Råmunddal, T.; Petursson, P.; Haraldsson, I.; Dworeck, C.; Odenstedt, J.; Ioaness, D.; Ravn-Fischer, A.; Wellin, P.; et al. Trends in Gender Differences in Cardiac Care and Outcome after Acute Myocardial Infarction in Western Sweden: A Report from the Swedish Web System for Enhancement of Evidence-Based Care in Heart Disease Evaluated According to Recommended Therapies (SWEDEHEART). *J. Am. Hear. Assoc.* **2015**, *4*, e001995. [CrossRef]
32. Radovanovic, D.; Nallamothu, B.K.; Seifert, B.; Bertel, O.; Eberli, F.; Urban, P.; Pedrazzini, G.; Rickli, H.; Stauffer, J.-C.; Windecker, S.; et al. Temporal trends in treatment of ST-elevation myocardial infarction among men and women in Switzerland between 1997 and 2011. *Eur. Hear. J. Acute Cardiovasc. Care* **2012**, *1*, 183–191. [CrossRef]
33. Ortolani, P.; Solinas, E.; Guastaroba, P.; Marino, M.; Casella, G.; Manari, A.; Piovaccari, G.; Ottani, F.; Varani, E.; Campo, G.; et al. Relevance of gender in patients with acute myocardial infarction undergoing coronary interventions. *J. Cardiovasc. Med.* **2013**, *14*, 421–429. [CrossRef]
34. Velders, M.A.; Boden, H.; van Boven, A.J.; van der Hoeven, B.L.; Heestermans, A.A.; Cannegieter, S.C.; Umans, V.A.; Jukema, J.W.; Hofma, S.H.; Schalij, M.J. Influence of Gender on Ischemic Times and Outcomes after ST-Elevation Myocardial Infarction. *Am. J. Cardiol.* **2012**, *111*, 312–318. [CrossRef]
35. Leurent, G.; Garlantézec, R.; Auffret, V.; Hacot, J.P.; Coudert, I.; Filippi, E.; Rialan, A.; Moquet, B.; Rouault, G.; Gilard, M.; et al. Gender differences in presentation, management and inhospital outcome in patients with ST-segment elevation myocardial infarction: Data from 5000 patients included in the ORBI prospective French regional registry. *Arch. Cardiovasc. Dis.* **2014**, *107*, 291–298. [CrossRef]

36. Asleh, R.; Manemann, S.M.; Weston, S.A.; Bielinski, S.J.; Chamberlain, A.M.; Jiang, R.; Gerber, Y.; Roger, V.L. Sex Differences in Outcomes after Myocardial Infarction in the Community. *Am. J. Med.* **2021**, *134*, 114–121. [CrossRef]
37. Bajaj, S. Gender Based Differences in Risk Factor Profile and Coronary Angiography of Patients Presenting with Acute Myocardial Infarction in North Indian Population. *J. Clin. Diagn. Res.* **2016**, *10*, OC05-7. [CrossRef]
38. Khraishah, H.; Alahmad, B.; Alfaddagh, A.; Jeong, S.Y.; Mathenge, N.; Kassab, M.B.; Kolte, D.; Michos, E.D.; Albaghdadi, M. Sex disparities in the presentation, management and outcomes of patients with acute coronary syndrome: Insights from the ACS QUIK trial. *Open Hear.* **2021**, *8*, e001470. [CrossRef]
39. Sajjadi, H.; Nasri, H.; Mehrabi, Y.; Etemad, K.; Ahmadi, A.; Soori, H. Current status of the clinical epidemiology of myocardial infarction in men and women: A national cross-sectional study in Iran. *Int. J. Prev. Med.* **2015**, *6*, 14. [CrossRef]
40. Nguyen, H.L.; Ha, D.A.; Phan, D.T.; Nguyen, Q.N.; Nguyen, V.L.; Nguyen, N.H.; Nguyen, H.; Goldberg, R.J. Sex Differences in Clinical Characteristics, Hospital Management Practices, and In-Hospital Outcomes in Patients Hospitalized in a Vietnamese Hospital with a First Acute Myocardial Infarction. *PLoS ONE* **2014**, *9*, e95631. [CrossRef]
41. Dreyer, R.P.; Beltrame, J.F.; Tavella, R.; Air, T.; Hoffmann, B.; Pati, P.K.; Di Fiore, D.; Arstall, M.; Zeitz, C. Evaluation of Gender Differences in Door-to-Balloon Time in ST-Elevation Myocardial Infarction. *Hear. Lung Circ.* **2013**, *22*, 861–869. [CrossRef]
42. Millett, E.R.C.; Peters, S.A.E.; Woodward, M. Sex differences in risk factors for myocardial infarction: Cohort study of UK Biobank participants. *BMJ* **2018**, *363*, k4247. [CrossRef]
43. Regitz-Zagrosek, V. Sex and gender differences in health: Science & Society Series on Sex and Science. *EMBO Rep.* **2012**, *13*, 596–603. [CrossRef]
44. Anand, S.S.; Islam, S.; Rosengren, A.; Franzosi, M.G.; Steyn, K.; Yusufali, A.H.; Keltai, M.; Diaz, R.; Rangarajan, S.; Yusuf, S. Risk factors for myocardial infarction in women and men: Insights from the INTERHEART study. *Eur. Hear. J.* **2008**, *29*, 932–940. [CrossRef] [PubMed]
45. Norhammar, A.; Stenestrand, U.; Lindback, J.; Wallentin, L. Women younger than 65 years with diabetes mellitus are a high-risk group after myocardial infarction: A report from the Swedish Register of Information and Knowledge about Swedish Heart Intensive Care Admission (RIKS-HIA). *Heart* **2008**, *94*, 1565–1570. [CrossRef] [PubMed]
46. Albrektsen, G.; Heuch, I.; Løchen, M.-L.; Thelle, D.S.; Wilsgaard, T.; Njølstad, I.; Bønaa, K.H. Lifelong Gender Gap in Risk of Incident Myocardial Infarction: The Tromsø Study. *JAMA Intern. Med.* **2016**, *176*, 1673–1679. [CrossRef] [PubMed]
47. Wilson, P.W. Established Risk Factors and Coronary Artery Disease: The Framingham Study. *Am. J. Hypertens.* **1994**, *7*, 7S–12S. [CrossRef] [PubMed]
48. Yusuf, S.; Hawken, S.; Ôunpuu, S.; Dans, T.; Avezum, A.; Lanas, F.; McQueen, M.; Budaj, A.; Pais, P.; Varigos, J.; et al. Effect of potentially modifiable risk factors associated with myocardial infarction in 52 countries (the INTERHEART study): Case-control study. *Lancet* **2004**, *364*, 937–952. [CrossRef]
49. Rapsomaniki, E.; Timmis, A.; George, J.; Pujades-Rodriguez, M.; Shah, A.D.; Denaxas, S.; White, I.R.; Caulfield, M.J.; Deanfield, J.E.; Smeeth, L.; et al. Blood pressure and incidence of twelve cardiovascular diseases: Lifetime risks, healthy life-years lost, and age-specific associations in 1·25 million people. *Lancet* **2014**, *383*, 1899–1911. [CrossRef]
50. Smilowitz, N.R.; Mahajan, A.M.; Roe, M.T.; Hellkamp, A.S.; Chiswell, K.; Gulati, M.; Reynolds, H.R. Mortality of Myocardial Infarction by Sex, Age, and Obstructive Coronary Artery Disease Status in the ACTION Registry–GWTG (Acute Coronary Treatment and Intervention Outcomes Network Registry–Get with the Guidelines). *Circ. Cardiovasc. Qual. Outcomes* **2017**, *10*, e003443. [CrossRef]
51. Manzo-Silberman, S.; Couturaud, F.; Charpentier, S.; Auffret, V.; El Khoury, C.; Le Breton, H.; Belle, L.; Marlière, S.; Zeller, M.; Cottin, Y.; et al. Influence of gender on delays and early mortality in ST-segment elevation myocardial infarction: Insight from the first French Metaregistry, 2005–2012 patient-level pooled analysis. *Int. J. Cardiol.* **2018**, *262*, 1–8. [CrossRef]
52. Zhang, Z.; Fang, J.; Gillespie, C.; Wang, G.; Hong, Y.; Yoon, P.W. Age-Specific Gender Differences in In-Hospital Mortality by Type of Acute Myocardial Infarction. *Am. J. Cardiol.* **2012**, *109*, 1097–1103. [CrossRef]
53. Lawesson, S.S.; Alfredsson, J.; Fredrikson, M.; Swahn, E. A gender perspective on short- and long term mortality in ST-elevation myocardial infarction—A report from the SWEDEHEART register. *Int. J. Cardiol.* **2013**, *168*, 1041–1047. [CrossRef]
54. Nohria, A.; Vaccarino, V.; Krumholz, H.M. Gender differences in mortality after myocardial infarction. Why women fare worse than men. *Cardiol. Clin.* **1998**, *16*, 45–57. [CrossRef]
55. Poon, S.; Goodman, S.G.; Yan, R.T.; Bugiardini, R.; Bierman, A.S.; Eagle, K.A.; Johnston, N.; Huynh, T.; Grondin, F.R.; Schenck-Gustafsson, K.; et al. Bridging the gender gap: Insights from a contemporary analysis of sex-related differences in the treatment and outcomes of patients with acute coronary syndromes. *Am. Hear. J.* **2012**, *163*, 66–73. [CrossRef]
56. Filardo, G.; Hamman, B.L.; Pollock, B.D.; da Graca, B.; Sass, D.M.; Phan, T.K.; Edgerton, J.; Prince, S.L.; Ring, W.S. Excess short-term mortality in women after isolated coronary artery bypass graft surgery. *Open Hear.* **2016**, *3*, e000386. [CrossRef]
57. Cenko, E.; van der Schaar, M.; Yoon, J.; Kedev, S.; Valvukis, M.; Vasiljevic, Z.; Ašanin, M.; Miličić, D.; Manfrini, O.; Badimon, L.; et al. Sex-Specific Treatment Effects after Primary Percutaneous Intervention: A Study on Coronary Blood Flow and Delay to Hospital Presentation. *J. Am. Hear. Assoc.* **2019**, *8*, e011190. [CrossRef]
58. Manfrini, O.; Yoon, J.; Van Der Schaar, M.; Kedev, S.; Vavlukis, M.; Stankovic, G.; Scarpone, M.; Miličić, D.; Vasiljevic, Z.; Badimon, L.; et al. Sex Differences in Modifiable Risk Factors and Severity of Coronary Artery Disease. *J. Am. Hear. Assoc.* **2020**, *9*, e017235. [CrossRef]

59. Guagliumi, G.; Capodanno, D.; Saia, F.; Musumeci, G.; Tarantini, G.; Garbo, R.; Tumminello, G.; Sirbu, V.; Coccato, M.; Fineschi, M.; et al. Mechanisms of Atherothrombosis and Vascular Response to Primary Percutaneous Coronary Intervention in Women Versus Men with Acute Myocardial Infarction: Results from the OCTAVIA study. *JACC Cardiovasc. Interv.* **2014**, *7*, 958–968. [CrossRef]
60. Daugherty, S.L.; Blair, I.V.; Havranek, E.P.; Furniss, A.; Dickinson, L.M.; Karimkhani, E.; Main, D.S.; Masoudi, F.A. Implicit Gender Bias and the Use of Cardiovascular Tests among Cardiologists. *J. Am. Hear. Assoc.* **2017**, *6*, e006872. [CrossRef]
61. Johnson, J.L.; Greaves, L.; Repta, R. Better science with sex and gender: Facilitating the use of a sex and gender-based analysis in health research. *Int. J. Equity Heal.* **2009**, *8*, 14. [CrossRef]
62. Connelly, P.J.; Azizi, Z.; Alipour, P.; Delles, C.; Pilote, L.; Raparelli, V. The Importance of Gender to Understand Sex Differences in Cardiovascular Disease. *Can. J. Cardiol.* **2021**, *37*, 699–710. [CrossRef]
63. Ski, C.F.; King-Shier, K.M.; Thompson, D.R. Gender, socioeconomic and ethnic/racial disparities in cardiovascular disease: A time for change. *Int. J. Cardiol.* **2014**, *170*, 255–257. [CrossRef]

Disclaimer/Publisher's Note: The statements, opinions and data contained in all publications are solely those of the individual author(s) and contributor(s) and not of MDPI and/or the editor(s). MDPI and/or the editor(s) disclaim responsibility for any injury to people or property resulting from any ideas, methods, instructions or products referred to in the content.

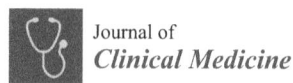

Review

Physical Activity and Diet in Older Women: A Narrative Review

Anna Vittoria Mattioli [1,2,*], Valentina Selleri [1,3], Giada Zanini [3], Milena Nasi [4], Marcello Pinti [3], Claudio Stefanelli [1,5], Francesco Fedele [1,6] and Sabina Gallina [1,7]

1. Istituto Nazionale per le Ricerche Cardiovascolari, 40126 Bologna, Italy
2. Department of Medical and Surgical Sciences for Children and Adults, University of Modena and Reggio Emilia, 41124 Modena, Italy
3. Department of Life Sciences, University of Modena and Reggio Emilia, 41125 Modena, Italy
4. Surgical, Medical and Dental Department of Morphological Sciences Related to Transplant, Oncology and Regenerative Medicine, University of Modena and Reggio Emilia, 41124 Modena, Italy
5. Department of Quality of Life, Alma Mater Studiorum, 40126 Bologna, Italy
6. Department of Clinical, Internal, Anesthesiology and Cardiovascular Sciences, Sapienza University of Rome, 00161 Rome, Italy
7. Department of Neuroscience, Imaging and Clinical Sciences, "G. D'Annunzio" University, 66100 Chieti, Italy
* Correspondence: annavittoria.mattioli@unimore.it

Abstract: Physical activity and diet are essential for maintaining good health and preventing the development of non-communicable diseases, especially in the older adults. One aspect that is often over-looked is the different response between men and women to exercise and nutrients. The body's response to exercise and to different nutrients as well as the choice of foods is different in the two sexes and is strongly influenced by the different hormonal ages in women. The present narrative review analyzes the effects of gender on nutrition and physical activity in older women. Understanding which components of diet and physical activity affect the health status of older women would help target non-pharmacological but lifestyle-related therapeutic interventions. It is interesting to note that this analysis shows a lack of studies dedicated to older women and a lack of studies dedicated to the interactions between diet and physical activity in women. Gender medicine is a current need that still finds little evidence.

Keywords: aging; women; nutrients; physical activity; long COVID; monitoring; vital signs

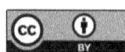

1. Introduction

Physical activity and diet are essential for maintaining good health and preventing the development of non-communicable diseases [1–3]. As a response to population ageing, different conceptual models such as active ageing, successful ageing or healthy ageing have been proposed to address the notion of ageing well [4]. However, women are less likely to engage in sports and physical activity due to high social pressures and stereotypes that force women to play numerous time-consuming roles in family, society and work [5,6]. This attitude in women has worsened during the recent pandemic leading to increase sedentary behaviours and subsequent loss of muscle [5–7]. During the global pandemic older adults' access to programs and services to facilitate the adoption of healthy lifestyles, such as gyms has been disrupted [8]. As a result, web-based interventions may represent a solution for helping older adults adopt and maintain a healthy lifestyle [8] The beneficial role of regular physical activity and structured exercise in health of older adults has been suggested by the World Health Organization [9]. The American College of Sports Medicine supported this suggestion in its guidelines published in 2022 [10]. More recently some manuscript underlined the popularity of fitness programs for older adults in the health and fitness industry at European and global level [11,12]. Women tend to have a longer life expectancy, however, while they live longer, women generally have worse health and more chronic diseases than men [13,14]. As a response to population ageing, different conceptual models such as active ageing, successful ageing or healthy ageing have been proposed to address the notion of ageing well [15].

Since physical activity and nutrition are directly related to the risk of chronic disease, it is essential to understand how these modifiable factors are related to health. The relationship between nutrition and health varies throughout life, with women having unique nutritional needs based on physiological and hormonal changes at various life times (e.g., menstruation, pregnancy, breastfeeding, menopause) [16]. However, women can experience deficiencies in their nutrition and micronutrient intake during periods of hormonal change in their lives. These deficiencies can affect aspects of your lifestyle such as sleep patterns and general quality of life and, in the long term, can impact your risk of developing chronic diseases [16–18].

Furthermore, physical activity must be associated with a balanced energy intake and the choice of the right foods to achieve the expected results and preserve health. It is conceivable that the choice of foods to be taken in subjects who perform regular physical activity is different in women and in men [13,19]. It is well known that the absorption and bioavailability of nutrients are different between women and men and this must influence the choice of diet at different stages of life [16,20]. The favorable effects of diet on human health are mediated by various nutrients, among these phenolic compounds are among the most widespread and well-known phytochemicals in plants and are found in many foods and drinks, such as fruit, vegetables and chocolate, as well as in coffee, tea, beer and wine [20,21]. Phenolic compounds of plant origin influence health through an antioxidant and anti-inflammatory action, this effect is different for men and women [20,21]. It is interesting to note that most of the studies analyze the differences in the choice of foods in relation to the different stages of life: young, adult and older adults. Whereas, only a few manuscripts have analyzed gender differences in dietary choice, although it is known that the different hormonal phases in women mainly influence the exposure to the risk of chronic diseases and that diet is a determining factor in the development of chronic non-communicable diseases [5,22,23].

2. Methods

Our search strategy was designed to inform this Review relating to gender differences in diet and physical activity in older healthy subjects. We searched MEDLINE, Scopus and Web of Science. In brief, we used a combination of terms relating to older adults (e.g., "elderly women", "older women", "older adult" and "longevity") and lifestyle habits (e.g., "food", "nutrients", "physical activity"). In all these combinations the terms "women", "sex", "gender" and "diet" were mandatory. For studies to be included in this Review, they had to: (i) report on primary research, (ii) be published in peer-reviewed journals, (iii) be written in English and include data on gender differences analysis, or on factors associated with wellbeing in older women. Due to the fact that very little data are available we included papers published in the last 10 years.

The present narrative review briefly analyzes the effects of gender on nutrition and physical activity in older women and suggests future prospective for prevention of chronic disease in women. Understanding which components of diet and physical activity affect the health status of older women would help target non-pharmacological but lifestyle-related therapeutic interventions.

3. Results

Among 632 citations obtained at November 2022, articles that were considered to contain the most important and novel data on the effects of gender on nutrition and physical activity in older women were included in this narrative review. Due to the very limited number of manuscripts that focused on older women we included also manuscript that analyzed gender differences in adult subjects. The analysis of original manuscript (excluding review) showed that the great majority of them focused on vitamin D (101 manuscript) and sarcopenic obesity or obesity (57 manuscript). Only few manuscripts analyzed the relationship between food and physical activity in older adult (56 original manuscript) and only 16 included a specific analysis by sex or gender. The great majority of studies analyzed middle-aged women or pre-menopausal women and included a wide range of age.

4. Discussion

4.1. Vitamin D Deficiency

The first aspect that emerges in the studies carried out on older women is the objective of evaluating the concentration of vitamin D with the women's health status. A low vitamin D status is a very common condition worldwide, and several studies from basic science to clinical applications have highlighted a strong association with chronic diseases, as well as acute conditions [24]. Estimates of the prevalence of 25 (OH)D levels < 50 nmol/L (or 20 ng/mL) have been reported as 24% (US), 37% (Canada), and 40% (Europe) [25,26]. However, the concentrations of Vit D undergo important variations in relation to sun exposure, skin color, and absorption capacities which are influenced by the intestinal microbiota. Furthermore, it may vary by age, with lower levels in childhood and the older adults [25,26], and also ethnicity in different regions, for example, European Caucasians show lower rates of vitamin D deficiency compared with nonwhite individuals [26].

A very recent manuscript evaluated whether the role of physical activity and vitamin D in sarcopenia, obesity, and sarcopenic obesity was different between men and women. They found that low physical activity was significantly associated with higher odds of sarcopenia in women only (OR = 1.70, 95% CI:1.18, 2.46, p < 0.01). Vitamin D deficiency was only associated with sarcopenia in men (OR = 1.85, 95% CI: 1.27, 2.69, p < 0.01). Low physical activity was significantly associated with obesity, sarcopenia, and sarcopenic obesity only in participants with serum 25 (OH)D < 20 ng/mL. This manuscript by Jia S et al. underline some differences between men and women about the role of vitamin D and PA in obesity and sarcopenia. Authors also underlined that the relationship between PA and sarcopenia was modified by serum vitamin D status. These findings highlighted the need to supplement vitamin D in individuals with physical inactivity and provide different interventions strategies to sarcopenia in men and women [27].

Many peri- and postmenopausal women are deficient in or have low levels of vitamin D and magnesium. Vitamin D is essential for bone health, as well as preventing muscle weakness, protecting against falls, and providing immune support [28]. Usually, women are more likely to take dietary supplements than men, but when we analyze the use of supplements and sports drinks in people physically active this difference disappears [16]. However, no studies have analyzed the differences between physically active women and men in response to supplement components. This gap could be responsible for the lower efficacy of supplements and reflect on less health care in women [9]. Recently, Cui et al. address the various issues related to the complex relationship between food and sports with attention to the nutrients necessary to perform sports in the best physical conditions and to obtain optimal results [19]. The relevant point explored by Cui et al. was the roles of each nutritional component that can be divided into: the protection of articular cartilage, improving muscle quality, regulating endocrine, weight control, prevention of anemia, increasing energy storage and utilization, and enhancing immune function [19]. These functions are extremely important in the older adults and must be considered when addressing the diet in older adults by specifying the differences that exist between women and men.

4.2. Sarcopenia and Sarcopenic Obesity

The second topic that dominates the analysis of studies dedicated to adult women is sarcopenia and sarcopenic obesity (Figure 1). Although the role of physical exercise in the prevention of fractures is recognized, there are still few studies that correlate nutrition and physical activity with respect to sarcopenic obesity and bone fragility. The UK Women's Cohort Study investigated associations between food and nutrient intakes and hip fracture risk in, evaluated the role of body mass index (BMI) as a potential effect modifier. The study included 26,318 UK women, ages 35–69 years, and 822 hip fracture cases were identified. Results of the study suggest that the potential roles of some foods and nutrients in hip fracture prevention. Particularly protein, tea and coffee seem to play a role in prevention of hip fractures in underweight women. Specifically, every additional cup of tea or coffee per day was associated with a 4% lower risk of hip fracture (HR (95% CI): 0.96 (0.92, 1.00)). A 25 g/day increment of dietary protein intake was also associated with a 14% lower risk of hip fracture (0.86 (0.73, 1.00)) [29].

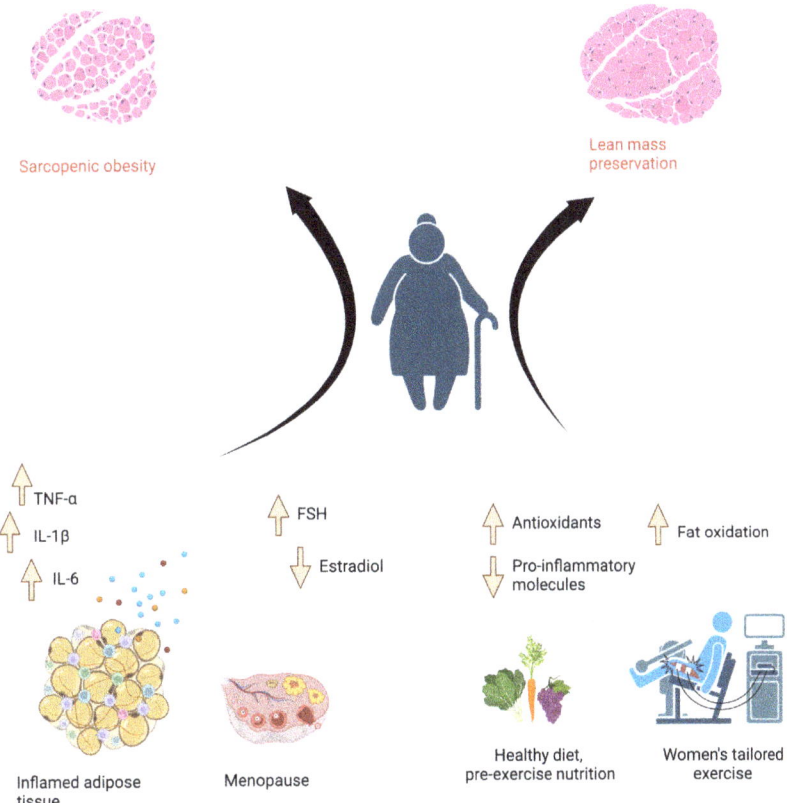

Figure 1. Factors that influence the development of sarcopenic obesity. Red, blue and yellow dots represent the pro-inflammatory cytokines TNF-α, IL-1β and IL-6 released by inflamed adipose tissue.

This study has the merit of having highlighted a specific role of nutrients in the prevention of fractures in older women beyond the concentration of Vit D. A decisive role on the development of fractures and also on cardiovascular risk is attributed to sarcopenic obesity. Sarcopenia is a geriatric syndrome, characterized by progressive decline in muscle strength and generalized loss of skeletal muscle mass [30]. The sarcopenic muscles display heterogeneity in fiber size, atrophy of type 2 (fast-twitch) myofibers, accumulation of intramuscular fat and connective tissue with a decreased oxidative capacity. All these conditions lead to an age-related decline in functions. Moreover, during sarcopenia there is also the loss of satellite cell, which compromises the recovery capacity of sarcopenic muscles in response to injury [31]. During adulthood, satellite cells main function is to sustain skeletal muscle regenerative capacity. The consequence of satellite cell aging is the loss of skeletal muscle regenerative capacity, which is pronounced in the sarcopenic muscle. The aging environment leads to the accumulation of cellular stressors that culminate in irreversible changes to the satellite cell [31]. For this reason, "inflammaging", a local and a systemic chronic low-grade inflammation that arises with aging, may contribute to muscle decline by impairing stem cell function and accelerating cellular senescence. Also obesity is recognized as a state of chronic inflammation with increased circulating pro-inflammatory cytokines tumour necrosis factor (TNF)-α, interleukin (IL)-1β and IL-6 [32,33]. In animal models of chronic, local or systemic inflammation, with high levels of IL-6 and TNF-α respectively, satellite cell proliferation decreases [34] and skeletal muscle becomes atrophic [35]. It is possible that in chronic inflammation the normal coordination between macrophages and muscle satellite cells is impaired and contributes to impaired satellite cell function.

Pro-inflammatory cytokines have been found to affect gene expression of satellite cells and muscle regeneration, contributing to age- and obesity-dependent decline in muscle function. During women midlife there are drastic hormonal changes due to ovarian aging and the consequent onset of menopausal. This transition phase includes a decline in the estradiol serum concentration and elevation of follicle-stimulating hormone (FSH) levels. Hormonal changes start approximately 5 years before and continue years after the final menstrual period. Muscle and bone mass decline with aging, increasing the risk for sarcopenia and osteoporosis in later life. Both these conditions are tightly related to aging and estrogen depletion and consequently to menopausal transition [36]. A few studies also suggest that menopausal hormonal changes influence the decline in lean mass (LM) among middle-aged women. Hormonal changes seem to be the major contributors to the changes in muscle and bone tissue in women undergoing menopausal transition. The preventive role of estrogens in cardiovascular disease (CVD) may depend not only on their role in the regulation of body fat distribution but also on their antioxidant effect [37,38]. Also changes in body composition, including an increase in total adiposity and a redistribution of fat with an increase in abdominal/visceral fat accumulation occur during the transition to menopause. Fat redistribution is reflected in the presence of intermuscular adipose tissue (IMAT) [39,40]. IMCLs are found in mitochondria where they increase ROS formation, resulting in the apoptosis/autophagy of muscle cells. Thus, it is considered as one of the potential mechanisms of obesity-mediated sarcopenia pathogenesis [41]. IMAT releases pro-inflammatory cytokines resulting in muscle local inflammation. Moreover, postmenopausal women have large amount of non-contractile muscle tissue, such as intramuscular fat, compared to younger women [42]. For these reasons, IMAT is a significant predictor of both muscle and mobility function in older adults and the relationship of increased levels of IMAT and decreased strength and muscle quality is reported in several studies [43–45].

Adipose tissue is the major metabolic and endocrine organ, containing adipocytes but also nerve tissue, connective tissue, and immune cells, such as resident eosinophils, Breg cells, CD4 T cells, Treg cells, iNKT cells, and M2 macrophages which balance local inflammation [46–49]. Recent studies have shown that most endocrine factors associated with muscle aging, such as sex steroids, glucocorticoids and thyroid hormones may regulate some muscle mitochondrial processes, including mitochondrial quality control (MQC) pathways, OXPHOS activity, redox balance, and apoptotic signaling [50–52]. The negative effect of chronically elevated levels of inflammatory cytokines on muscle mitochondrial function may underlie the well-known association between low-grade inflammation and sarcopenia. Further investigations are needed to understand the complex interaction and relationship among mitochondrial dysfunction, inflammation and sarcopenia.

4.3. Physical Activity and Nutrients in Women

It has been reported that the timing of nutrient consumption can influence the metabolism in women. To date, 95% of our nutrient timing recommendations originate from studies conducted in men. The timing of nutrient consumption during exercise directly affects performance, fatigue recovery, fat oxidation and energy expenditure [53]. Interestingly, women often exercise on an empty stomach, driven by a desire to "burn fat". However, evidence indicates that for women in particular, fasted exercise can attenuate fat oxidation [54]. Alternatively, exercising on a full stomach will result in a higher total daily energy expenditure and increased fat oxidation and, indirectly, improve body composition. A recent analysis suggests that consuming a bolus of protein before exercise, instead of consuming a bolus of carbohydrates, significantly increases energy expenditure and improves fat oxidation after exercise for aerobic exercise, the high intensity interval training and resistance training [55]. When this approach is combined with resistance training, it appears that pre-exercise nutrition may be more effective for women to see improvements in strength and lean body mass, than post-exercise nutrition [55].

Therefore, it is necessary that women adopt an adequate diet when engaging in physical activity and sports and it is mandatory to identify which nutrients are more suitable for women than for men. Furthermore, the different hormonal phases of a woman's life further influence her state of health. It is plausible that gender differences influence the response to food in athletes and also in subjects who perform physical activity [56]. This aspect is not always addressed in studies that explore the effects of diet and food resulting in an important lack of knowledge considering that nutrition plays a fundamental role in maintaining health. In a previous manuscript we stressed the need to teach gender medicine in medical schools in order to optimize the prescription of physical activity for prevention and therapy [57].

Expanding lifespan is not associated with robust health for all during aging, and there has been a substantial increase in age-associated morbidity. The research field on healthy aging has focused to identify risk factors affecting health and quality of life and to provide evidence of effective and acceptable interventions [58]. As previously written, nutritional needs vary greatly between and within age groups and between genders, therefore, general dietary recommendations may not be optimal for the entire population. In November 2019 the WHO introduced the definition of Sustainable Healthy Diets. These are dietary patterns that promote individuals' health and well-being; have low environmental impact; are accessible, affordable, safe and equitable; and are culturally acceptable. The aims of Sustainable Healthy Diets are to (a) promote optimal growth and development and support physical, mental, and social well-being at all life stages for present and future generations; (b) contribute to preventing all forms of malnutrition (i.e., undernutrition, micronutrient deficiency, overweight and obesity); (c) reduce the risk of diet-related NCDs; (d) support the preservation of biodiversity and planetary health [59]. Increasing age is associated with many physiological changes that increase the risk of undernutrition, affecting up to 22% of individuals, with subsequent physical and cognitive impairments, including reduced bone and muscle mass, increased frailty, diminished cognitive function and ability to care for oneself, and thus a higher risk of becoming dependent on care [60]. The mechanisms by which diet affects aging are not well understood, but it seems likely that a wide range of dietary factors counteract molecular damage (e.g., inflammation, oxidative stress and endothelial dysfunction) and mitigate associated functional changes that are induced in aging [61,62]. In addition, several studies have demonstrated the crucial role that gut microbiota plays in maintaining human health. As a model of healthy aging, centenarians have different gut microbiota from ordinary older people. The core microbiome of centenarians in various countries has shown some common characteristics, which are worth further exploration [63]. It is quite difficult to identify a specific diet that is effective in the older woman, a personalized approach is needed. A recent article by Sun and coworkers assessed the effects of whey protein (WP) or WP hydrolysate (WPH) combined with an energy-restricted diet (ERD) on weight reduction and muscle preservation in older women with overweight and obesity [64]. Weight loss is important for older adults with obesity, but a conventionally adopted low-calorie diet is likely to exacerbate the age-related sarcopenia. In older adults the mortality risks of sarcopenia may outweigh the potential benefits of weight loss [65]. Sun and co-workers found that an energy-restricted diet significantly decreased body weight and fat mass, with more noticeable results in the WPH group [64]. Tischmann L and coworkers evaluated long-term effects of soy nut consumption on vascular function and cardiometabolic risk markers in healthy older men and women [66]. They concluded that longer-term soy nut intake as part of a healthy diet improved endothelial function, and LDL-cholesterol concentrations suggesting mechanisms by which an increased soy food intake beneficially affects CVD risk in older adults [66].

Cubas-Basterrechea et al. evaluated the adherence to Mediterranean Diet (MedDiet) in older subjects and found an inverse relationship was established between adherence to the MedDiet and the prevalence of Metabolic syndrome [67]. Scientific evidence supported the beneficial effects of MedDiet consumption in older subjects related to longevity, quality of life, and disease prevention [68]. The MedDiet is rich in bioactive components such as antioxidants (vitamins C and E, among others), fibre, and phytosterols (from vegetables, fruits, legumes, nuts, whole grains, olive oil, and wine), and provide the correct balance of polyunsaturated fatty acids (omega-6 vs. omega-3) through regular consumption of fish, seafood, and nuts, along with high consumption of monounsaturated fats (e.g., olive oil) and low consumption of saturated fats (e.g., meat) [69,70]. The MedDiet has important and proven benefits in the prevention of chronic non-communicable diseases and promotes longevity. There is no evidence that any component of the diet is more effective in older women than in men. This requires further investigations from the perspective of a gender approach to disease prevention.

Many manuscripts underlined the critical role of physical activity, exercise training, and cardiorespiratory fitness (CRF) in the primary and secondary prevention of cardiovascular disease [71–73]. The very recent "Clinical practice statement of the ASPC" defined exercise training, as a subcategory of physical activity (PA), as any structured exercise regimen with the objective of improving or maintaining CRF, muscle strength, health, functional independence, athletic performance, or combinations thereof. Aerobic capacity or CRF is typically expressed as $mLO_2/kg/min$ or metabolic equivalents (METs; 1 MET = 3.5 mL/kg/min) and can be directly determined using gas-exchange measurements or estimated from the attained treadmill speed, percent grade, and duration (minutes) or the cycle ergometer workload, expressed as kilogram meters per minute [74]. Patients with higher fitness and a major CVD risk factor, such as diabetes, obesity, hypertension, or dyslipidemia, generally had a better prognosis those without these risk factors but with low fitness [75]. Kokkinos et al. analyzed a cohort of U.S. veterans and a very diverse population regardless of age, sex, race, and ethnicity, supporting the importance of CRF across various U.S. populations, with no increased risk at very high CRF [75]. However, physicians should be aware that CRF is modifiable with an increase in physical activity. It is known that individuals with low CRF levels who regularly engage in physical activity or exercise can significantly reduce the risk of mortality compared to individuals who remain physically inactive and have low CRF levels [76]. A prolonged period of sedentary behaviour and inactivity in older individuals accelerates the deterioration of skeletal muscle health, including loss of muscle mass and function. Decreased muscle mass in older adults is associated with increased mortality and reduced quality of life [77].

After the pandemic some article explore the effects of Diet and of physical activity on immune system assuming that a healthy diet and a regular physical activity contribute to a stronger immune response and a reduction in systemic inflammatory status [49,78,79]. Clinical studies underline that vitamins and folate, polysaccharides and dietary fiber, lipids, peptides, and natural polyphenols are important for the body's immune system against viruses [78,79]. Natural polyphenols (flavonoids, phenolic acids, stilbenes, lignans) exert known anti-inflammatory, antimicrobial and antioxidant activities, have antiviral capacity, prevent digestion issues and reduce the risk of chronic diseases. Specifically, against the SARS-CoV-2 Virus, they act by inhibiting viral replication, disrupting viral spike protein and inhibiting the SARS-CoV-2 protease [80–82]. Reactive oxygen species play a crucial role in the inflammatory response. Therefore, compound with antioxidant properties have been used to reduce the cytokine storm induced by virus infection [79,83]. To date, antioxidant therapies are being considered to improve muscle responses in patients suffering from long COVID [84–86]. Interestingly, some of the long-standing COVID immunological and systemic features suggest signs of accelerated or premature aging and may aggravate pre-existing age-associated degenerative conditions, such as sarcopenia and cognitive decline [81,82]. There is currently a lack of specific treatments for long COVID. Patient management it is mainly based on symptomatic treatments and recommendations for conducting a healthy lifestyle. Several food supplements and natural bioactive substances have been tested for their potential to counter the long-COVID [85–87].

Global epidemiological trends demonstrate that women have almost double the lifetime rates of anxiety and depression compared to men and increased subclinical rates of symptoms of these disorders [75,85,86]. Women with obesity are more likely to become depressed and report symptoms of depression at a younger age compared to males [88,89]. Depression and stress lead to unhealthy nutritional habits such as cravings [89–91]. A craving for calorie-dense, energy-dense foods can lead to weight gain or obesity. Men and women experience food cravings differently. Women are much more likely to be craving for food (28% compared to 13% of men) and report negative feelings for indulging in cravings, while men are less likely to crave food and report positive feelings associated with cravings [91]. Food energy density is believed to be the strongest predictor of cravings in overweight and obese adults. An energy restriction study found that 75% of coveted foods were chocolate, salty snacks, ice cream, or sugary baked goods [92]. Consuming large quantities of energy-dense foods is not only problematic in terms of nutrient intake, but also in terms of energy balance [90,91]. Today, an increase in physical activity and a healthy diet is suggested in the recovery actions of the unhealthy lifestyle developed during COVID-19.

4.4. Monitoring of Vital Parameters

Another aspect that is becoming increasingly important is the autonomous and home monitoring of vital parameters. The 5 vital signs identified by the WHO are heart rate, respiratory rate, oxygen saturation, blood pressure and body temperature. Alterations of 1 or more parameters indicate disease [92]. The early detection of changes in vital signs typically correlates with faster detection of changes in the cardiopulmonary status of the patients [93]. Some vital signs can be influenced by common age-related pathologies, including hypertension, atherosclerosis, and arrhythmias. Atherosclerotic disease can further increase pulse pressure, which, in conjunction with a high resting heart rate, causes mechanical stress and damage to the endothelium. Finally, the stress response further promotes atherosclerosis. Atherosclerosis can reduce the flexibility of the arteries, contributing to the development of hypertension and the increase of blood pressure with age [92,94]. Similarly, some arrhythmias, i.e., atrial fibrillation increase with age. Monitoring heart beat allow the early diagnosis of heart rhythm abnormalities with the possibility of a more rapid and effective intervention [95,96]. Different devices can be used for the measurement of vital sign, however it is important that they are validated instruments and that provide adequate measurements. In the older adults, the control of vital parameters is important both at rest and during physical exercise.

4.5. Strengths and Limitations of the Study

The strength of the present literature review was to highlight a paucity of studies devoted to the analysis of diet and exercise in older women. It is known that gender medicine complains of a lack of studies dedicated to the differences between men and women and, although there has been an increase in the perception of this need, a gap still persists.

The limitation of the study is due to the difficulty of identifying articles analyzing outcomes in older women. While studies of menopausal women abound, older women are an underrepresented population in clinical trials.

5. Conclusions

It is the general opinion of experts and confirmed by numerous studies that good nutrition and regular physical activity are milestones for counteracting the effects of aging. However, the analysis of the recent literature does not highlight studies in which these two aspects are evaluated together in older women. Gender medicine needs an increase in studies dedicated to women who consider the different phases of hormonal transition. These aspects must be investigated in view of the increase in life span. We need to identify personalized pathways for older women to reduce the risk of chronic disease and improve the quality of life.

Author Contributions: A.V.M., M.P. and M.N. conceived of the idea at the basis of the article, A.V.M., M.N., V.S., G.Z., M.P., C.S., F.F. and S.G. developed the different part of the manuscript and performed the final supervision. All authors have read and agreed to the published version of the manuscript.

Funding: Valentina Selleri received a fellowship from the Istituto Nazionale per le Ricerche Cardiovascolari (INRC). Donazione Anna Maria Ruvinetti.

Institutional Review Board Statement: Not applicable.

Informed Consent Statement: Not applicable.

Data Availability Statement: Not applicable.

Conflicts of Interest: The authors declare no conflict of interest.

References

1. Nozaki, K.; Hamazaki, N.; Kamiya, K.; Kariya, H.; Uchida, S.; Noda, T.; Ueno, K.; Maekawa, E.; Matsunaga, A.; Yamaoka-Tojo, M.; et al. Sex Differences in Frequency of Instrumental Activities of Daily Living after Cardiac Rehabilitation and Its Impact on Outcomes in Patients with Heart Failure. *J. Cardiovasc. Dev. Dis.* **2022**, *9*, 289. [CrossRef] [PubMed]
2. Nasi, M.; Patrizi, G.; Pizzi, C.; Landolfo, M.; Boriani, G.; Cas, A.D.; Cicero, A.F.; Fogacci, F.; Rapezzi, C.; Sisca, G.; et al. The role of physical activity in individuals with cardiovascular risk factors: An opinion paper from Italian Society of Cardiology-Emilia Romagna-Marche and SIC-Sport. *J. Cardiovasc. Med.* **2019**, *20*, 631–639. [CrossRef] [PubMed]
3. da Silveira, M.P.; da Silva Fagundes, K.K.; Bizuti, M.R.; Starck, É.; Rossi, R.C.; de Resende e Silva, D.T. Physical exercise as a tool to help the immune system against COVID-19: An integrative review of the current literature. *Clin. Exp. Med.* **2021**, *21*, 15–284. [CrossRef] [PubMed]
4. Foster, L.; Walker, A. Active Ageing across the Life Course: Towards a Comprehensive Approach to Prevention. *Biomed. Res. Int.* **2021**, *2021*, 6650414. [CrossRef] [PubMed]
5. Vogel, B.; Acevedo, M.; Appelman, Y.; Merz, C.N.B.; Chieffo, A.; Figtree, G.A.; Guerrero, M.; Kunadian, V.; Lam, C.S.P.; Maas, A.H.E.M.; et al. The Lancet women and cardiovascular disease Commission: Reducing the global burden by 2030. *Lancet* **2021**, *397*, 2385–2438. [CrossRef]
6. Mattioli, A.V.; Sciomer, S.; Moscucci, F.; Maiello, M.; Cugusi, L.; Gallina, S.; Dei Cas, A.; Lombardi, C.; Pengo, M.; Parati, G.; et al. Cardiovascular prevention in women: A narrative review from the Italian Society of Cardiology working groups on 'Cardiovascular Prevention, Hypertension and peripheral circulation' and on 'Women Disease'. *J. Cardiovasc. Med.* **2019**, *20*, 575–583. [CrossRef]
7. Coppi, F.; Nasi, M.; Farinetti, A.; Manenti, A.; Gallina, S.; Mattioli, A.V. Physical activity, sedentary behaviour, and diet in menopausal women: Comparison between COVID19 "first wave" and "second wave" of pandemic in Italy. *Prog. Nutr.* **2021**, *23*, 11755. [CrossRef]
8. Astley, C.; Clarke, R.; Cartledge, S.; Beleigoli, A.; Du, H.; Gallagher, C.; Millington, S.; Hendriks, J.M. Remote cardiac rehabilitation services and the digital divide: Implications for elderly populations during the COVID-19 pandemic. *Eur. J. Cardiovasc. Nurs.* **2021**, *20*, 521–523. [CrossRef]
9. Bull, F.C.; Al-Ansari, S.S.; Biddle, S.; Borodulin, K.; Buman, M.P.; Cardon, G.; Carty, C.; Chaput, J.-P.; Chastin, S.; Chou, R.; et al. World Health Organization 2020 guidelines on physical activity and sedentary behaviour. *Br. J. Sports Med.* **2020**, *54*, 1451–1462. [CrossRef]
10. Liguori, G.; Feito, Y.; Fountaine, C.; Roy, B.A.; American College of Sports Medicine. *ACSM's Guidelines for Exercise Testing and Prescription*, 11th ed.; Wolters Kluwer Health: Philadelphia, PA, USA, 2021.
11. Kercher, V.M.; Kercher, K.; Bennion, T.; Levy, P.; Alexander, C.; Amaral, P.C.; Li, Y.-M.; Han, J.; Liu, Y.; Wang, R.; et al. 2022 Fitness Trends from Around the Globe. *ACSM's Health Fit. J.* **2022**, *26*, 21–37. [CrossRef]
12. Batrakoulis, A. European survey of fitness trends for 2020. *ACSM's Health Fit. J.* **2019**, *23*, 28–35. [CrossRef]
13. Badimon, L.; Vilahur, G.; Padro, T. Nutraceuticals and atherosclerosis: Human trials. *Cardiovasc Ther.* **2010**, *28*, 202–215. [CrossRef] [PubMed]
14. Austad, S.N.; Fischer, K.E. Sex differences in lifespan. *Cell Metab.* **2016**, *23*, 1022–1033. [CrossRef] [PubMed]
15. Peterson, J.R.; Baumgartner, D.A.; Austin, S.L. Healthy ageing in the far North:perspectives and prescriptions. *Int. J. Circumpolar Health* **2020**, *79*, 1735036. [CrossRef] [PubMed]
16. Bailey, R.L.; Dog, T.L.; Smith-Ryan, A.E.; Das, S.K.; Baker, F.C.; Madak-Erdogan, Z.; Hammond, B.R.; Sesso, H.D.; Eapen, A.; Mitmesser, S.H.; et al. Sex Differences Across the Life Course: A Focus on Unique Nutritional and Health Considerations among Women. *J. Nutr.* **2022**, *152*, 1597–1610. [CrossRef]

17. Gernand, A.D.; Schulze, K.J.; Stewart, C.P.; West, K.P.; Christian, P. Micronutrient deficiencies in pregnancy worldwide: Health effects and prevention. *Nat. Rev. Endocrinol.* **2016**, *12*, 274–289. [CrossRef]
18. Potischman, N.; Freudenheim, J.L. Biomarkers of nutritional exposure and nutritional status: An overview. *J. Nutr.* **2003**, *133*, 873S–874S. [CrossRef]
19. Cui, P.; Li, M.; Yu, M.; Liu, Y.; Ding, Y.; Liu, W.; Liu, J. Advances in sports food: Sports nutrition, food manufacture, opportunities and challenges. *Food Res. Int.* **2022**, *157*, 111258. [CrossRef]
20. Campesi, I.; Marino, M.; Cipolletti, M.; Romani, A.; Franconi, F. Put "gender glasses" on the effects of phenolic compounds on cardiovascular function and diseases. *Eur. J. Nutr.* **2018**, *57*, 2677–2691. [CrossRef]
21. Truzzi, M.L.; Ballerini Puviani, M.; Tripodi, A.; Toni, S.; Farinetti, A.; Nasi, M.; Mattioli, A.V. Mediterranean Diet as a model of sustainable, resilient and healthy diet. *Prog. Nutr.* **2020**, *22*, 388–394. [CrossRef]
22. D'Archivio, M.; Santangelo, C.; Silenzi, A.; Scazzocchio, B.; Varì, R.; Masella, R. Dietary EVOO Polyphenols and Gut Microbiota Interaction: Are There Any Sex/Gender Influences? *Antioxidants* **2022**, *11*, 1744. [CrossRef] [PubMed]
23. Mattioli, A.V.; Toni, S.; Coppi, F.; Farinetti, A. Practical tips for prevention of cardiovascular disease in women after quarantine for COVID-19 disease. *Acta Biomed.* **2020**, *91*, e2020127. [CrossRef] [PubMed]
24. Amrein, K.; Scherkl, M.; Hoffmann, M.; Neuwersch-Sommeregger, S.; Köstenberger, M.; Berisha, A.T.; Martucci, G.; Pilz, S.; Malle, O. Vitamin D deficiency 2.0: An update on the current status worldwide. *Eur. J. Clin. Nutr.* **2020**, *74*, 1498–1513. [CrossRef] [PubMed]
25. Cashman, K.D.; Dowling, K.G.; Škrabáková, Z.; Gonzalez-Gross, M.; Valtueña, J.; De Henauw, S.; Moreno, L.; Damsgaard, C.T.; Michaelsen, K.F.; Mølgaard, C.; et al. Vitamin D deficiency in Europe: Pandemic? *Am. J. Clin. Nutr.* **2016**, *103*, 1033–1044. [CrossRef] [PubMed]
26. Cashman, K.D. Vitamin D deficiency: Defining, prevalence, causes, and strategies of addressing. *Calcif. Tissue Int.* **2019**, *106*, 14–29. [CrossRef] [PubMed]
27. Jia, S.; Zhao, W.; Hu, F.; Zhao, Y.; Ge, M.; Xia, X.; Yue, J.; Dong, B. Sex differences in the association of physical activity levels and vitamin D with obesity, sarcopenia, and sarcopenic obesity: A cross-sectional study. *BMC Geriatr.* **2022**, *22*, 898. [CrossRef]
28. Roberts, S.B.; Silver, R.E.; Das, S.K.; Fielding, R.A.; Gilhooly, C.H.; Jacques, P.F.; Kelly, J.M.; Mason, J.B.; McKeown, N.M.; Reardon, M.A.; et al. Healthy aging-nutrition matters: Start early and screen often. *Adv. Nutr.* **2021**, *12*, 1438–1448. [CrossRef]
29. Webster, J.; Greenwood, D.C.; Cade, J.E. Foods, nutrients and hip fracture risk: A prospective study of middle-aged women. *Clin. Nutr.* **2022**, *41*, 2825–2832. [CrossRef]
30. Delmonico, M.J.; Harris, T.B.; Lee, J.-S.; Visser, M.; Nevitt, M.; Kritchevsky, S.B.; Tylavsky, F.A.; Newman, A.B. Alternative definitions of sarcopenia, lower extremity performance, and functional impairment with aging in older men and women. *J. Am. Geriatr. Soc.* **2007**, *55*, 769–774. [CrossRef]
31. Sousa-Victor, P.; Gutarra, S.; García-Prat, L.; Rodriguez-Ubreva, J.; Ortet, L.; Ruiz-Bonilla, V.; Jardí, M.; Ballestar, E.; González, S.; Serrano, A.L.; et al. Geriatric muscle stem cells switch reversible quiescence into senescence. *Nature* **2014**, *506*, 316–321. [CrossRef]
32. Akhmedov, D.; Berdeaux, R. The effects of obesity on skeletal muscle regeneration. *Front. Physiol.* **2013**, *4*, 371. [CrossRef] [PubMed]
33. Florez, H.; Troen, B.R. Fat and inflammaging: A dual path to unfitness in elderly people? *J. Am. Geriatr. Soc.* **2008**, *56*, 558–560. [CrossRef] [PubMed]
34. Langen, R.C.; Schols, A.M.W.J.; Kelders, M.C.J.M.; van der Velden, J.L.J.; Wouters, E.F.M.; Janssen-Heininger, Y.M.W. Muscle wasting and impaired muscle regeneration in a murine model of chronic pulmonary inflammation. *Am. J. Respir. Cell Mol. Biol.* **2006**, *35*, 689–696. [CrossRef] [PubMed]
35. Bodell, P.W.; Kodesh, E.; Haddad, F.; Zaldivar, F.P.; Cooper, D.M.; Adams, G.R. Skeletal muscle growth in young rats is inhibited by chronic exposure to IL-6 but preserved by concurrent voluntary endurance exercise. *J. Appl. Physiol.* **2008**, *106*, 443–453. [CrossRef] [PubMed]
36. Sjoblom, S.; Suuronen, J.; Rikkonen, T.; Honkanen, R.; Kröger, H.; Sirola, J. Relationship between postmenopausal osteoporosis and the components of clinical sarcopenia. *Maturitas* **2013**, *75*, 175–180. [CrossRef]
37. Pansini, F.; Cervellati, C.; Guariento, A.; Stacchini, M.A.; Castaldini, C.; Bernardi, A.; Pascale, G.; Bonaccorsi, G.; Patella, A.; Bagni, B.; et al. Oxidative stress, body fat composition, and endocrine status in pre- and postmenopausal women. *Menopause* **2008**, *15*, 112–118. [CrossRef]
38. Barbieri, E.; Sestili, P. Reactive oxygen species in skeletal muscle signaling. *J. Signal Transduct.* **2012**, *2012*, 982794. [CrossRef]
39. Coen, P.M.; Goodpaster, B.H. Role of intramyocelluar lipids in human health. *Trends Endocrinol. Metab.* **2012**, *23*, 391–398. [CrossRef]
40. Ritter, O.; Jelenik, T.; Roden, M. Lipid-mediated muscle insulin resistance: Different fat, different pathways? *J. Mol. Med.* **2015**, *93*, 831–843. [CrossRef]
41. Marzetti, E.; Calvani, R.; Cesari, M.; Buford, T.W.; Lorenzi, M.; Behnke, B.J.; Leeuwenburgh, C. Mitochondrial dysfunction and sarcopenia of aging: From signaling pathways to clinical trials. *Int. J. Biochem. Cell Biol.* **2013**, *45*, 2288–2301. [CrossRef]
42. Khadilkar, S.S. Musculoskeletal Disorders and Menopause. *J. Obstet. Gynecol. India* **2019**, *69*, 99–103. [CrossRef] [PubMed]
43. Health AgingBody Composition Study; Delmonico, M.J.; Harris, T.B.; Visser, M.; Park, S.W.; Conroy, M.B.; Velasquez-Mieyer, P.; Boudreau, R.; Manini, T.M.; Nevitt, M.; et al. Longitudinal study of muscle strength, quality, and adipose tissue infiltration. *Am. J. Clin. Nutr.* **2009**, *90*, 1579–1585. [PubMed]

44. Zoico, E.; Rossi, A.; Di Francesco, V.; Sepe, A.; Olioso, D.; Pizzini, F.; Fantin, F.; Bosello, O.; Cominacini, L.; Harris, T.B.; et al. Adipose tissue infiltration in skeletal muscle of healthy elderly men: Relationships with body composition, insulin resistance, and inflammation at the systemic and tissue level. *J. Gerontol. A Biol. Sci. Med. Sci.* **2010**, *65*, 295–299. [CrossRef] [PubMed]
45. Addison, O.; Marcus, R.L.; LaStayo, P.C.; Ryan, A.S. Intermuscular fat: A review of the consequences and causes. *Int. J. Endocrinol.* **2014**, *2014*, 309570. [CrossRef]
46. Kalinkovich, A.; Livshits, G. Sarcopenic obesity or obese sarcopenia: A cross talk between age-associated adipose tissue and skeletal muscle inflammation as a main mechanism of the pathogenesis. *Ageing Res. Rev.* **2017**, *35*, 200–221. [CrossRef]
47. Schipper, H.S.; Prakken, B.; Kalkhoven, E.; Boes, M. Adipose tissue-resident immune cells: Key players in immunometabolism. *Trends Endocrinol. Metab.* **2012**, *23*, 407–415. [CrossRef]
48. Mattioli, A.V.; Pinti, M.; Farinetti, A.; Nasi, M. Obesity risk during collective quarantine for the COVID-19 epidemic. *Obes. Med.* **2020**, *20*, 100263. [CrossRef]
49. De Gaetano, A.; Solodka, K.; Zanini, G.; Selleri, V.; Mattioli, A.V.; Nasi, M.; Pinti, M. Molecular Mechanisms of mtDNA-Mediated Inflammation. *Cells* **2021**, *10*, 2898. [CrossRef]
50. Weber, K.; Brück, P.; Mikes, Z.; Küpper, J.H.; Klingenspor, M.; Wiesner, R.J. Glucocorticoid hormone stimulates mitochondrial biogenesis specifically in skeletal muscle. *Endocrinology* **2002**, *143*, 177–184. [CrossRef]
51. Weitzel, J.M.; Iwen, K.A. Coordination of mitochondrial biogenesis by thyroid hormone. *Mol. Cell Endocrinol.* **2011**, *342*, 1–7. [CrossRef]
52. Guo, W.; Wong, S.; Li, M.; Liang, W.; Liesa, M.; Serra, C.; Jasuja, R.; Bartke, A.; Kirkland, J.L.; Shirihai, O.; et al. Testosterone plus low-intensity physical training in late life improves functional performance, skeletal muscle mitochondrial biogenesis, and mitochondrial quality control in male mice. *PLoS ONE* **2012**, *7*, e51180. [CrossRef] [PubMed]
53. Kerksick, C.M.; Arent, S.; Schoenfeld, B.J.; Stout, J.R.; Campbell, B.; Wilborn, C.D.; Taylor, L.; Kalman, D.; Smith-Ryan, A.E.; Kreider, R.B.; et al. International Society of Sports Nutrition position stand: Nutrient timing. *J. Int. Soc. Sports Nutr.* **2017**, *14*, 33. [CrossRef] [PubMed]
54. Henderson, G.C.; Alderman, B.L. Determinants of resting lipid oxidation in response to a prior bout of endurance exercise. *J. Appl. Physiol.* **2014**, *116*, 95–103. [CrossRef] [PubMed]
55. Wingfield, H.L.; Smith-Ryan, A.E.; Melvin, M.N.; Roelofs, E.J.; Trexler, E.T.; Hackney, A.C.; Weaver, M.A.; Ryan, E.D. The acute effect of exercise modality and nutrition manipulations on post-exercise resting energy expenditure and respiratory exchange ratio in women: A randomized trial. *Sports Med. Open* **2015**, *1*, 11. [CrossRef] [PubMed]
56. Tam, R.; Beck, K.L.; Manore, M.M.; Giford, J.; Flood, V.M.; O'Connor, H. Effectiveness of education interventions designed to improve nutrition knowledge in athletes: A systematic review. *Sports Med.* **2019**, *49*, 1769–1786. [CrossRef]
57. Mattioli, A.V.; Nasi, M.; Pinti, M.; Palumbo, C. Teaching Gender Differences at Medical School Could Improve the Safety and Efficacy of Personalized Physical Activity Prescription. *Front. Cardiovasc. Med.* **2022**, *9*, 919257. [CrossRef]
58. Wickramasinghe, K.; Mathers, J.C.; Wopereis, S.; Marsman, D.S.; Griffiths, J.C. From lifespan to healthspan: The role of nutrition in healthy ageing. *J. Nutr. Sci.* **2020**, *9*, e33. [CrossRef]
59. World Health Organization. Ending Inappropriate Promotion of Commercially Available Complementary Foods for Infants and Young Children between 6 and 36 Months in Europe. 2019. Available online: http://www.euro.who.int/en/health-topics/disease-prevention/nutrition/publications/2019/ending-inappropriate-promotion-of-commercially-available-complementary-foods-for-infants-and-young-children-between-6-and-36-months-in-europe-2019 (accessed on 10 September 2022).
60. World Health Organization. Essential Nutrition Actions: Mainstreaming Nutrition through the Life-Course. 2019. Available online: https://www.who.int/nutrition/publications/essential-nutrition-actions-2019/en/ (accessed on 30 January 2020).
61. Malcomson, F.C.; Mathers, J.C. Nutrition and ageing. *Subcell. Biochem.* **2018**, *90*, 373–424.
62. López-Otín, C.; Blasco, M.A.; Partridge, L.; Serrano, M.; Kroemer, G. The hallmarks of aging. *Cell* **2013**, *153*, 1194–1217. [CrossRef]
63. Shi, X.; Ma, T.; Sakandar, H.A.; Menghe, B.; Sun, Z. Gut microbiome and aging nexus and underlying mechanism. *Appl. Microbiol. Biotechnol.* **2022**, *106*, 5349–5358. [CrossRef]
64. Sun, Y.; Ling, C.; Liu, L.; Zhang, J.; Wang, J.; Tong, X.; Hidayat, K.; Chen, M.; Chen, X.; Zhou, H.; et al. Effects of Whey Protein or Its Hydrolysate Supplements Combined with an Energy-Restricted Diet on Weight Loss: A Randomized Controlled Trial in Older Women. *Nutrients* **2022**, *14*, 4540. [CrossRef] [PubMed]
65. Coker, R.H.; Miller, S.; Schutzler, S.; Deutz, N.; Wolfe, R.R. Whey protein and essential amino acids promote the reduction of adipose tissue and increased muscle protein synthesis during caloric restriction-induced weight loss in elderly, obese individuals. *Nutr. J.* **2012**, *11*, 105. [CrossRef] [PubMed]
66. Tischmann, L.; Adam, T.C.; Mensink, R.P.; Joris, P.J. Longer-term soy nut consumption improves vascular function and cardiometabolic risk markers in older adults: Results of a randomized, controlled cross-over trial. *Clin. Nutr.* **2022**, *41*, 1052–1058. [CrossRef] [PubMed]
67. Cubas-Basterrechea, G.; Elío, I.; Alonso, G.; Otero, L.; Gutiérrez-Bardeci, L.; Puente, J.; Muñoz-Cacho, P. Adherence to the Mediterranean Diet Is Inversely Associated with the Prevalence of Metabolic Syndrome in Older People from the North of Spain. *Nutrients* **2022**, *14*, 4536. [CrossRef]
68. Dominguez, L.J.; Di Bella, G.; Veronese, N.; Barbagallo, M. Impact of Mediterranean diet on chronic non-communicable diseases and longevity. *Nutrients* **2021**, *13*, 2028. [CrossRef]
69. Barbouti, A.; Goulas, V. Dietary antioxidants in the Mediterranean diet. *Antioxidants* **2021**, *10*, 1213. [CrossRef]

70. Mattioli, A.V.; Francesca, C.; Mario, M.; Alberto, F. Fruit and vegetables in hypertensive women with asymptomatic peripheral arterial disease. *Clin. Nutr. ESPEN* **2018**, *27*, 110–112. [CrossRef]
71. Sanchis-Gomar, F.; Lavie, C.J.; Marín, J.; Perez-Quilis, C.; Eijsvogels, T.M.H.; O'Keefe, J.H.; Perez, M.V.; Blair, S.N. Exercise effects on cardiovascular disease: From basic aspects to clinical evidence. *Cardiovasc. Res.* **2022**, *118*, 2253–2266. [CrossRef]
72. Paolisso, P.; Bergamaschi, L.; Saturi, G.; D'Angelo, E.C.; Magnani, I.; Toniolo, S.; Stefanizzi, A.; Rinaldi, A.; Bartoli, L.; Angeli, F.; et al. Secondary Prevention Medical Therapy and Outcomes in Patients with Myocardial Infarction with Non-Obstructive Coronary Artery Disease. *Front. Pharmacol.* **2020**, *10*, 1606. [CrossRef]
73. Lavie, C.; Sanchis-Gomar, F.; Ozemek, C. Fit Is It for Longevity Across Populations. *J. Am. Coll. Cardiol.* **2022**, *80*, 610–612. [CrossRef]
74. Franklin, B.A.; Eijsvogels, T.M.H.; Pandey, A.; Quindry, J.; Toth, P.P. Physical activity, cardiorespiratory fitness, and cardiovascular health: A clinical practice statement of the ASPC Part I: Bioenergetics, contemporary physical activity recommendations, benefits, risks, extreme exercise regimens, potential maladaptations. *Am. J. Prev. Cardiol.* **2022**, *12*, 100424. [CrossRef] [PubMed]
75. Kokkinos, P.; Faselis, C.; Samuel, I.B.H.; Pittaras, A.; Doumas, M.; Murphy, R.; Heimall, M.S.; Sui, X.; Zhang, J.; Myers, J. Cardiorespiratory fitness and mortality risk across the spectra of age, race, and sex. *J. Am. Coll. Cardiol.* **2022**, *80*, 598–609. [CrossRef] [PubMed]
76. Imboden, M.T.; Harber, M.P.; Whaley, M.H.; Finch, W.H.; Bishop, D.L.; Fleenor, B.S.; Kaminsky, L.A. The association between the change in directly measured cardiorespiratory fitness across time and mortality risk. *Prog. Cardiovasc. Dis.* **2019**, *62*, 157–162. [CrossRef] [PubMed]
77. Park, S.; Chang, Y.; Wolfe, R.R.; Kim, I.Y. Prevention of Loss of Muscle Mass and Function in Older Adults during COVID-19 Lockdown: Potential Role of Dietary Essential Amino Acids. *Int. J. Environ. Res. Public Health* **2022**, *19*, 8090. [CrossRef]
78. Mattioli, A.V.; Sciomer, S.; Maffei, S.; Gallina, S. Lifestyle and Stress Management in Women during COVID-19 Pandemic: Impact on Cardiovascular Risk Burden. *Am. J. Lifestyle Med.* **2021**, *15*, 356–359. [CrossRef]
79. Tosato, M.; Ciciarello, F.; Zazzara, M.B.; Pais, C.; Savera, G.; Picca, A.; Galluzzo, V.; Coelho-Júnior, H.J.; Calvani, R.; Marzetti, E.; et al. Nutraceuticals and Dietary Supplements for Older Adults with Long COVID-19. *Clin. Geriatr. Med.* **2022**, *38*, 565–591. [CrossRef]
80. Biancatelli, R.M.L.C.; Berrill, M.; Catravas, J.D.; Marik, P.E. Quercetin and Vitamin C: An Experimental, Synergistic Therapy for the Prevention and Treatment of SARS-CoV-2 Related Disease (COVID-19). *Front. Immunol.* **2020**, *11*, 1451. [CrossRef]
81. Hoffmann, M.; Kleine-Weber, H.; Schroeder, S.; Krüger, N.; Herrler, T.; Erichsen, S.; Schiergens, T.S.; Herrler, G.; Wu, N.-H.; Nitsche, A.; et al. SARS-CoV-2 Cell Entry Depends on ACE2 and TMPRSS2 and Is Blocked by a Clinically Proven Protease Inhibitor. *Cell* **2020**, *181*, 271–280.e8. [CrossRef]
82. Ayivi, R.D.; Ibrahim, S.A.; Colleran, H.L.; Silva, R.C.; Williams, L.L.; Galanakis, C.M.; Fidan, H.; Tomovska, J.; Siddiqui, S.A. COVID-19: Human immune response and the influence of food ingredients and active compounds. *Bioact. Compd. Health Dis.* **2021**, *4*, 100–148. [CrossRef]
83. Lo Tartaro, D.; Neroni, A.; Paolini, A.; Borella, R.; Mattioli, M.; Fidanza, L.; Quong, A.; Petes, C.; Awong, G.; Douglas, S.; et al. Molecular and cellular immune features of aged patients with severe COVID-19 pneumonia. *Commun. Biol.* **2022**, *5*, 590. [CrossRef]
84. Maeng, L.Y.; Coppi, L.; Nasi, M.; Pinti, M.; Gallina, S. Long COVID: A New Challenge for Prevention of Obesity in Women. *Am. J. Lifestyle Med.* **2022**, in press. [CrossRef]
85. Luo, P.; Liu, D.; Li, J. Pharmacological perspective: Glycyrrhizin may be an efficacious therapeutic agent for COVID-19. *Int. J. Antimicrob. Agents* **2020**, *55*, 105995. [CrossRef] [PubMed]
86. Rychter, A.M.; Hryhorowicz, S.; Słomski, R.; Dobrowolska, A.; Krela-Kaźmierczak, I. Antioxidant effects of vitamin E and risk of cardiovascular disease in women with obesity—A narrative review. *Clin Nutr.* **2022**, *41*, 1557–1565. [CrossRef] [PubMed]
87. Galanakis, C.M.; Aldawoud, T.M.S.; Rizou, M.; Rowan, N.J.; Ibrahim, S.A. Food ingredients and active compounds against the coronavirus disease (COVID-19) pandemic: A comprehensive review. *Foods* **2020**, *9*, 1701. [CrossRef] [PubMed]
88. Maeng, L.Y.; Milad, M.R. Sex differences in anxiety disorders: Interactions between fear, stress, and gonadal hormones. *Horm. Behav.* **2015**, *76*, 106–117. [CrossRef]
89. Bucciarelli, V.; Nasi, M.; Bianco, F.; Seferovic, J.; Ivkovic, V.; Gallina, S.; Mattioli, A.V. Depression pandemic and cardiovascular risk in the COVID-19 era and long COVID syndrome: Gender makes a difference. *Trends Cardiovasc. Med.* **2022**, *32*, 12–17. [CrossRef]
90. Gilhooly, C.H.; Das, S.K.; Golden, J.K.; McCrory, M.A.; Dallal, G.E.; Saltzman, E.; Kramer, F.M.; Roberts, S.B. Food cravings and energy regulation: The characteristics of craved foods and their relationship with eating behaviors and weight change during 6 months of dietary energy restriction. *Int. J. Obes.* **2007**, *31*, 1849–1858. [CrossRef]
91. Lafay, L.; Thomas, F.; Mennen, L.; Charles, M.A.; Eschwege, E.; Borys, J.M.; Basdevant, A. Gender differences in the relation between food cravings and mood in an adult community: Results from the Fleurbaix Laventie ville Santé Study. *Int. J. Eat. Disord.* **2001**, *29*, 195–204. [CrossRef]
92. Cooper, R.J.; Schriger, D.L.; Flaherty, H.L.; Lin, E.J.; Hubbell, K.A. Effect of vital signs on triage decisions. *Ann. Emerg. Med.* **2002**, *39*, 223–232. [CrossRef]
93. Chester, J.G.; Rudolph, J.L. Vital signs in older patients: Age-related changes. *J. Am. Med. Dir. Assoc.* **2011**, *12*, 337–343. [CrossRef]
94. Lakatta, E.G.; Levy, D. Arterial and cardiac aging: Major shareholders in cardiovascular disease enterprises: Part I: Aging arteries: A "set up" for vascular disease. *Circulation* **2003**, *107*, 139–146. [CrossRef] [PubMed]

95. Ball, J.; Carrington, M.J.; McMurray, J.J.; Stewart, S. Atrial fibrillation: Profile and burden of an evolving epidemic in the 21st century. *Int. J. Cardiol.* **2013**, *167*, 1807–1824. [CrossRef] [PubMed]
96. Samol, A.; Masin, M.; Gellner, R.; Otte, B.; Pavenstädt, H.J.; Ringelstein, E.B.; Reinecke, H.; Waltenberger, J.; Kirchhof, P. Prevalence of unknown atrial fibrillation in patients with risk factors. *Europace* **2013**, *15*, 657–662. [CrossRef] [PubMed]

Disclaimer/Publisher's Note: The statements, opinions and data contained in all publications are solely those of the individual author(s) and contributor(s) and not of MDPI and/or the editor(s). MDPI and/or the editor(s) disclaim responsibility for any injury to people or property resulting from any ideas, methods, instructions or products referred to in the content.

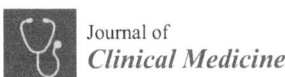

Review

The Impact of Physical Activity and Inactivity on Cardiovascular Risk across Women's Lifespan: An Updated Review

Valentina Bucciarelli [1], Anna Vittoria Mattioli [2,3], Susanna Sciomer [4], Federica Moscucci [4], Giulia Renda [5] and Sabina Gallina [5,*]

1. Cardiovascular Sciences Department, Azienda Ospedaliero—Universitaria delle Marche, 60126 Ancona, Italy; valentina.bucciarelli@ospedaliriuniti.marche.it
2. Department of Medical and Surgical Sciences for Children and Adults, University of Modena and Reggio Emilia, 41124 Modena, Italy
3. National Institute for Cardiovascular Research-INRC, 40126 Bologna, Italy
4. Department of Clinical and Internal Medicine, Anesthesiology and Cardiovascular Sciences, University of Rome 'Sapienza', Policlinico Umberto I, 49971 Rome, Italy
5. Department of Neuroscience, Imaging and Clinical Sciences, University of Chieti-Pescara, 66100 Chieti, Italy; giulia.renda@unich.it
* Correspondence: sgallina@unich.it; Tel.: +39-0871-41512

Abstract: Physical inactivity (PI) represents a significant, modifiable risk factor that is more frequent and severe in the female population worldwide for all age groups. The physical activity (PA) gender gap begins early in life and leads to considerable short-term and long-term adverse effects on health outcomes, especially cardiovascular (CV) health. Our review aims to highlight the prevalence and mechanisms of PI across women's lifespan, describing the beneficial effects of PA in many physiological and pathological clinical scenarios and underlining the need for more awareness and global commitment to promote strategies to bridge the PA gender gap and limit PI in current and future female generations.

Keywords: physical inactivity; physical activity; cardiovascular risk; women; gender medicine

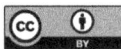

1. Introduction

Cardiovascular disease (CVD) is the leading cause of morbidity and mortality in the female population [1]. There are substantial gender differences in the pathophysiology of CVD, principally related to estrogen's protective anti-inflammatory and anti-apoptotic role [2]. Besides traditional CV risk factors, there is an evolving group of risk factors specific to the female gender, including autoimmune disease, breast cancer treatment, cardio-metabolic gestational disorders, and menopause [3,4]. Physical inactivity (PI) is defined as an insufficient physical activity (PA) level to meet present PA recommendations for age and represents a significant modifiable traditional CV risk factor still hard to counteract. This occurs regardless of the abundance of scientific evidence supporting PA as one of the most effective non-pharmacological therapies in primary and secondary CV prevention, with an outstanding effect on vascular homeostasis [5–10]. Furthermore, the role of regular PA in preventing and treating non-communicable diseases (NCDs) has been widely demonstrated. The data from a prospective cohort of adults from the United States (63% women) indicated the nearly maximum association with lower mortality achievable by completing, during middle and late adulthood, 150–300 min per week of vigorous PA, 300–600 min per week of moderate PA, or an equivalent combination of both [11,12]. PA showed robust beneficial associations with different mental health conditions, including anxiety and depression, both in the general population and in women, across all lifespans [13–17].

Although the efforts made by the leading international scientific societies to promote adherence to a correct lifestyle, including a healthy diet, adequate levels of PA, and a concomitant reduction in PI, the latest World Health Organization (WHO) records highlighted that, worldwide, 1 in 4 adults and 3 in 4 adolescents (aged 11–17 years) still do not currently meet the global recommendations for PA, with higher levels of PI in economically developed countries [18]. The global costs of PI to healthcare systems are exorbitant, estimated at INT$53.8 billion in 2013 and will reach a cost of INT$520 billion by 2030 if the prevalence of PI does not change [19]. Moreover, globally, PI causes 7.2% of all-cause deaths and 7.6% of CVD deaths, with the more significant relative burden in high-income countries [20]. In women older than 30, the population risk of CVD associated with PI seems to exceed that of other risk factors [21]. The economic burden of PI is disproportionately spread across regions, with the highest economic cost occurring among high-income countries, which account for 70% of expenditure on treatment for illnesses related to PI [22]. On the other hand, a strong association between PA and the risk of developing CVD has been extensively described, with a median risk reduction of CV risk more significant in women than men [23]. Moreover, the level of global CV risk does not alter the inverse connection between PA and incident CVD in women, suggesting that the promotion of PA is essential, regardless of subjective CV risk [24]. Finally, PA in women can be a protective factor in the etiology of many non-traditional CV risk factors, i.e., cardio-metabolic gestational disorders, autoimmune diseases, breast cancer, and breast-cancer-related treatments [25–27].

Regardless of the abovementioned outstanding positive effects of PA in women, according to the WHO data PI is more frequent and severe in the female population for all age groups, with a global average of 31.7% for inactive women vs. 23.4% for inactive men [18,28].

Going deeper into the statistical details, the latest National Health Interview Survey (NHIS) data about the levels of PA in the civilian non-institutionalized population of the United States (U.S.) suggested that the prevalence of PI decreased from 40.5% (1998) to 25.6% (2018), with a concomitant increase in meeting the recommended high aerobic PA levels from 26.0% (1998) to 37.4% (2018). However, the prevalence of PI in 2018 was still higher in women (27.8%) than in men (23.2%), and the prevalence of high aerobic PA levels remained lower in women (33%) than in men (42%) [29].

In Europe, about 35.4% of adults, predominantly from southern European countries, were inactive in 2016; in particular, regular PA decreases with age: only 1 in 4 adults older than 55 years old exercises at least once a week. In line with U.S. data, fewer women than men are active in Europe, especially in the youngest age group of 15 to 24 years old (73% of active men compared with 58% of active women) [30].

There are several multifaceted obstacles to women's participation in PA and sports that can be divided into three main categories: economic and socio-cultural barriers, practical barriers, and knowledge barriers. Among the significant economic and socio-cultural barriers are the wrong belief that sport is masculine and exclusive, low female self-esteem, parents' disagreement with sport, the fear of scholastic failure, family care, and housework. Practical obstacles include poverty, lack of financial resources, scarcity of leisure time, and scarcity of accessible, safe, and appropriate facilities. Finally, knowledge barriers include the need for more knowledge about the benefits of PA [31,32].

The PA gender gap begins early in life and may have short-term and long-term adverse effects on health outcomes, especially regarding CV status [33].

This paper aims to provide an up-to-date review of the evidence of PI and the benefits of PA in the female population throughout all women's life stages, underlining the need for global commitment to endorse strategies to bridge the PA gender gap, overcome barriers to women's participation to PA, and limit PI in current and future female generations (Figure 1).

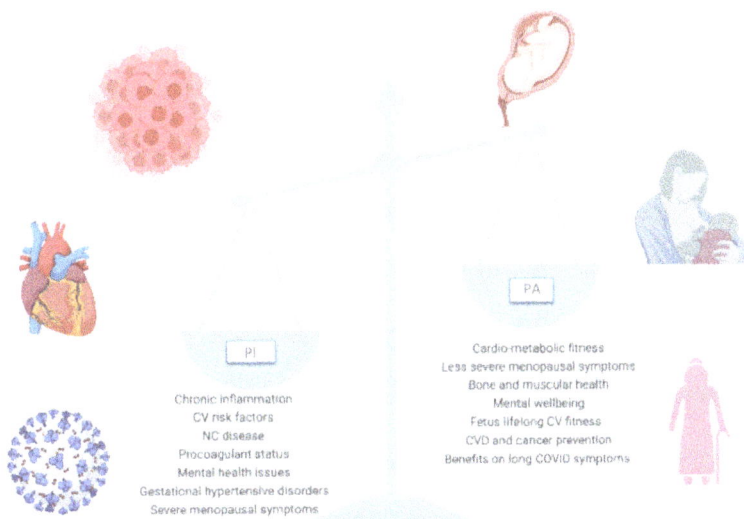

Figure 1. Physical activity (PA) benefits compared with physical inactivity (PI) adverse effects throughout women's life stages and across different clinical scenarios. Abbreviations: CV, cardiovascular; NC, non-communicable; CVD, cardiovascular disease.

2. Physical Activity and Inactivity in Infancy and Adolescence

2.1. Benefits of Physical Activity

In children and adolescents, regular PA provides many benefits regarding CV and cardio-metabolic fitness, bone health, mental well-being, and cognitive outcomes. Young people represent 24% of the worldwide population, and investing in their health is crucial, as childhood PA can affect adult health, with a biological and behavioral carry-over effect into adulthood regarding the global health status and a fitter lifestyle [34–36].

In 1989, Blair et al. proposed a model for the health consequences of childhood PA, suggesting that three main benefits derive from sufficient childhood PA: 1. improvement in childhood health status; 2. improvement in childhood quality of life; 3. improvement in adult health status. All three could significantly delay the onset of chronic disease and maintain sufficient activity in adulthood [37]. Much scientific evidence supports these hypotheses and confirms PA's significant positive effect on cardiorespiratory fitness (CRF), body composition, insulin resistance, and CVD risk factors in childhood. Several observational studies documented the dose–response relations between PA and health, suggesting that the higher the PA, the greater the health benefit. However, experimental evidence suggests that even limited amounts of PA, especially if aerobic-based and of moderate or vigorous intensity, can provide great health benefits, especially in high-risk adolescents (i.e., obese with high blood pressure) [38]. It is well known that CRF is a good predictor of CV health starting from childhood, as higher levels of CRF in this period correlate to a better CV profile in adulthood. Data from the Healthy Lifestyle in Europe by Nutrition in Adolescence (HELENA) study, in a population of 3528 adolescents from 10 European centers, confirmed the strong association between CRF and the ideal CV health index, according to the American Heart Association (AHA) indicators, and suggested that a CRF cutoff level of 40–47 mL/kg/min for boys and 35–42 mL/kg/min for girls is associated with a better CV health profile [39]. Other data from the HELENA database demonstrated that vigorous PA, rather than low-intensity PA, is effective in preventing obesity in adolescents, being negatively associated with indices of fat mass and positively associated with markers of muscle mass; in contrast, both average PA and at least moderate PA reduce total and central body fat in youth [40,41]. Moreover, higher vigorous

PA (≥30 min/day) and lower sedentary behavior (<2 h/day) have a protective effect on cardio-metabolic risk factors [42]. Another sub-analysis from the HELENA database showed a negative association between PA and markers of insulin resistance, with low CRF modifying this relationship, especially in female adolescents [43]. A systematic review by Janssen et al. examined the relationship between PA and global health in school-aged children and young adults. The authors concluded that even if the results from many observational studies suggest a direct relationship between the amount of PA and the relevance of health benefits, several experimental studies revealed that even a limited volume of PA can have substantial health benefits in the young population at high CV risk. Regarding the type of PA, it seems that aerobic PA is successful at controlling blood pressure within both sexes, even if the effects of the volume and intensity of PA on blood pressure and the effect of age on the relationship between PA and blood pressure are still to be clarified [38]. The beneficial effects of PA on metabolic and psychological status have been confirmed even in children with type 1 diabetes [44]. Furthermore, moderate-to-vigorous PA is also associated with better sleep efficiency, the latter being associated with higher levels of CRF and a more favorable cardio-metabolic profile, as confirmed by a systematic review by Saunders et al. [45–47].

2.2. Sedentary Behavior and Physical Inactivity Disadvantages

PI in childhood and adolescence is related to unfavorable health adaptations that start from childhood and follow children and adolescents throughout adulthood, leading to higher composite risk factor scores for CVD and a potential decline in CV health [48,49]. PI in children and adolescents leads to increased morbidity since many of the chronic conditions of adults, including early atheromatosis, start in childhood [50].

According to several prospective studies, changes in body fatness are associated with PI; in particular, in children, an inverse relationship between the level of fatness and energy expenditure has been described, suggesting that the latter profoundly impacts the development of obesity [51]. Other adverse health habits have been correlated with PI, such as higher fat intake and cigarette smoking, according to data from the Cardiovascular Risk in Young Finns Study, suggesting that the covariance of PI with other negative health habits in youth affects the development of CVD later in life [52]. Exposure to CV risk factors early in life may influence vascular health, causing modifications to the development of structural and functional vascular changes, i.e., increased intima–media thickness and pulse wave velocity, which are related to early atherosclerosis [53,54]. PI seems to be associated with the accumulation of numerous harmful habits in adulthood, with the strongest association documented in females [52,55]. Consistent with the latest epidemiological data, most adolescents do not meet current PA guidelines, with a trend relatively stable over the past decade [56]. The latest WHO records reported that, in 2018, across 26 European Union Member States, only 17.6% of boys and 9.6% of girls met the recommendation regarding PA, with Portugal, France, and Italy reporting the lowest prevalence of PA among adolescents. An important consideration is that PA prevalence in pediatrics is inversely proportional to age, with the achievement of the recommended amount of daily PA ranging from 24% in children aged 11 to 19% at age 13 and 15% at age 15 [57].

Furthermore, in most countries, girls are less physically active than boys, with a prevalence of recommended levels of PA less than 20% in female adolescents and a subsequent further increase in PI into adulthood [58–61]. The causes for this gender disparity in PA involvement are still poorly understood [5]. Family support appears to be a consistent factor associated with the PA of both male and female adolescents; in contrast, low self-esteem, lack of interest and awareness about the role of PA, time limitations, scarcity of economic resources, and parental authority seem to influence girls' participation in PA, especially in low-income countries [62,63]. Ricardo et al. have recently examined records from the Global School-Based Student Health Survey, collected among adolescents from 13 to 17 years old from 64 Global South countries between 2010 and 2020. The pooled ratio for all countries showed that boys presented a PA prevalence 1.58 times higher than that of girls on average, with the highest absolute and relative inequalities in high-income countries [64].

2.3. Proposal for Intervention

As stated in the 2020 WHO guidelines, school-age youth (5–17 years) should participate daily in 60 min or more of moderate-to-vigorous PA (MVPA), mostly aerobic; activities focused on musculoskeletal strength should be incorporated at least 3 days a week. Sedentary behavior (SB, defined as any waking behavior characterized by an energy expenditure of ≤ 1.5 metabolic equivalents while in a sitting, reclining, or lying posture) should be limited as much as possible, especially in terms of recreational screen time [65,66].

The "PI pandemic" should be prevented from early childhood, as there is no doubt that early lifestyle-related factors significantly influence individual's biological risk factor profile, and childhood appears to be the most appropriate period for positive lifestyle adoption. Schools should offer children curriculums concentrated on the harmful effects of PI and on the positive effects of PA, and should strongly encourage physical practices to ensure that the recommendations for daily PA are embraced and met in student populations and to reduce SB [67]. Physical education teachers should be conscious of their central role in limiting gender inequality, endorsing activities potentially appealing for female students, and eliminating heterosexism and homophobia [68]. According to the latest evidence from systematic reviews, the most successful school-based interventions among adolescents to reduce PI used whole-of-school methodologies combining curricular activities with the broader school environment and the local community [69]. Moreover, playing on sports teams and participating in physical exercise classes may contribute more to global activity in girls [70]. However, these interventions demonstrated only minor results when PA was assessed quantitatively, i.e., using an accelerometer [71,72]. School-based interventions should promote PA programs that institutional teams will be determined to implement and that the involved adolescents are encouraged to support. PA initiatives should focus on the specific requests and necessities of adolescents. In this regard, a study by James et al. explored the recommendations made by a group of teenagers from secondary schools to improve PA engagement, highlighting a significant gap between the most proposed activities and the adolescents' needs. According to adolescents' suggestions, the activities should be cheaper, more locally accessible, and specific to teenagers, with a broader choice of proposed activities. Teenage girls stressed their need to engage in enjoyable activities that should not be competitive but friendly and entertaining. Moreover, both boys and girls strongly agree on the need for increased opportunities to participate in more unstructured activities [73]. Finally, it is crucial to offer sufficient education on gender equality for teachers and students, and future research is needed to further clarify the role of all the social and environmental factors potentially related to PI, to propose new approaches to overcome the inactivity phenomenon from the first decades of life.

3. Physical Activity and Inactivity in Pre-Pregnancy, Pregnancy, and Post-Pregnancy Period

3.1. Benefits of Physical Activity

The AHA statement on women's CV health underlines the importance of lifestyle interventions in the "Life's Simple 7", a list of the 7 most important health factors (diet, PA, non-smoking, body mass index, blood pressure, lipids, and glycemia), recently revised to "Life's Essential 8", incorporating sleep health as the 8th metric [74]. Among the abovementioned CV health metrics, PA can counteract CV risk factors before, during, and after pregnancy, and according to the latest evidence, the improvement in maternal cardio-metabolic health is reflected in the cardio-metabolic health of the fetus and future offspring [75,76]. The exposure of a fetus or neonate to specific risk factors, namely, developmental programming, can influence the development of CVD in later life. Much evidence has confirmed that maternal CV risk factors can influence both endothelial and glucose homeostasis in offspring, increasing the risk of developing early endothelial dysfunction and insulin resistance. In contrast, hypertensive disorders of pregnancy (HDP) can affect maternal health and fetal growth, which are, in turn, associated with increased CV risk later in life [77–79]. Moreover, it seems that CV risk factors, both micro- and macro-vascular, track from mother to child, regardless of environmental exposures and pregnancy complications, causing an adverse CV profile in the offspring at a 6- to -9 year follow-up [80].

There are several benefits of PA for maternal cardio-metabolic health including positive vascular remodeling and angiogenesis, improved endothelial function and arterial stiffness, reduced oxidative stress, and decreased levels of inflammatory cytokines and cortisol [81,82]. A greater amount of leisure-time PA in the first trimester of pregnancy leads to a lower risk of adverse pregnancy outcomes (APOs) [83]. Additionally, women who exercise as recommended have a 30% lower risk of developing HDP, including gestational hypertension and pre-eclampsia, and experience a reduced CV risk profile in perimenopause [81,84]. PA has also been associated with a meaningful reduction in gestational weight gain and post-gestational weight retention, both related to a higher risk of short- and long-term CV events, especially in women with a history of gestational diabetes and HDP [85–87]. Finally, PA causes a decline in the odds and severity of maternal mental issues, i.e., anxiety and prenatal depression, related to an increased risk of new CVD within 24 months postpartum. Moreover, PA significantly improves the maternal quality of life, along with reduced stress and cortisol levels, both associated with lower maternal oxidative stress and a better long-term metabolic environment of the offspring [82,88,89]. Furthermore, PA improves fertility and assisted reproductive therapy outcomes, as well as metabolic profile in polycystic ovary syndrome, which is recognized as the leading cause of anovulatory infertility [90,91].

3.2. Sedentary Behavior and Physical Inactivity Disadvantages

A statement from the American Heart Association (AHA) on women's CV health and its influence on pregnancy complications has been recently published [92]. According to the latest statistics, less than 1% of young adults of reproductive age have optimal CV health, and almost 1 in 5 births experiences an APO, with a substantial increase in cases over the past decade, especially regarding HDP [93,94].

A recent study by Silva-Jose et al. showed that although in the last 15 years there has been a substantial intensification in physical practice in the pregnant population, the current levels are still very far from the international recommendations [95]. Even if more than two-thirds of pregnant women participate in some type of recreational PA, the percentage of pregnant women exercising at the recommended level is still low, ranging from 15 to 27.3% [96,97]. Recent data from a Swedish epidemiological study showed a correlation between longer sedentary time during pregnancy and the increase in blood loss during delivery/postpartum, as well as worse self-rated health during pregnancy [97]. Pregnancy determines several physiological, cardio-metabolic adaptations in the mother, essential to support fetal development. In women with pre-pregnancy elevated cardio-metabolic risk factors, mainly exacerbated by PI, these phenomena may indicate the occurrence of APOs [98,99]. APOs are strongly related to the risk of subsequent CVD and long-term kidney disease, and the pre-pregnancy period could be involved in the pathophysiology of APOs [98,100]. For example, women with obesity and abnormal pre-pregnancy blood pressure, as well as women with pre-pregnancy insulin resistance or a family history of diabetes, are more likely to develop pre-eclampsia or gestational hypertension or gestational diabetes, respectively, compared with women without these conditions [101,102]. Among APOs, HDP seems to be associated with an increased risk of atherosclerotic CVD, hemorrhagic stroke, and heart failure. In contrast, gestational diabetes, preterm delivery, placental abruption, miscarriages or stillbirths, and the presence of anomalies in the weight of the newborn seem to be associated with an increased risk of atherosclerotic CVD [98]. The association between APOs and the risk of subsequent CVD is so important that the 2011 AHA guidelines for the prevention of CVD in women recommends including a history of APOs in the CVD risk evaluation in women. Moreover, APOs should be considered CV risk enhancers in evaluating statin prescriptions for CVD prevention [103,104]. Additional studies are needed to assess the impact of different levels of sedentary time on pregnancy outcomes [97].

3.3. Proposal for Intervention

The 2020 WHO guidelines on PA and SB recommend that all pregnant women, without contraindication, should do at least 150 min of moderate-intensity aerobic PA throughout the week, with a variety of aerobic and muscle-strengthening activities, replacing sedentary time with PA of any intensity, including light intensity [105,106].

Similarly, many governments have developed guidelines for PA during pregnancy, recently summarized in a review by Hayman et al., highlighting the remarkable concordance in the recommendations offered worldwide [107].

All women's healthcare providers should absorb and adopt the guidelines and efficiently support safe involvement in PA before, during, and after pregnancy, with effective lifestyle counseling that should start in the pre-conceptional period and continue during the postpartum months and beyond, as PA represents an investment in future CV health, especially during the menopausal transition [98,108].

4. Physical Activity and Inactivity in Perimenopause and Beyond

4.1. Benefits of Physical Activity

Menopause is considered one of the emergent non-modifiable CV risk factors in the female population, being associated with a decline in ovarian hormone concentrations that leads to cardio-metabolic negative adaptations and increased inflammatory status [2,109]. The noticeable changes in cardio-metabolic health observed in this scenario may be partially explained by modifiable lifestyle factors such as PI [110]. In this regard, PA represents a valuable tool to counteract these undesirable adaptations, especially if women exercise with a high level of adherence to a fitness program. Moreover, PA can improve the immune-neuroendocrine profile and serum angiogenic properties during the menopausal transition [111–115]. Regarding aerobic exercise, continuous aerobic training and high-intensity aerobic interval training can elicit the same physiological benefits in terms of a reduction in plasma glucose, insulin, homeostasis model assessment-adiponectin, and insulin resistance and an increase in plasma high-density lipoprotein-cholesterol, adiponectin, and aerobic fitness [116]. Perimenopausal women can also benefit from regular strength training, which can help to improve bone density, reduce body fat, and build skeletal muscle mass, maintaining adequate physical performance [117–119]. Both aerobic and resistance training, alone or in combination, can improve CRF and muscular strength in this population [120]. Moreover, a moderate-to-intense PA is crucial to protect or ameliorate cognitive health through body movement [121]. Finally, a recent study by Wu et al. suggests a strong negative correlation between PA and the severity of menopausal symptoms, with higher PA levels correlated with a better perceived health status [122].

4.2. Sedentary Behavior and Physical Inactivity Disadvantages

Despite the abovementioned and well-known health benefits, few adults, and fewer older adults, especially in the postmenopausal female population, meet recommended guidelines [123]. Furthermore, older women seem generally more sedentary and less active than older men [124].

In this population, SB has been associated with metabolic disorders, obesity, CVD, cancer, mortality, and psychological distress, as well as with adverse changes in coagulation homeostasis and severe menopausal symptoms [125,126]. Therefore, reducing sedentary activity provides an alternative strategy to reduce the risk of CVD and CVD-related mortality [108,127,128]. Further attention should be paid to supporting menopausal women in maintaining an adequate level of spontaneous PA when they regularly exercise, as it seems that the involvement in a planned program of physical exercise may result in a decline in spontaneous PA, which in turn reduces the positive effects of exercise on lipid profile [129,130]. The baseline spontaneous PA and leptin-to-fat-mass ratio of postmenopausal women involved in exercise training seem to be negative and independently correlated with a subsequent reduction in spontaneous PA [131].

4.3. Proposal for Intervention

The 2020 WHO guidelines on PA and SB recommend that adults and older adults with chronic conditions should perform at least 150–300 min of moderate-intensity aerobic PA, or at least 75–150 min of vigorous-intensity aerobic PA, or an equivalent combination of moderate- and vigorous-intensity activity throughout the week for substantial health benefits [105].

Every woman needs to find an enjoyable activity that fits into her daily lifestyle [132,133]. Menopausal women should aim for 30 min of moderate-intensity PA every day, i.e., walking, jogging, swimming, cycling, dancing, and gardening. Other beneficial activities include strength training and balance exercises, which are especially important as women age which can increase the risk of falls. Healthcare professionals should actively promote PA as a cheap and effective therapy free of side effects in menopausal women, taking into account both known facilitators (i.e., program adaption, gratification, and setting) and strategies to overcome barriers to PA participation (i.e., lack of social and economic support and exercise experience) in order to improve women's adherence to fitness programs [134,135]. In this sense, the positive effects of PA should be optimized according to women's life habits. For instance, the evening execution of a walking program may lead to better positive effects in terms of body composition improvement, potentially linked to spontaneous dietary habit modification [136]. Increased sedentary time should also be strongly discouraged as a negative compensatory adaptive response to exercise training [131].

5. Physical Activity and Inactivity in CVD

5.1. Benefits of Physical Activity

The inverse association between PA and CVD has been extensively validated, especially in high-risk subgroups, including patients with metabolic syndrome, current smokers, and older adults.

This positive relationship has also been confirmed in the female population, as shown by Paynter et al. in the WHI-OS (Women's Health Initiative Observational Study), demonstrating that recreational PA was the only lifestyle factor independently associated with incident CVD when added to traditional risk factor models [137]. PA seems to be similarly effective in preventing CVD among women with varying levels of global CV risk [24]. Even light-to-moderate PA is associated with lower coronary heart disease rates in women, and higher daily life movement has been independently associated with a lower CV risk in older women [138]. Combining different PA interventions is the most effective way to reduce CV risk factors in women [139].

5.2. Sedentary Behavior and Physical Inactivity Disadvantages

Current records from clinical trials suggest that PA alone is not enough to reduce the risk of CVD, especially in older adults, as both PI and SB negatively influence CV health status, especially in older women, regardless of the level and intensity of PA [127]. Data from the Women's Health Initiative confirmed the presence of a linear connection between more significant amounts of sedentary time and mortality risk after controlling for multiple potential confounders [140]. In the same population, prolonged sitting time was associated with increased CVD risk in postmenopausal women without a history of CVD, independent of leisure-time PA [141].

Moreover, Ekelund et al. described a statistically significant higher risk of death for sedentary times of 9.5 or more hours daily [127,142,143]. On the other hand, lower sedentary time is associated with lower all-cause mortality [144]. High sedentary time and long mean bout duration have been associated in a dose–response manner with increased CV risk in a subcohort from Women's Health Initiative [126]. Moreover, a positive correlation between prolonged SB periods and worsening arterial stiffness, a well-known prognostic marker for CVD, has been recently highlighted in a population of 1125 women from the Physical Activity and Health in Older Women Study, with more prolonged bouts of SB being associated with higher levels of arterial stiffness [145]. Patients with CVD exhibit considerably higher amounts of SB than healthy controls and show low engagement in moderate-to-vigorous PA even following specific cardiac rehabilitation programs [146].

Duran et al. demonstrated, in a population of 149 patients with acute coronary syndrome (30.2% women), that during the first month post-discharge there is a significant tendency to accumulate high volumes of sedentary time, with most patients showing slight improvement over time [147]. This negative lifestyle adaptation is associated with a worse long-term prognosis among patients with acute coronary syndrome as high SB, mainly when associated with low PA, strongly correlates with poor cardiorespiratory fitness [148]. Incremental tertiles of time-varying SB also correlate with an increased risk of incident HF in postmenopausal women, according to the data from the Women's Health Initiative Observational Study by LaMonte et al. [149].

5.3. Proposal for Intervention

The latest guidelines on CVD prevention in clinical practice, endorsed by the European Society of Cardiology, suggest that every patient with atherosclerotic CVD events or with a history of heart failure should participate in a medically supervised, structured, and exercise-based cardiac rehabilitation program that should start as soon as possible after the initial CV event. The program should be tailored to each patient and include both aerobic and resistance exercises [150–152]. A specific tool, namely, the EXPERT tool (Exercise Prescription in Everyday Practice and Rehabilitation Training), has been proposed to optimize exercise training. Home-based telemonitoring and telehealth interventions have been suggested to increase rates of participation. The efforts of every clinician should be focused on the improvement of adherence to a rehabilitation program and on specific interventions aimed at reducing SB, i.e., the use of an interactive accelerometer equipped with cloud-based services to store and monitor patient's habitual activity online in order to create a patient's habitual activity and SB profile, which can be supervised over long periods of time [152–155].

6. Current Evidence on Physical Activity and Inactivity in the COVID-19 Pandemic

It has been widely demonstrated that the health policy reactions to the COVID-19 pandemic, with lockdown and significant movement restrictions, caused widespread effects on CV risk. The significant limitation of economic and social activities has led to unemployment, increased sedentary time, social isolation, and increased incidence of mental health issues, all of which are well-recognized risk factors for CVD and associated with worsening CV outcomes [156]. The pandemic has been a stressful time for everyone, especially for women when juggling work and home life. Women are often expected to be the primary caretakers for their families, and with the extra stress of the pandemic, it has been even more difficult for them to manage.

Many studies demonstrated that women of all ages were significantly less physically active than men during COVID-19 and reported more barriers and fewer facilitators to PA than men, with a significant worsening in psychological health. On the other hand, women who engaged in more PA had improved mental health scores [157–160].

Given these premises, home-based PA programs for the prevention of PI and SB during the COVID-19 era have been strongly suggested as powerful tools to preserve both general and CV well-being and mental health, especially in women who were severely affected by emotional stress and anxiety, with a potentially devastating impact on CV risk burden [161–167].

Recently, the "Long COVID syndrome" or "post-acute sequelae of COVID-19" (PASC) is emerging in clinical practice. This condition occurs 3 or more weeks after the original infection and is characterized by symptoms lasting for at least 2 months, with no other explanation, in subjects who have had a severe, moderate, or mild form of COVID-19, mainly females [168–172]. The persistence of SARS-CoV-2 symptoms severely affects functional and emotional status, as well as leisure-time PA, especially in the female population, limiting PA participation and decreasing both CV health and quality of life [173–175].

PASC has been associated with more than 100 symptoms, including fatigue, anxiety, depression, sleep disorders, and CV symptoms and complications, including palpitations, chest pain, and dyspnea, the latter being reported in 5–29% of COVID-19 survivors [176]. Furthermore, independent of symptom burden, women with PASC seem to experience a worsening in vascular health, with higher levels of blood pressure and central arterial stiffness [177]. The latest consensus statement by the American Academy of Physical Medicine and Rehabilitation highlighted that PI is strongly correlated with CV morbidity and mortality, more severe COVID-19, and risk of PASC [178]. The authors recommend exercise training as an effective intervention to improve both mental health issues and CV complications, paying attention to minimizing or avoiding post-exertional symptom exacerbation (PESE), which has been extensively described in this population [179–183].

7. Conclusions and Future Directions

PI represents a real global emergency as it significantly affects general and CV well-being, especially in women that are globally more inactive compared with men. Gender differences in terms of PA are tangible and exist across all age groups and clinical scenarios. The equal opportunity for everyone to be active from a young age and maintain activity should be provided worldwide and would represent an actual investment in short- and long-term global health.

Many studies confirmed that increasing PA in the population would reduce working-age mortality and morbidity and increase productivity, with significant economic gains for the economy worldwide, especially in high-income countries [184]. Moreover, pre-pregnancy and pregnancy CV health should be considered a central target to improve women's lifelong health but also the health of the birthing individuals over their life course [92]. Recently, the latest global status report on PA by the WHO highlighted that, although national guidelines to fight NCDs and PI have increased in recent years, currently only 72% of policies are reported to be supported or applied. Moreover, it seems that only just over 50% of countries have planned a mass participation PA event or a national communications campaign about PA in the last 2 years. Governments should help break down barriers to women's participation in sport, promoting different regulations to provide everyone with access to PA and suitable infrastructures to ease protected access and privacy in facilities. Schools and universities, sports societies, non-governmental associations, and local initiatives can also play an essential role in accelerating this revolution, spreading the need for gender equality in PA and promoting projects focused on the existing barriers to women's awareness of and access to PA, and claiming more space and involvement for women in sport. Proposed activities should be tailored to the specific requests and necessities of the female population of every age.

Health education messages supplied to mobile devices, focused on the role of an active lifestyle on CV fitness, promoting the WHO's guidelines on PA levels, and explaining the adverse effects of PI and SB by captivating visual content may constitute an effective tool to improve health literacy, especially in the youngest population [185].

Strategies to reduce the gender gap should be highlighted in efforts to increase PA levels in all age groups and in all countries, from childhood to old age, to achieve radical changes at every level through multidisciplinary and cross-sectoral collaboration to increase levels of PA in current and future generations, as stated in the WHO Global Action Plan on PA 2018–2030 [64,186].

Author Contributions: Conceptualization, V.B., A.V.M., S.S., F.M., G.R. and S.G.; writing—original draft preparation, V.B. and A.V.M.; writing—review and editing, V.B., A.V.M. and S.G.; supervision, S.G.; project administration, V.B., A.V.M. and S.G. All authors have read and agreed to the published version of the manuscript.

Funding: This research received no external funding.

Institutional Review Board Statement: Not applicable.

Informed Consent Statement: Not applicable.

Data Availability Statement: Not applicable.

Conflicts of Interest: The authors declare no conflict of interest.

References

1. Tsao, C.W.; Aday, A.W.; Almarzooq, Z.I.; Anderson, C.A.; Arora, P.; Avery, C.L.; Baker-Smith, C.M.; Beaton, A.Z.; Boehme, A.K.; Buxton, A.E.; et al. Heart Disease and Stroke Statistics—2023 Update: A Report From the American Heart Association. *Circulation* **2023**, *147*, e93–e621. [CrossRef] [PubMed]
2. Salerni, S.; Di Francescomarino, S.; Cadeddu, C.; Acquistapace, F.; Maffei, S.; Gallina, S. The different role of sex hormones on female cardiovascular physiology and function: Not only oestrogens. *Eur. J. Clin. Investig.* **2015**, *45*, 634–645. [CrossRef]
3. Garcia, M.; Mulvagh, S.L.; Bairey Merz, C.N.; Buring, J.E.; Manson, J.E. Cardiovascular Disease in Women: Clinical Perspectives. *Circ. Res.* **2016**, *118*, 1273–1293. [CrossRef]
4. Cho, L.; Davis, M.; Elgendy, I.; Epps, K.; Lindley, K.J.; Mehta, P.K.; Michos, E.D.; Minissian, M.; Pepine, C.; Vaccarino, V.; et al. Summary of Updated Recommendations for Primary Prevention of Cardiovascular Disease in Women: JACC State-of-the-Art Review. *J. Am. Coll. Cardiol.* **2020**, *75*, 2602–2618. [CrossRef]
5. Soto-Lagos, R.; Cortes-Varas, C.; Freire-Arancibia, S.; Energici, M.-A.; McDonald, B. How Can Physical Inactivity in Girls Be Explained? A Socioecological Study in Public, Subsidized, and Private Schools. *Int. J. Environ. Res. Public Health* **2022**, *19*, 9304. [CrossRef]
6. Kohl, H.W., 3rd; Craig, C.L.; Lambert, E.V.; Inoue, S.; Alkandari, J.R.; Leetongin, G.; Kahlmeier, S. The pandemic of physical inactivity: Global action for public health. *Lancet* **2012**, *380*, 294–305. [CrossRef]
7. Tremblay, M.S.; Aubert, S.; Barnes, J.D.; Saunders, T.J.; Carson, V.; Latimer-Cheung, A.E.; Chastin, S.F.; Altenburg, T.M.; Chinapaw, M.J. Sedentary Behavior Research Network (SBRN)—Terminology Consensus Project process and outcome. *Int. J. Behav. Nutr. Phys. Act.* **2017**, *14*, 75. [CrossRef] [PubMed]
8. Riccioni, G.; Scotti, L.; Guagnano, M.T.; Bosco, G.; Bucciarelli, V.; Di Ilio, E.; Speranza, L.; Martini, F.; Bucciarelli, T. Physical exercise reduces synthesis of ADMA, SDMA, and L-Arg. *Front. Biosci. (Elite Ed.)* **2015**, *7*, 417–422. [CrossRef] [PubMed]
9. Gao, J.; Pan, X.; Li, G.; Chatterjee, E.; Xiao, J. Physical Exercise Protects Against Endothelial Dysfunction in Cardiovascular and Metabolic Diseases. *J. Cardiovasc. Transl. Res.* **2022**, *15*, 604–620. [CrossRef]
10. Falone, S.; Mirabilio, A.; Passerini, A.; Izzicupo, P.; Cacchio, M.; Gallina, S.; Baldassarre, A.D.; Amicarelli, F. Aerobic Performance and Antioxidant Protection in Runners. *Int. J. Sports Med.* **2009**, *30*, 782–788. [CrossRef] [PubMed]
11. Reiner, M.; Niermann, C.; Jekauc, D.; Woll, A. Long-term health benefits of physical activity—A systematic review of longitudinal studies. *BMC Public Health* **2013**, *13*, 813. [CrossRef]
12. Lee, D.H.; Rezende, L.F.; Joh, H.-K.; Keum, N.; Ferrari, G.; Rey-Lopez, J.P.; Rimm, E.B.; Tabung, F.K.; Giovannucci, E.L. Long-Term Leisure-Time Physical Activity Intensity and All-Cause and Cause-Specific Mortality: A Prospective Cohort of US Adults. *Circulation* **2022**, *146*, 523–534. [CrossRef]
13. Singh, B.; Olds, T.; Curtis, R.; Dumuid, D.; Virgara, R.; Watson, A.; Szeto, K.; O'Connor, E.; Ferguson, T.; Eglitis, E.; et al. Effectiveness of physical activity interventions for improving depression, anxiety and distress: An overview of systematic reviews. *Br. J. Sports Med.* **2023**; online ahead of print. [CrossRef]
14. De Cocker, K.; Biddle, S.J.H.; Teychenne, M.J.; Bennie, J.A. Is all activity equal? Associations between different domains of physical activity and depressive symptom severity among 261,121 European adults. *Depress. Anxiety* **2021**, *38*, 950–960. [CrossRef]
15. Dugan, S.A.; Bromberger, J.; Segawa, E.; Avery, E.; Sternfeld, B. Association between Physical Activity and Depressive Symptoms: Midlife Women in SWAN. *Med. Sci. Sports Exerc.* **2015**, *47*, 335–342. [CrossRef] [PubMed]
16. Azar, D.; Ball, K.; Salmon, J.; Cleland, V.J. Physical activity correlates in young women with depressive symptoms: A qualitative study. *Int. J. Behav. Nutr. Phys. Act.* **2010**, *7*, 3. [CrossRef]
17. Meng, Y.; Luo, Y.; Qin, S.; Xu, C.; Yue, J.; Nie, M.; Fan, L. The effects of leisure time physical activity on depression among older women depend on intensity and frequency. *J. Affect. Disord.* **2021**, *295*, 822–830. [CrossRef]
18. World Health Organization. *World Health Organization Global Action Plan on Physical Activity 2018–2030: More Active People for a Healthier World*; World Health Organization: Geneva, Switzerland, 2018.
19. Santos, A.C.; Willumsen, J.; Meheus, F.; Ilbawi, A.; Bull, F.C. The cost of inaction on physical inactivity to public health-care systems: A population-attributable fraction analysis. *Lancet Glob. Health* **2023**, *11*, e32–e39. [CrossRef] [PubMed]

20. Katzmarzyk, P.T.; Friedenreich, C.; Shiroma, E.J.; Lee, I.-M. Physical inactivity and non-communicable disease burden in low-income, middle-income and high-income countries. *Br. J. Sports Med.* **2022**, *56*, 101–106. [CrossRef] [PubMed]
21. Brown, W.J.; Pavey, T.; Bauman, A.E. Comparing population attributable risks for heart disease across the adult lifespan in women. *Br. J. Sports Med.* **2015**, *49*, 1069–1076. [CrossRef]
22. Milton, K.; Gomersall, S.R.; Schipperijn, J. Let's get moving: The Global Status Report on Physical Activity 2022 calls for urgent action. *J. Sport Health Sci.* **2023**, *12*, 5–6. [CrossRef]
23. Shiroma, E.J.; Lee, I.M. Physical activity and cardiovascular health: Lessons learned from epidemiological studies across age, gender, and race/ethnicity. *Circulation* **2010**, *122*, 743–752. [CrossRef]
24. Chomistek, A.K.; Cook, N.R.; Rimm, E.B.; Ridker, P.M.; Buring, J.E.; Lee, I.M. Physical Activity and Incident Cardiovascular Disease in Women: Is the Relation Modified by Level of Global Cardiovascular Risk? *J. Am. Heart Assoc.* **2018**, *7*, 12. [CrossRef]
25. Sandborg, J.; Migueles, J.H.; Söderström, E.; Blomberg, M.; Henriksson, P.; Löf, M. Physical Activity, Body Composition, and Cardiometabolic Health during Pregnancy: A Compositional Data Approach. *Med. Sci. Sports Exerc.* **2022**, *54*, 2054–2063. [CrossRef]
26. Di Giuseppe, D.; Bottai, M.; Askling, J.; Wolk, A. Physical activity and risk of rheumatoid arthritis in women: A population-based prospective study. *Thromb. Haemost.* **2015**, *17*, 40. [CrossRef] [PubMed]
27. Xu, Y.; Rogers, C.J. Physical Activity and Breast Cancer Prevention: Possible Role of Immune Mediators. *Front. Nutr.* **2020**, *7*, 557997. [CrossRef] [PubMed]
28. Guthold, R.; Stevens, G.A.; Riley, L.M.; Bull, F.C. Worldwide trends in insufficient physical activity from 2001 to 2016: A pooled analysis of 358 population-based surveys with 1.9 million participants. *Lancet Glob. Health* **2018**, *6*, e1077–e1086. [CrossRef]
29. Whitfield, G.P.; Hyde, E.T.; Carlson, S.A. Participation in Leisure-Time Aerobic Physical Activity Among Adults, National Health Interview Survey, 1998–2018. *J. Phys. Act. Health* **2021**, *18*, S25–S36. [CrossRef] [PubMed]
30. European Commission. Special Eurobarometer SP525: Sport and Physical Activity. 2022. Available online: https://europa.eu/eurobarometer/surveys/detail/2668 (accessed on 21 September 2022).
31. Donoso, B.; Reina, A.; Alvarez-Sotomayor, A. Women and competitive sport: Perceived barriers to equality. *Cult. Cienc. Deporte* **2022**, *17*, 54.
32. Moreno-Llamas, A.; García-Mayor, J.; De la Cruz-Sánchez, E. Gender inequality is associated with gender differences and women participation in physical activity. *J. Public Health* **2022**, *44*, e519–e526. [CrossRef]
33. Cla, T. Time to tackle the physical activity gender gap. *Lancet Public Health* **2019**, *4*, e360.
34. Boreham, C.; Riddoch, C. The physical activity, fitness and health of children. *J. Sports Sci.* **2001**, *19*, 915–929. [CrossRef]
35. Loprinzi, P.D.; Cardinal, B.J.; Loprinzi, K.L.; Lee, H. Benefits and Environmental Determinants of Physical Activity in Children and Adolescents. *Obes. Facts* **2012**, *5*, 597–610. [CrossRef]
36. van Sluijs, E.M.; Ekelund, U.; Crochemore-Silva, I.; Guthold, R.; Ha, A.; Lubans, D.; Oyeyemi, A.L.; Ding, D.; Katzmarzyk, P.T. Physical activity behaviours in adolescence: Current evidence and opportunities for intervention. *Lancet* **2021**, *398*, 429–442. [CrossRef]
37. Blair, S.N. Exercise and Fitness in Childhood: Implications for a Lifetime of Health. In *Perspectives in Exercise Science and Sports Medicine, vol.2: Youth, Exercise and Sport*; Gisolfi, C.V., Lamb, D.R., Eds.; Benchmark Press: Indianapolis, IN, USA, 1989; pp. 401–430.
38. Janssen, I.; LeBlanc, A.G. Systematic review of the health benefits of physical activity and fitness in school-aged children and youth. *Int. J. Behav. Nutr. Phys. Act.* **2010**, *7*, 40. [CrossRef]
39. Ruiz, J.R.; Huybrechts, I.; Cuenca-García, M.; Artero, E.G.; Labayen, I.; Meirhaeghe, A.; Vicente-Rodriguez, G.; Polito, A.; Manios, Y.; González-Gross, M.; et al. Cardiorespiratory fitness and ideal cardiovascular health in European adolescents. *Heart* **2015**, *101*, 766–773. [CrossRef]
40. Moliner-Urdiales, D.; on behalf of the HELENA Study Group; Ruiz, J.R.; Ortega, F.B.; Rey-Lopez, J.P.; Vicente-Rodriguez, G.; España-Romero, V.; Munguía-Izquierdo, D.; Castillo, M.J.; Sjöström, M.; et al. Association of objectively assessed physical activity with total and central body fat in Spanish adolescents: The HELENA Study. *Int. J. Obes.* **2009**, *33*, 1126–1135. [CrossRef] [PubMed]
41. Jiménez-Pavón, D.; Fernández-Vázquez, A.; Alexy, U.; Pedrero, R.; Cuenca-García, M.; Polito, A.; Vanhelst, J.; Manios, Y.; Kafatos, A.; Molnar, D.; et al. Association of objectively measured physical activity with body components in European adolescents. *BMC Public Health* **2013**, *13*, 667. [CrossRef] [PubMed]
42. Rendo-Urteaga, T.; de Moraes, A.C.F.; Collese, T.S.; Manios, Y.; Hagströmer, M.; Sjöström, M.; Kafatos, A.; Widhalm, K.; Vanhelst, J.; Marcos, A.; et al. The combined effect of physical activity and sedentary behaviors on a clustered cardio-metabolic risk score: The Helena study. *Int. J. Cardiol.* **2015**, *186*, 186–195. [CrossRef]
43. Jiménez-Pavón, D.; Ruiz, J.R.; Ortega, F.B.; Martínez-Gómez, D.; Moreno, S.; Urzanqui, A.; Gottrand, F.; Molnár, D.; Castillo, M.J.; Sjöström, M.; et al. Physical activity and markers of insulin resistance in adolescents: Role of cardiorespiratory fitness levels—The HELENA study. *Pediatr. Diabetes* **2013**, *14*, 249–258. [CrossRef]
44. Absil, H.; Baudet, L.; Robert, A.; Lysy, P.A. Benefits of physical activity in children and adolescents with type 1 diabetes: A systematic review. *Diabetes Res. Clin. Pract.* **2019**, *156*, 107810. [CrossRef]
45. Saunders, T.J.; Gray, C.E.; Poitras, V.J.; Chaput, J.-P.; Janssen, I.; Katzmarzyk, P.T.; Olds, T.; Gorber, S.C.; Kho, M.E.; Sampson, M.; et al. Combinations of physical activity, sedentary behaviour and sleep: Relationships with health indicators in school-aged children and youth. *Appl. Physiol. Nutr. Metab.* **2016**, *41*, S283–S293. [CrossRef]

46. Fonseca, A.P.L.M.; de Azevedo, C.V.M.; Santos, R.M.R. Sleep and health-related physical fitness in children and adolescents: A systematic review. *Sleep Sci.* **2021**, *14*, 357–365. [CrossRef] [PubMed]
47. Ekstedt, M.; Nyberg, G.; Ingre, M.; Marcus, C. Sleep, physical activity and BMI in six to ten-year-old children measured by accelerometry: A cross-sectional study. *Int. J. Behav. Nutr. Phys. Act.* **2013**, *10*, 1–10. [CrossRef]
48. Tanha, T.; Wollmer, P.; Thorsson, O.; Karlsson, M.K.; Lindén, C.; Andersen, L.B.; Dencker, M. Lack of physical activity in young children is related to higher composite risk factor score for cardiovascular disease. *Acta Paediatr.* **2011**, *100*, 717–721. [CrossRef]
49. Gooding, H.C.; Ning, H.; Perak, A.M.; Allen, N.; Lloyd-Jones, D.; Moore, L.L.; Singer, M.R.; de Ferranti, S.D. Cardiovascular health decline in adolescent girls in the NGHS cohort, 1987–1997. *Prev. Med. Rep.* **2020**, *20*, 101276. [CrossRef]
50. Wilson, D. *Is Atherosclerosis a Pediatric Disease?* Feingold, K.R., Anawalt, B., Blackman, M.R., Boyce, A., Chrousos, G., Corpas, E., de Herder, W.W., Dhatariya, K., Dungan, K., Hofland, J., et al., Eds.; MDText.com Inc.: South Dartmouth, MA, USA, 2020.
51. Ortega, F.B.; Ruiz, J.R.; Castillo, M.J. Physical activity, physical fitness, and overweight in children and adolescents: Evidence from epidemiologic studies. *Endocrinol. Nutr. (Engl. Ed.)* **2013**, *60*, 458–469. [CrossRef] [PubMed]
52. Raitakari, O.T.; Porkka, K.V.; Taimela, S.; Telama, R.; Räsänen, L.; Viikari, J.S. Effects of persistent physical activity and inactivity on coronary risk factors in children and young adults. The Cardiovascular Risk in Young Finns Study. *Am. J. Epidemiol.* **1994**, *140*, 195–205. [CrossRef]
53. Aatola, H.; Hutri-Kähönen, N.; Juonala, M.; Viikari, J.S.; Hulkkonen, J.; Laitinen, T.; Taittonen, L.; Lehtimäki, T.; Raitakari, O.T.; Kahonen, M. Lifetime risk factors and arterial pulse wave velocity in adulthood: The cardiovascular risk in young Finns study. *Hypertension* **2010**, *55*, 806–811. [CrossRef]
54. Raitakari, O.T.; Juonala, M.; Kähönen, M.; Taittonen, L.; Laitinen, T.; Mäki-Torkko, N.; Järvisalo, M.J.; Uhari, M.; Jokinen, E.; Rönnemaa, T.; et al. Cardiovascular risk factors in childhood and carotid artery intima-media thickness in adulthood: The Cardiovascular Risk in Young Finns Study. *JAMA* **2003**, *290*, 2277–2283. [CrossRef]
55. Lounassalo, I.; Hirvensalo, M.; Palomäki, S.; Salin, K.; Tolvanen, A.; Pahkala, K.; Rovio, S.; Fogelholm, M.; Yang, X.; Hutri-Kähönen, N.; et al. Life-course leisure-time physical activity trajectories in relation to health-related behaviors in adulthood: The Cardiovascular Risk in Young Finns study. *BMC Public Health* **2021**, *21*, 533. [CrossRef]
56. Reilly, J.J.; Barnes, J.; Gonzalez, S.; Huang, W.Y.; Manyanga, T.; Tanaka, C.; Tremblay, M.S. Recent Secular Trends in Child and Adolescent Physical Activity and Sedentary Behavior Internationally: Analyses of Active Healthy Kids Global Alliance Global Matrices 1.0 to 4.0. *J. Phys. Act. Health* **2022**, *19*, 729–736. [CrossRef]
57. Inchley, J.; Currie, D.; Budisavljevic, S.; Torsheim, T.; Jastad, A.; Cosma, A. *Spotlight on Adolescent Health and Well-Being. Findings from the 2017/2018 Health Behaviour in School-Aged Children (HBSC) Survey in Europe and Canada*; International Report. Key findings; WHO Regional Office for Europe: Copenhagen, Denmark, 2020; Volume 1.
58. Guthold, R.; Stevens, G.A.; Riley, L.M.; Bull, F.C. Global trends in insufficient physical activity among adolescents: A pooled analysis of 298 population-based surveys with 1.6 million participants. *Lancet Child. Adolesc. Health* **2020**, *4*, 23–35. [CrossRef] [PubMed]
59. Sallis, J.F.; Bull, F.; Guthold, R.; Heath, G.W.; Inoue, S.; Kelly, P.; Oyeyemi, A.L.; Perez, L.G.; Richards, J.; Hallal, P.C. Progress in physical activity over the Olympic quadrennium. *Lancet* **2016**, *388*, 1325–1336. [CrossRef]
60. Dumith, S.C.; Gigante, D.P.; Domingues, M.R.; Kohl, H.W., III. Physical activity change during adolescence: A systematic review and a pooled analysis. *Int. J. Epidemiol.* **2011**, *40*, 685–698. [CrossRef]
61. Kwan, M.Y.; Cairney, J.; Faulkner, G.; Pullenayegum, E. Physical Activity and Other Health-Risk Behaviors During the Transition Into Early Adulthood: A Longitudinal Cohort Study. *Am. J. Prev. Med.* **2012**, *42*, 14–20. [CrossRef]
62. Wenthe, P.J.; Janz, K.F.; Levy, S.M. Gender similarities and differences in factors associated with adolescent moderate-vigorous physical activity. *Pediatr. Exerc. Sci.* **2009**, *21*, 291–304. [CrossRef] [PubMed]
63. Onagbiye, S.O.; Tshwaro, R.M.T.; Barry, A.; Marie, Y. Physical Activity and Non-communicable Disease Risk Factors: Knowledge and Perceptions of Youth in a Low Resourced Community in the Western Cape. *Open Public Health J.* **2019**, *12*, 558–566. [CrossRef]
64. Ricardo, L.I.C.; Wendt, A.; Costa, C.D.S.; Mielke, G.I.; Brazo-Sayavera, J.; Khan, A.; Kolbe-Alexander, T.L.; Crochemore-Silva, I. Gender inequalities in physical activity among adolescents from 64 Global South countries. *J. Sport Health Sci.* **2022**, *11*, 509–520. [CrossRef] [PubMed]
65. Chaput, J.-P.; Willumsen, J.; Bull, F.; Chou, R.; Ekelund, U.; Firth, J.; Jago, R.; Ortega, F.B.; Katzmarzyk, P.T. 2020 WHO guidelines on physical activity and sedentary behaviour for children and adolescents aged 5–17 years: Summary of the evidence. *Int. J. Behav. Nutr. Phys. Act.* **2020**, *17*, 141. [CrossRef]
66. Andriyani, F.D.; Biddle, S.J.; Priambadha, A.A.; Thomas, G.; De Cocker, K. Physical activity and sedentary behaviour of female adolescents in Indonesia: A multi-method study on duration, pattern and context. *J. Exerc. Sci. Fit.* **2022**, *20*, 128–139. [CrossRef]
67. Mavrovouniotis, F. Inactivity in Childhood and Adolescence: A Modern Lifestyle Associated with Adverse Health Consequences. *Sport Sci. Rev.* **2012**, *21*, 75–99. [CrossRef]
68. Guerrero, M.A.; Puerta, L.G. Advancing Gender Equality in Schools through Inclusive Physical Education and Teaching Training: A Systematic Review. *Societies* **2023**, *13*, 64. [CrossRef]
69. Shackleton, N.; Jamal, F.; Viner, R.M.; Dickson, K.; Patton, G.; Bonell, C. School-Based Interventions Going Beyond Health Education to Promote Adolescent Health: Systematic Review of Reviews. *J. Adolesc. Health* **2016**, *58*, 382–396. [CrossRef] [PubMed]

70. Lenhart, C.M.; Hanlon, A.; Kang, Y.; Daly, B.P.; Brown, M.D.; Patterson, F. Gender Disparity in Structured Physical Activity and Overall Activity Level in Adolescence: Evaluation of Youth Risk Behavior Surveillance Data. *ISRN Public Health* **2012**, *2012*, 674936. [CrossRef]
71. van Sluijs, E.M.F.; McMinn, A.M.; Griffin, S.J. Effectiveness of interventions to promote physical activity in children and adolescents: Systematic review of controlled trials. *BMJ* **2007**, *335*, 703. [CrossRef] [PubMed]
72. Okely, A.D.; Lubans, D.R.; Morgan, P.J.; Cotton, W.; Peralta, L.; Miller, J.; Batterham, M.; Janssen, X. Promoting physical activity among adolescent girls: The Girls in Sport group randomized trial. *Int. J. Behav. Nutr. Phys. Act.* **2017**, *14*, 81. [CrossRef]
73. James, M.; Todd, C.; Scott, S.; Stratton, G.; McCoubrey, S.; Christian, D.; Halcox, J.; Audrey, S.; Ellins, E.; Anderson, S.; et al. Teenage recommendations to improve physical activity for their age group: A qualitative study. *BMC Public Health* **2018**, *18*, 372. [CrossRef]
74. Lloyd-Jones, D.M.; Allen, N.B.; Anderson, C.A.; Black, T.; Brewer, L.C.; Foraker, R.E.; Grandner, M.A.; Lavretsky, H.; Perak, A.M.; Sharma, G.; et al. Life's Essential 8: Updating and Enhancing the American Heart Association's Construct of Cardiovascular Health: A Presidential Advisory From the American Heart Association. *Circulation* **2022**, *146*, e18–e43. [CrossRef]
75. Nagpal, S.T.; Mottola, M.F. Physical activity throughout pregnancy is key to preventing chronic disease. *Reproduction* **2020**, *160*, R111–R118. [CrossRef]
76. Truzzi, M.L.; Ballerini Puviani, M.; Tripodi, A.; Toni, S.; Farinetti, A.; Nasi, M.; Mattioli, A.V. Mediterranean Diet as a model of sustainable, resilient and healthy diet. *Prog. Nutr.* **2020**, *22*, 388–394.
77. Sutton, E.F.; Gilmore, L.A.; Dunger, D.B.; Heijmans, B.T.; Hivert, M.F.; Ling, C.; Martinez, J.A.; Ozanne, S.E.; Simmons, R.A.; Szyf, M.; et al. Developmental programming: State-of-the-science and future directions-Summary from a Pennington Biomedical symposium. *Obesity (Silver Spring)* **2016**, *24*, 1018–1026. [CrossRef]
78. Palinski, W. Effect of Maternal Cardiovascular Conditions and Risk Factors on Offspring Cardiovascular Disease. *Circulation* **2014**, *129*, 2066–2077. [CrossRef]
79. Alexander, B.T.; Dasinger, J.H.; Intapad, S. Fetal Programming and Cardiovascular Pathology. *Compr. Physiol.* **2015**, *5*, 997–1025. [CrossRef] [PubMed]
80. Benschop, L.; Schalekamp-Timmermans, S.; van Lennep, J.E.R.; Jaddoe, V.W.; Steegers, E.A.; Ikram, M.K. Cardiovascular Risk Factors Track From Mother to Child. *J. Am. Heart Assoc.* **2018**, *7*, e009536. [CrossRef]
81. Witvrouwen, I.; Mannaerts, D.; Van Berendoncks, A.M.; Jacquemyn, Y.; Van Craenenbroeck, E.M. The Effect of Exercise Training During Pregnancy to Improve Maternal Vascular Health: Focus on Gestational Hypertensive Disorders. *Front. Physiol.* **2020**, *11*, 450. [CrossRef]
82. Cai, C.; Busch, S.; Wang, R.; Sivak, A.; Davenport, M.H. Physical activity before and during pregnancy and maternal mental health: A systematic review and meta-analysis of observational studies. *J. Affect. Disord.* **2022**, *309*, 393–403. [CrossRef] [PubMed]
83. Catov, J.M.; Parker, C.B.; Gibbs, B.B.; Bann, C.M.; Carper, B.; Silver, R.M.; Simhan, H.N.; Parry, S.; Chung, J.H.; Haas, D.M.; et al. Patterns of leisure-time physical activity across pregnancy and adverse pregnancy outcomes. *Int. J. Behav. Nutr. Phys. Act.* **2018**, *15*, 68. [CrossRef]
84. Clapp, J.F. Long-term outcome after exercising throughout pregnancy: Fitness and cardiovascular risk. *Am. J. Obstet. Gynecol.* **2008**, *199*, 489.e1–489.e6. [CrossRef] [PubMed]
85. Rich-Edwards, J.W.; Stuart, J.; Skurnik, G.; Roche, A.T.; Tsigas, E.; Fitzmaurice, G.M.; Wilkins-Haug, L.E.; Levkoff, S.E.; Seely, E.W. Randomized Trial to Reduce Cardiovascular Risk in Women with Recent Preeclampsia. *J. Women's Health* **2019**, *28*, 1493–1504. [CrossRef] [PubMed]
86. Jowell, A.R.; Sarma, A.A.; Michos, M.G.E.D.; Vaught, A.J.; Natarajan, P.; Powe, C.E.; Honigberg, M.C. Interventions to mitigate cardiovascular disease risk after adverse pregnancy outcomes: A review. *JAMA Cardiol.* **2022**, *7*, 346–355. [CrossRef]
87. Hamann, V.; Deruelle, P.; Enaux, C.; Deguen, S.; Kihal-Talantikite, W. Physical activity and gestational weight gain: A systematic review of observational studies. *BMC Public Health* **2022**, *22*, 1951. [CrossRef] [PubMed]
88. Ackerman-Banks, C.M.; Lipkind, H.S.; Palmsten, K.; Pfeiffer, M.; Gelsinger, C.; Ahrens, K.A. Association of Prenatal Depression With New Cardiovascular Disease Within 24 Months Postpartum. *J. Am. Hearth Assoc.* **2023**, *12*, e028133. [CrossRef] [PubMed]
89. Cattane, N.; Räikkönen, K.; Anniverno, R.; Mencacci, C.; Riva, M.A.; Pariante, C.M.; Cattaneo, A. Depression, obesity and their comorbidity during pregnancy: Effects on the offspring's mental and physical health. *Mol. Psychiatry* **2021**, *26*, 462–481. [CrossRef] [PubMed]
90. Brown, W.J.; Hayman, M.; Moran, L.J.; Redman, L.M.; Harrison, C.L. The Role of Physical Activity in Preconception, Pregnancy and Postpartum Health. *Semin. Reprod. Med.* **2016**, *34*, e28–e37. [CrossRef]
91. Moholdt, T.; Hawley, J.A. Maternal Lifestyle Interventions: Targeting Preconception Health. *Trends Endocrinol. Metab.* **2020**, *31*, 561–569. [CrossRef]
92. Khan, S.S.; Brewer, L.C.; Canobbio, M.M.; Cipolla, M.J.; Grobman, W.A.; Lewey, J.; Michos, E.D.; Miller, E.C.; Perak, A.M.; Wei, G.S.; et al. Optimizing Prepregnancy Cardiovascular Health to Improve Outcomes in Pregnant and Postpartum Individuals and Offspring: A Scientific Statement From the American Heart Association. *Circulation* **2023**, *147*, e76–e91. [CrossRef]
93. Freaney, P.M.; Harrington, K.; Molsberry, R.; Perak, A.M.; Wang, M.C.; Grobman, W.; Greenland, P.; Allen, N.B.; Capewell, S.; O'flaherty, M.; et al. Temporal Trends in Adverse Pregnancy Outcomes in Birthing Individuals Aged 15 to 44 Years in the United States, 2007 to 2019. *J. Am. Heart Assoc.* **2022**, *11*, e025050. [CrossRef]

94. Perak, A.M.; Ning, H.; Khan, S.S.; Van Horn, L.V.; Grobman, W.A.; Lloyd-Jones, D.M. Cardiovascular Health Among Pregnant Women, Aged 20 to 44 Years, in the United States. *J. Am. Heart Assoc.* **2020**, *9*, e015123. [CrossRef]
95. Silva-Jose, C.; Sánchez-Polán, M.; Barakat, R.; Gil-Ares, J.; Refoyo, I. Level of Physical Activity in Pregnant Populations from Different Geographic Regions: A Systematic Review. *J. Clin. Med.* **2022**, *11*, 4638. [CrossRef]
96. Kuhrt, K.; Hezelgrave, N.L.; Shennan, A.H. Exercise in pregnancy. *Obstet. Gynaecol.* **2015**, *17*, 281–287. [CrossRef]
97. Meander, L.; Lindqvist, M.; Mogren, I.; Sandlund, J.; West, C.E.; Domellöf, M. Physical activity and sedentary time during pregnancy and associations with maternal and fetal health outcomes: An epidemiological study. *BMC Pregnancy Childbirth* **2021**, *21*, 166. [CrossRef] [PubMed]
98. Parikh, N.I.; Gonzalez, J.M.; Anderson, C.A.; Judd, S.E.; Rexrode, K.M.; Hlatky, M.A.; Gunderson, E.P.; Stuart, J.J.; Vaidya, D. Adverse Pregnancy Outcomes and Cardiovascular Disease Risk: Unique Opportunities for Cardiovascular Disease Prevention in Women: A Scientific Statement from the American Heart Association. *Circulation* **2021**, *143*, e902–e916. [CrossRef] [PubMed]
99. Leskinen, T.; Stenholm, S.; Heinonen, O.J.; Pulakka, A.; Aalto, V.; Kivimäki, M.; Vahtera, J. Change in physical activity and accumulation of cardiometabolic risk factors. *Prev. Med.* **2018**, *112*, 31–37. [CrossRef]
100. Barrett, P.M.; McCarthy, F.P.; Kublickiene, K.; Cormican, S.; Judge, C.; Evans, M.; Kublickas, M.; Perry, I.J.; Stenvinkel, P.; Khashan, A.S. Faculty Opinions recommendation of Adverse Pregnancy Outcomes and Long-term Maternal Kidney Disease: A Systematic Review and Meta-analysis. *JAMA Netw. Open* **2020**, *3*, e1920964. [CrossRef] [PubMed]
101. ACOG Practice Bulletin No. 190: Gestational Diabetes Mellitus. *Obstet. Gynecol.* **2018**, *131*, e49–e64.
102. Duckitt, K.; Harrington, D. Risk factors for pre-eclampsia at antenatal booking: Systematic review of controlled studies. *BMJ* **2005**, *330*, 565. [CrossRef]
103. Mosca, L.; Benjamin, E.J.; Berra, K.; Bezanson, J.L.; Dolor, R.J.; Lloyd-Jones, D.M.; Newby, L.K.; Piña, I.L.; Roger, V.L.; Shaw, L.J.; et al. Effectiveness-Based Guidelines for the Prevention of Cardiovascular Disease in Women—2011 Update: A Guideline From the American Heart Association. *Circulation* **2011**, *123*, 1243–1262. [CrossRef]
104. Grundy, S.M.; Stone, N.J.; Bailey, A.L.; Beam, C.; Birtcher, K.K.; Blumenthal, R.S.; Braun, L.T.; De Ferranti, S.; Faiella-Tommasino, J.; Forman, D.E.; et al. 2018 AHA/ACC/AACVPR/AAPA/ABC/ACPM/ADA/AGS/APhA/ASPC/NLA/PCNA Guideline on the Management of Blood Cholesterol: A Report of the American College of Cardiology/American Heart Association Task Force on Clinical Practice Guidelines. *Circulation* **2019**, *139*, e1082–e1143.
105. Bull, F.C.; Al-Ansari, S.S.; Biddle, S.; Borodulin, K.; Buman, M.P.; Cardon, G.; Carty, C.; Chaput, J.P.; Chastin, S.; Chou, R.; et al. World Health Organization 2020 guidelines on physical activity and sedentary behaviour. *Br. J. Sports Med.* **2020**, *54*, 1451–1462. [CrossRef]
106. Savvaki, D.; Taousani, E.; Goulis, D.G.; Tsirou, E.; Voziki, E.; Douda, H.; Nikolettos, N.; Tokmakidis, S.P. Guidelines for exercise during normal pregnancy and gestational diabetes: A review of international recommendations. *Hormones* **2018**, *17*, 521–529. [CrossRef] [PubMed]
107. Hayman, M.; Brown, W.J.; Brinson, A.; Budzynski-Seymour, E.; Bruce, T.; Evenson, K.R. Public health guidelines for physical activity during pregnancy from around the world: A scoping review. *Br. J. Sports Med.* **2022**. [CrossRef] [PubMed]
108. Sternfeld, B.; Dugan, S. Physical Activity and Health During the Menopausal Transition. *Obstet. Gynecol. Clin. N. Am.* **2011**, *38*, 537–566. [CrossRef]
109. Mattioli, A.V.; Moscucci, F.; Sciomer, S.; Maffei, S.; Nasi, M.; Pinti, M.; Bucciarelli, V.; Dei Cas, A.; Parati, G.; Ciccone, M.M.; et al. Cardiovascular prevention in women: An update by the Italian Society of Cardiology working group on 'Prevention, hypertension and peripheral disease'. *J. Cardiovasc. Med. (Hagerstown)* **2023**, *24* (Suppl. S2), e147–e155. [CrossRef]
110. Centers for Disease, C. and Prevention, Trends in leisure-time physical inactivity by age, sex, and race/ethnicity--United States, 1994-2004. *MMWR Morb. Mortal Wkly. Rep.* **2005**, *54*, 991–994.
111. Bucciarelli, V.; Bianco, F.; Mucedola, F.; Di Blasio, A.; Izzicupo, P.; Tuosto, D.; Ghinassi, B.; Bucci, I.; Napolitano, G.; Di Baldassarre, A.; et al. Effect of Adherence to Physical Exercise on Cardiometabolic Profile in Postmenopausal Women. *Int. J. Environ. Res. Public Health* **2021**, *18*, 656. [CrossRef]
112. Izzicupo, P.; D'Amico, M.A.; Bascelli, A.; Di Fonso, A.; D'angelo, E.; Di Blasio, A.; Bucci, I.; Napolitano, G.; Gallina, S.; Di Baldassarre, A. Walking training affects dehydroepiandrosterone sulfate and inflammation independent of changes in spontaneous physical activity. *Menopause* **2013**, *20*, 455–463. [CrossRef]
113. Izzicupo, P.; Ghinassi, B.; D'Amico, M.A.; Di Blasio, A.; Gesi, M.; Napolitano, G.; Gallina, S.; Di Baldassarre, A. Effects of ACE I/D Polymorphism and Aerobic Training on the Immune–Endocrine Network and Cardiovascular Parameters of Postmenopausal Women. *J. Clin. Endocrinol. Metab.* **2013**, *98*, 4187–4194. [CrossRef]
114. Izzicupo, P.; D'amico, M.A.; Di Blasio, A.; Napolitano, G.; Nakamura, F.Y.; Di Baldassarre, A.; Ghinassi, B. Aerobic Training Improves Angiogenic Potential Independently of Vascular Endothelial Growth Factor Modifications in Postmenopausal Women. *Front. Endocrinol.* **2017**, *8*, 363. [CrossRef]
115. Di Blasio, A.; Izzicupo, P.; Di Baldassarre, A.; Gallina, S.; Bucci, I.; Giuliani, C.; Di Santo, S.; Di Iorio, A.; Ripari, P.; Napolitano, G. Walking training and cortisol to DHEA-S ratio in postmenopause: An intervention study. *Women Health* **2018**, *58*, 387–402. [CrossRef]
116. Di Blasio, A.; Izzicupo, P.; D'angelo, E.; Melanzi, S.; Bucci, I.; Gallina, S.; Di Baldassarre, A.; Napolitano, G. Effects of Patterns of Walking Training on Metabolic Health of Untrained Postmenopausal Women. *J. Aging Phys. Act.* **2014**, *22*, 482–489. [CrossRef]

117. Gudmundsdottir, S.L.; Flanders, W.D.; Augestad, L.B. Physical activity and cardiovascular risk factors at menopause: The Nord-Trøndelag health study. *Climacteric* **2013**, *16*, 438–446. [CrossRef]
118. Hyvarinen, M.; Juppi, H.K.; Taskinen, S.; Karppinen, J.E.; Karvinen, S.; Tammelin, T.H.; Kovanen, V.; Aukee, P.; Kujala, U.M.; Rantalainen, T.; et al. Metabolic health, menopause, and physical activity-a 4-year follow-up study. *Int. J. Obes. (Lond.)* **2022**, *46*, 544–554. [CrossRef]
119. Juppi, H.-K.; Sipilä, S.; Cronin, N.J.; Karvinen, S.; Karppinen, J.E.; Tammelin, T.H.; Aukee, P.; Kovanen, V.; Kujala, U.M.; Laakkonen, E.K. Role of Menopausal Transition and Physical Activity in Loss of Lean and Muscle Mass: A Follow-Up Study in Middle-Aged Finnish Women. *J. Clin. Med.* **2020**, *9*, 1588. [CrossRef]
120. Khalafi, M.; Sakhaei, M.H.; Maleki, A.H.; Rosenkranz, S.K.; Pourvaghar, M.J.; Fang, Y.; Korivi, M. Influence of exercise type and duration on cardiorespiratory fitness and muscular strength in post-menopausal women: A systematic review and meta-analysis. *Front. Cardiovasc. Med.* **2023**, *10*, 1190187. [CrossRef] [PubMed]
121. Di Blasio, A.; Bucci, I.; Napolitano, G.; Melanzi, S.; Izzicupo, P.; Di Donato, F.; Tonizzo, C.; D'Angelo, E.; Ricci, G.; Ripari, P. Characteristics of spontaneous physical activity and executive functions in postmenopause. *Minerva Med.* **2013**, *104*, 61–74. [PubMed]
122. Wu, S.; Shi, Y.; Zhao, Q.; Men, K. The relationship between physical activity and the severity of menopausal symptoms: A cross-sectional study. *BMC Women's Health* **2023**, *23*, 212. [CrossRef] [PubMed]
123. Tsao, C.W.; Aday, A.W.; Almarzooq, Z.I.; Alonso, A.; Beaton, A.Z.; Bittencourt, M.S.; Boehme, A.K.; Buxton, A.E.; Carson, A.P.; Commodore-Mensah, Y.; et al. Heart Disease and Stroke Statistics—2022 Update: A Report From the American Heart Association. *Circulation* **2022**, *145*, e153–e639. [CrossRef]
124. Lee, Y.-S. Gender Differences in Physical Activity and Walking Among Older Adults. *J. Women Aging* **2005**, *17*, 55–70. [CrossRef] [PubMed]
125. Izzicupo, P.; Di Blasio, A.; Di Credico, A.; Gaggi, G.; Vamvakis, A.; Napolitano, G.; Ricci, F.; Gallina, S.; Ghinassi, B.; Di Baldassarre, A. The Length and Number of Sedentary Bouts Predict Fibrinogen Levels in Postmenopausal Women. *Int. J. Environ. Res. Public Health* **2020**, *17*, 3051. [CrossRef]
126. Bellettiere, J.; LaMonte, M.J.; Evenson, K.R.; Rillamas-Sun, E.; Kerr, J.; Lee, I.M.; Di, C.; Rosenberg, D.E.; Stefanick, M.L.; Buchner, D.M.; et al. Sedentary behavior and cardiovascular disease in older women: The Objective Physical Activity and Cardiovascular Health (OPACH) Study. *Circulation* **2019**, *139*, 1036–1046. [CrossRef]
127. Dogra, S.; Ashe, M.C.; Biddle, S.J.H.; Brown, W.J.; Buman, M.P.; Chastin, S.; Gardiner, P.A.; Inoue, S.; Jefferis, B.J.; Oka, K.; et al. Sedentary time in older men and women: An international consensus statement and research priorities. *Br. J. Sports Med.* **2017**, *51*, 1526–1532. [CrossRef]
128. Paolisso, P.; Bergamaschi, L.; Saturi, G.; D'Angelo, E.C.; Magnani, I.; Toniolo, S.; Stefanizzi, A.; Rinaldi, A.; Bartoli, L.; Angeli, F.; et al. Secondary Prevention Medical Therapy and Outcomes in Patients With Myocardial Infarction With Non-Obstructive Coronary Artery Disease. *Front. Pharmacol.* **2019**, *10*, 1606. [CrossRef]
129. Di Blasio, A.; Ripari, P.; Bucci, I.; Di Donato, F.; Izzicupo, P.; D'Angelo, E.; Di Nenno, B.; Taglieri, M.; Napolitano, G. Walking training in postmenopause: Effects on both spontaneous physical activity and training-induced body adaptations. *Menopause* **2012**, *19*, 23–32. [CrossRef]
130. Di Blasio, A.; Bucci, I.; Ripari, P.; Giuliani, C.; Izzicupo, P.; Di Donato, F.; D'angelo, E.; Napolitano, G. Lifestyle and high density lipoprotein cholesterol in postmenopause. *Climacteric* **2014**, *17*, 37–47. [CrossRef] [PubMed]
131. Di Blasio, A.; Di Donato, F.; Di Santo, S.; Bucci, I.; Izzicupo, P.; Di Baldassarre, A.; Gallina, S.; Bergamin, M.; Ripari, P.; Napolitano, G. Aerobic physical exercise and negative compensation of non-exercise physical activity in post-menopause: A pilot study. *J. Sports Med. Phys. Fit.* **2018**, *58*, 1497–1508. [CrossRef]
132. Cugusi, L.; Manca, A.; Serpe, R.; Romita, G.; Bergamin, M.; Cadeddu, C.; Solla, P.; Mercuro, G. Effects of a mini-trampoline rebounding exercise program on functional parameters, body composition and quality of life in overweight women. *J. Sports Med. Phys. Fit.* **2018**, *58*, 287–294. [CrossRef]
133. Cugusi, L.; Manca, A.; Bergamin, M.; Di Blasio, A.; Yeo, T.J.; Crisafulli, A.; Mercuro, G. Zumba Fitness and Women's Cardiovascular Health: A systematic review. *J. Cardiopulm. Rehabil. Prev.* **2019**, *39*, 153–160. [CrossRef]
134. Thomas, A.; Daley, A.J. Women's views about physical activity as a treatment for vasomotor menopausal symptoms: A qualitative study. *BMC Women's Health* **2020**, *20*, 203. [CrossRef] [PubMed]
135. Fricke, A.; Rauff, E.; Fink, P.W.; Lark, S.D.; Rowlands, D.S.; Shultz, S.P. Perceptions of a 12-week mini-trampoline exercise intervention for postmenopausal women. *J. Sport Exerc. Sci.* **2023**, *1*, 53–59.
136. Di Blasio, A.; Di Donato, F.; Mastrodicasa, M.; Fabrizio, N.; Di Renzo, D.; Napolitano, G.; Petrella, V.; Gallina, S.; Ripari, P. Effects of the time of day of walking on dietary behaviour, body composition and aerobic fitness in post-menopausal women. *J. Sports Med. Phys. Fit.* **2010**, *50*, 196–201.
137. Paynter, N.P.; LaMonte, M.J.; Manson, J.E.; Martin, L.W.; Phillips, L.S.; Ridker, P.M.; Robinson, J.G.; Cook, N.R. Comparison of Lifestyle-Based and Traditional Cardiovascular Disease Prediction in a Multiethnic Cohort of Nonsmoking Women. *Circulation* **2014**, *130*, 1466–1473. [CrossRef] [PubMed]
138. Lee, I.M. Physical activity and coronary heart disease in women: Is "no pain, no gain" passe? *JAMA* **2001**, *285*, 1447–1454. [CrossRef] [PubMed]

139. Akgöz, A.D.; Ozer, Z.; Gözüm, S. The effect of lifestyle physical activity in reducing cardiovascular disease risk factors (blood pressure and cholesterol) in women: A systematic review. *Health Care Women Int.* **2021**, *42*, 4–27. [CrossRef]
140. Seguin, R.; Buchner, D.M.; Liu, J.; Allison, M.; Manini, T.; Wang, C.Y.; Manson, J.E.; Messina, C.R.; Patel, M.J.; Moreland, L.; et al. Sedentary behavior and mortality in older women: The Women's Health Initiative. *Am. J. Prev. Med.* **2014**, *46*, 122–135. [CrossRef]
141. Chomistek, A.K.; Manson, J.E.; Stefanick, M.L.; Lu, B.; Sands-Lincoln, M.; Going, S.B.; Garcia, L.; Allison, M.A.; Sims, S.T.; LaMonte, M.J.; et al. Relationship of Sedentary Behavior and Physical Activity to Incident Cardiovascular Disease. *JACC* **2013**, *61*, 2346–2354. [CrossRef]
142. Ekelund, U.; Steene-Johannessen, J.; Brown, W.J.; Fagerland, M.W.; Owen, N.; Powell, K.E.; Bauman, A.; Lee, I.-M. Does physical activity attenuate, or even eliminate, the detrimental association of sitting time with mortality? A harmonised meta-analysis of data from more than 1 million men and women. *Lancet* **2016**, *388*, 1302–1310. [CrossRef]
143. Ekelund, U.; Tarp, J.; Steene-Johannessen, J.; Hansen, B.H.; Jefferis, B.; Fagerland, M.W.; Whincup, P.; Diaz, K.M.; Hooker, S.P.; Chernofsky, A.; et al. Dose-response associations between accelerometry measured physical activity and sedentary time and all cause mortality: Systematic review and harmonised meta-analysis. *BMJ* **2019**, *366*, l4570. [CrossRef]
144. Länsitie, M.; Kangas, M.; Jokelainen, J.; Venojärvi, M.; Timonen, M.; Keinänen-Kiukaanniemi, S.; Korpelainen, R. Cardiovascular disease risk and all-cause mortality associated with accelerometer-measured physical activity and sedentary time—A prospective population-based study in older adults. *BMC Geriatr.* **2022**, *22*, 729. [CrossRef] [PubMed]
145. Du, L.; Li, G.; Ren, P.; He, Q.; Pan, Y.; Chen, S.; Zhang, X. Associations between objectively measured patterns of sedentary behaviour and arterial stiffness in Chinese community-dwelling older women. *Eur. J. Cardiovasc. Nurs.* **2023**, *22*, 374–381. [CrossRef] [PubMed]
146. Bakker, E.A.; van Bakel, B.M.; Aengevaeren, W.R.; Meindersma, E.P.; Snoek, J.A.; Waskowsky, W.M.; van Kuijk, A.A.; Jacobs, M.M.; Hopman, M.T.; Thijssen, D.H.; et al. Sedentary behaviour in cardiovascular disease patients: Risk group identification and the impact of cardiac rehabilitation. *Int. J. Cardiol.* **2021**, *326*, 194–201. [CrossRef] [PubMed]
147. Duran, A.T.; Garber, C.E.; Cornelius, T.; Schwartz, J.E.; Diaz, K.M. Patterns of Sedentary Behavior in the First Month After Acute Coronary Syndrome. *J. Am. Heart Assoc.* **2019**, *8*, e011585. [CrossRef]
148. Vasankari, V.; Halonen, J.; Vasankari, T.; Anttila, V.; Airaksinen, J.; Sievänen, H.; Hartikainen, J. Physical activity and sedentary behaviour in secondary prevention of coronary artery disease: A review. *Am. J. Prev. Cardiol.* **2021**, *5*, 100146. [CrossRef] [PubMed]
149. LaMonte, M.J.; Larson, J.C.; Manson, J.E.; Bellettiere, J.; Lewis, C.E.; LaCroix, A.Z.; Bea, J.W.; Johnson, K.C.; Klein, L.; Noel, C.A.; et al. Association of Sedentary Time and Incident Heart Failure Hospitalization in Postmenopausal Women. *Circ. Heart Fail.* **2020**, *13*, e007508. [CrossRef]
150. Visseren, F.L.; Mach, F.; Smulders, Y.M.; Carballo, D.; Koskinas, K.C.; Bäck, M.; Benetos, A.; Biffi, A.; Boavida, J.M.; Capodanno, D.; et al. 2021 ESC Guidelines on cardiovascular disease prevention in clinical practice. *Eur. Heart J.* **2021**, *42*, 3227–3337. [CrossRef]
151. Abreu, A.; Frederix, I.; Dendale, P.; Janssen, A.; Doherty, P.; Piepoli, M.F.; Völler, H.; on behalf of the Secondary Prevention and Rehabilitation Section of EAPC Reviewers: Marco Ambrosetti; Davos, C.H. Standardization and quality improvement of secondary prevention through cardiovascular rehabilitation programmes in Europe: The avenue towards EAPC accreditation programme: A position statement of the Secondary Prevention and Rehabilitation Section of the European Association of Preventive Cardiology (EAPC). *Eur. J. Prev. Cardiol.* **2021**, *28*, 496–509. [CrossRef]
152. Bjarnason-Wehrens, B.; McGee, H.; Zwisler, A.-D.; Piepoli, M.F.; Benzer, W.; Schmid, J.-P.; Dendale, P.; Pogosova, N.-G.V.; Zdrenghea, D.; Niebauer, J.; et al. Cardiac rehabilitation in Europe: Results from the European Cardiac Rehabilitation Inventory Survey. *Eur. J. Prev. Cardiol.* **2010**, *17*, 410–418. [CrossRef] [PubMed]
153. Hansen, D.; Dendale, P.; Coninx, K.; Vanhees, L.; Piepoli, M.F.; Niebauer, J.; Cornelissen, V.; Pedretti, R.; Geurts, E.; Ruiz, G.R.; et al. The European Association of Preventive Cardiology Exercise Prescription in Everyday Practice and Rehabilitative Training (EXPERT) tool: A digital training and decision support system for optimized exercise prescription in cardiovascular disease. Concept, definitions and construction methodology. *Eur. J. Prev. Cardiol.* **2017**, *24*, 1017–1031. [CrossRef]
154. Resurreccion, D.; Moreno-Peral, P.; Gómez-Herranz, M.; Rubio-Valera, M.; Pastor, L.; De Almeida, J.M.C.; Motrico, E. Factors associated with non-participation in and dropout from cardiac rehabilitation programmes: A systematic review of prospective cohort studies. *Eur. J. Cardiovasc. Nurs.* **2019**, *18*, 38–47. [CrossRef]
155. Hamilton, S.J.; Mills, B.; Birch, E.M.; Thompson, S.C. Smartphones in the secondary prevention of cardiovascular disease: A systematic review. *BMC Cardiovasc. Disord.* **2018**, *18*, 25. [CrossRef]
156. Bucciarelli, V.; Nasi, M.; Bianco, F.; Seferovic, J.; Ivkovic, V.; Gallina, S.; Mattioli, A.V. Depression pandemic and cardiovascular risk in the COVID-19 era and long COVID syndrome: Gender makes a difference. *Trends Cardiovasc. Med.* **2022**, *32*, 12–17. [CrossRef]
157. Nienhuis, C.P.; Lesser, I.A. The Impact of COVID-19 on Women's Physical Activity Behavior and Mental Well-Being. *Int. J. Environ. Res. Public Health* **2020**, *17*, 9036. [CrossRef]
158. Okuyama, J.; Seto, S.; Fukuda, Y.; Funakoshi, S.; Amae, S.; Onobe, J.; Izumi, S.; Ito, K.; Imamura, F. Mental Health and Physical Activity among Children and Adolescents during the COVID-19 Pandemic. *Tohoku J. Exp. Med.* **2021**, *253*, 203–215. [CrossRef] [PubMed]
159. Coronado, P.J.; Fasero, M.; Otero, B.; Sanchez, S.; de la Viuda, E.; Ramirez-Polo, I.; Llaneza, P.; Mendoza, N.; Baquedano, L. Health-related quality of life and resilience in peri- and postmenopausal women during COVID-19 confinement. *Maturitas* **2021**, *144*, 4–10. [CrossRef] [PubMed]

160. Kaygısız, B.B.; Topcu, Z.G.; Meriç, A.; Gözgen, H.; Çoban, F. Determination of exercise habits, physical activity level and anxiety level of postmenopausal women during COVID-19 pandemic. *Health Care Women Int.* **2020**, *41*, 1240–1254. [CrossRef] [PubMed]
161. Ricci, F.; Izzicupo, P.; Moscucci, F.; Sciomer, S.; Maffei, S.; Di Baldassarre, A.; Mattioli, A.V.; Gallina, S. Recommendations for Physical Inactivity and Sedentary Behavior During the Coronavirus Disease (COVID-19) Pandemic. *Front. Public Health* **2020**, *8*, 199. [CrossRef]
162. Mattioli, A.V.; Sciomer, S.; Maffei, S.; Gallina, S. Lifestyle and Stress Management in Women During COVID-19 Pandemic: Impact on Cardiovascular Risk Burden. *Am. J. Lifestyle Med.* **2021**, *15*, 356–359. [CrossRef] [PubMed]
163. Mattioli, A.V.; Coppi, F.; Gallina, S. Importance of physical activity during and after the SARS-CoV-2/COVID-19 pandemic: A strategy for women to cope with stress. *Eur. J. Neurol.* **2021**, *28*, e78–e79. [CrossRef]
164. Davenport, M.H.; Meyer, S.; Meah, V.L.; Strynadka, M.C.; Khurana, R. Moms Are Not OK: COVID-19 and Maternal Mental Health. *Front. Glob. Women's Health* **2020**, *1*, 1. [CrossRef]
165. Moscucci, F.; Gallina, S.; Bucciarelli, V.; Aimo, A.; Pelà, G.; Cadeddu-Dessalvi, C.; Nodari, S.; Maffei, S.; Meloni, A.; Deidda, M.; et al. Impact of COVID-19 on the cardiovascular health of women: A review by the Italian Society of Cardiology Working Group on 'gender cardiovascular diseases'. *J. Cardiovasc. Med.* **2023**, *24* (Suppl. S1), e15–e23. [CrossRef]
166. De Gaetano, A.; Solodka, K.; Zanini, G.; Selleri, V.; Mattioli, A.V.; Nasi, M.; Pinti, M. Molecular Mechanisms of mtDNA-Mediated Inflammation. *Cells* **2021**, *10*, 2898. [CrossRef] [PubMed]
167. Mattioli, A.V.; Selleri, V.; Zanini, G.; Nasi, M.; Pinti, M.; Stefanelli, C.; Fedele, F.; Gallina, S. Physical Activity and Diet in Older Women: A Narrative Review. *J. Clin. Med.* **2022**, *12*, 81. [CrossRef] [PubMed]
168. Nabavi, N. Long covid: How to define it and how to manage it. *BMJ* **2020**, *370*, m3489. [CrossRef]
169. Mattioli, A.V.; Coppi, F.; Nasi, M.; Pinti, M.; Gallina, S. Long COVID: A New Challenge for Prevention of Obesity in Women. *Am. J. Lifestyle Med.* **2023**, *17*, 164–168. [CrossRef] [PubMed]
170. Yelin, D.; Wirtheim, E.; Vetter, P.; Kalil, A.C.; Bruchfeld, J.; Runold, M.; Guaraldi, G.; Mussini, C.; Gudiol, C.; Pujol, M.; et al. Long-term consequences of COVID-19: Research needs. *Lancet Infect. Dis.* **2020**, *20*, 1115–1117. [CrossRef]
171. World Health Organization. Post COVID-19 Condition (Long COVID). 2022. Available online: https://www.who.int/europe/news-room/fact-sheets/item/post-covid-19-condition (accessed on 28 March 2022).
172. Hanson, S.W.; Abbafati, C.; Aerts, J.G.; Al-Aly, Z.; Ashbaugh, C.; Ballouz, T.; Blyuss, O.; Bobkova, P.; Bonsel, G.; Borzakova, S.; et al. Estimated Global Proportions of Individuals With Persistent Fatigue, Cognitive, and Respiratory Symptom Clusters Following Symptomatic COVID-19 in 2020 and 2021. *JAMA* **2022**, *328*, 1604–1615.
173. Carter, S.J.; Baranauskas, M.N.; Raglin, J.S.; Pescosolido, B.A.; Perry, B.L. Functional Status, Mood State, and Physical Activity Among Women With Post-Acute COVID-19 Syndrome. *Int. J. Public Health* **2022**, *67*, 1604589. [CrossRef]
174. Gil, S.; Gualano, B.; de Araújo, A.L.; de Oliveira Júnior, G.N.; Damiano, R.F.; Pinna, F.; Imamura, M.; Rocha, V.; Kallas, E.; Batistella, L.R.; et al. Post-acute sequelae of SARS-CoV-2 associates with physical inactivity in a cohort of COVID-19 survivors. *Sci. Rep.* **2023**, *13*, 215. [CrossRef]
175. Wright, J.; Astill, S.L.; Sivan, M. The Relationship between Physical Activity and Long COVID: A Cross-Sectional Study. *Int. J. Environ. Res. Public Health* **2022**, *19*, 5093. [CrossRef]
176. Hayes, L.D.; Ingram, J.; Sculthorpe, N.F. More Than 100 Persistent Symptoms of SARS-CoV-2 (Long COVID): A Scoping Review. *Front. Med. (Lausanne)* **2021**, *8*, 750378. [CrossRef]
177. Nandadeva, D.; Skow, R.J.; Stephens, B.Y.; Grotle, A.-K.; Georgoudiou, S.; Barshikar, S.; Seo, Y.; Fadel, P.J. Cardiovascular and Cerebral Vascular Health in Females with Post-Acute Sequelae of COVID-19 (PASC). *Am. J. Physiol. Circ. Physiol.* **2023**, *324*, H713–H720. [CrossRef] [PubMed]
178. Whiteson, J.H.; Azola, A.; Barry, J.T.; Bartels, M.N.; Blitshteyn, S.; Fleming, T.K.; McCauley, M.D.; Neal, J.D.; Pillarisetti, J.; Sampsel, S.; et al. Multi-disciplinary collaborative consensus guidance statement on the assessment and treatment of cardiovascular complications in patients with post-acute sequelae of SARS-CoV-2 infection (PASC). *PM R* **2022**, *14*, 855–878. [CrossRef] [PubMed]
179. Tabacof, L.; Tosto-Mancuso, J.; Wood, J.; Cortes, M.; Kontorovich, A.; McCarthy, D.; Rizk, D.; Rozanski, G.; Breyman, E.; Nasr, L.; et al. Post-acute COVID-19 Syndrome Negatively Impacts Physical Function, Cognitive Function, Health-Related Quality of Life, and Participation. *Am. J. Phys. Med. Rehabil.* **2022**, *101*, 48–52. [CrossRef]
180. Bellan, M.; Soddu, D.; Balbo, P.E.; Baricich, A.; Zeppegno, P.; Avanzi, G.C.; Baldon, G.; Bartolomei, G.; Battaglia, M.; Battistini, S.; et al. Respiratory and Psychophysical Sequelae Among Patients With COVID-19 Four Months After Hospital Discharge. *JAMA Netw. Open* **2021**, *4*, e2036142. [CrossRef] [PubMed]
181. Fugazzaro, S.; Contri, A.; Esseroukh, O.; Kaleci, S.; Croci, S.; Massari, M.; Facciolongo, N.C.; Besutti, G.; Iori, M.; Salvarani, C.; et al. Rehabilitation Interventions for Post-Acute COVID-19 Syndrome: A Systematic Review. *Int. J. Environ. Res. Public Health* **2022**, *19*, 5185. [CrossRef]
182. Schwendinger, F. Exercise as medicine in post-COVID-19: A call to action. *Sport. Exerc. Med.* **2022**, *70*. [CrossRef]
183. Twomey, R.; DeMars, J.; Franklin, K.; Culos-Reed, S.N.; Weatherald, J.; Wrightson, J.G. Chronic Fatigue and Postexertional Malaise in People Living With Long COVID: An Observational Study. *Phys. Ther.* **2022**, *102*, pzac005. [CrossRef]
184. Hafner, M.; Yerushalmi, E.; Stepanek, M.; Phillips, W.; Pollard, J.; Deshpande, A.; Whitmore, M.; Millard, F.; Subel, S.; Van Stolk, C. Estimating the global economic benefits of physically active populations over 30 years (2020–2050). *Br. J. Sports Med.* **2020**, *54*, 1482–1487. [CrossRef]

185. Climie, R.; Fuster, V.; Empana, J.-P. Health Literacy and Primordial Prevention in Childhood—An Opportunity to Reduce the Burden of Cardiovascular Disease. *JAMA Cardiol.* **2020**, *5*, 1323. [CrossRef]
186. Guthold, R.; Willumsen, J.; Bull, F.C. What is driving gender inequalities in physical activity among adolescents? *J. Sport Health Sci.* **2022**, *11*, 424–426. [CrossRef]

Disclaimer/Publisher's Note: The statements, opinions and data contained in all publications are solely those of the individual author(s) and contributor(s) and not of MDPI and/or the editor(s). MDPI and/or the editor(s) disclaim responsibility for any injury to people or property resulting from any ideas, methods, instructions or products referred to in the content.

Review

Gender Effect on Clinical Profiles, Pharmacological Treatments and Prognosis in Patients Hospitalized for Heart Failure

Luca Fazzini [1], Mattia Casati [1], Alessandro Martis [1], Ferdinando Perra [1], Paolo Rubiolo [1], Martino Deidda [1,2,*], Giuseppe Mercuro [1] and Christian Cadeddu Dessalvi [1]

1. Department of Medical Sciences and Public Health, University of Cagliari, 09124 Cagliari, Italy; luca.fazzini10@gmail.com (L.F.); mattiacasati1996@gmail.com (M.C.); amartismed@gmail.com (A.M.); ferdinando.perra@gmail.com (F.P.); paolo.f.rubiolo@gmail.com (P.R.); giuseppemercuro@gmail.com (G.M.); cadedduc@unica.it (C.C.D.)
2. Sassu Cardiologic Center, Cittadella Universitaria, 09033 Sardinia, Italy
* Correspondence: martino.deidda@tiscali.it

Abstract: Heart failure (HF) is a significant disease affecting 1–2% of the general population. Despite its general aspects, HF, like other cardiovascular diseases, presents various gender-specific aspects in terms of etiology, hemodynamics, clinical characteristics, therapy, and outcomes. As is well known, HF with preserved ejection fraction more frequently affects females, with diabetes and arterial hypertension representing the most critical determinants of HF. On the other hand, women are traditionally underrepresented in clinical trials and are often considered undertreated. However, it is not clear whether such differences reflect cultural behaviors and clinical inertia or if they indicate different clinical profiles and the impact of sex on hard clinical outcomes. We aimed to review the sex-related differences in patients affected by HF.

Keywords: acute heart failure; gender medicine; pharmacological treatments; prognosis

1. Introduction

Heart failure (HF) is a prevalent and progressive clinical syndrome characterized by cardinal symptoms and typical signs. It arises from structural and functional abnormalities in the heart, leading to elevated intracardiac pressures or inadequate cardiac output, both at rest and during exercise.

The classification of HF has been delineated into distinct phenotypes based on left ventricular ejection fraction (LVEF): HF with reduced EF (HFrEF) with an $EF \leq 40\%$, HF with mildly reduced fraction (HFmrEF) with an EF ranging from 41% to 49%, and HF with preserved EF (HFpEF) with an EF greater than 50% [1].

Noteworthy gender disparities exist within the HF spectrum. HFrEF predominantly affects men, while women are more predisposed to HFpEF due to distinct comorbidities such as hypertensive heart disease (more prevalent in females) and diabetes. Additionally, sex-specific pathophysiological factors, including pregnancy-related disorders, nulliparity, loss of estrogen, premature menopause, and consequences of breast cancer treatments such as chemotherapy and radiotherapy-induced cardiomyopathy, contribute to these differences [1–4].

2. Gender Differences in Risk Factors for Heart Failure

There is a growing body of evidence highlighting the significance of gender differences in the epidemiology, pathophysiology, treatment, and outcomes of various diseases, and cardiovascular disease (CVD) is no exception. Sex differences refer to biology-related distinctions between women and men, stemming from diverse sex chromosomes, sex-specific gene expressions of autosomes, sex hormones, and their respective impacts on organ systems. Concurrently, gender differences result from sociocultural processes, encompassing distinct behaviors, exposure to specific environmental influences, dietary patterns, lifestyles, stress, and variations in attitudes toward treatments and prevention between women and men [5].

Furthermore, women face sex-specific risk factors for HF, particularly associated with complications arising from pregnancy [4].

Epidemiological studies indicate that diabetes mellitus (DM) presents a more potent risk factor for CVD in women compared to men [6]. As reported by Kautzky-Willer et al., sex hormones play a significant role in influencing energy metabolism, body composition, vascular function, and inflammatory responses [7]. Indeed, endocrine imbalances are associated with unfavorable cardiometabolic traits, evident in women with androgen excess or men with hypogonadism [7]. While in men, DM is often diagnosed at a younger age and lower body mass index (BMI), obesity, a prominent risk factor, is more prevalent in women [7] (Figure 1).

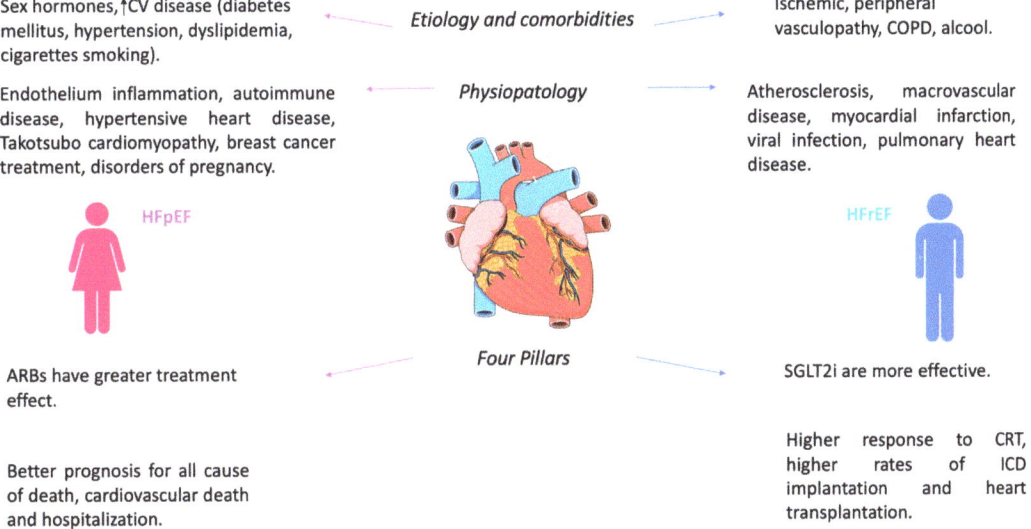

Figure 1. Main gender differences in clinical profile, pharmacological treatment, and prognosis in patients hospitalized for heart failure. COPD: chronic obstructive pulmonary disease. ARBs: angiotensin receptor blockers. SGLT2i: sodium-glucose co-transporter 2 inhibitor. CRT: cardiac resynchronization therapy. ICD: implantable cardioverter defibrillator.

Therefore, crucial parameters to consider include BMI, with normal values ranging from 18.5 kg/m^2 to 24.99 kg/m^2, and waist circumference, with reference values of <80 cm in women and <94 cm in men. The Framingham study showed that women with obesity have an increased risk of coronary heart disease (CHD) of 64% compared to 46% among men with obesity [8].

Furthermore, in the realm of pregnancy-related risk factors for HF, conditions such as gestational diabetes and preeclampsia are at the forefront. The INTERHEART study pointed out that gestational diabetes heightens the likelihood of developing type 2 diabetes and experiencing a myocardial infarction [9]. Similarly, preeclampsia increases the risk of hypertension, coronary artery disease, stroke, and HF for up to four decades following the pregnancy.

Evidence suggests that the evolution of lifetime blood pressure (BP) varies between women and men, potentially leading to an increased CVD risk at lower BP thresholds [5]. Generally, the diagnosis and treatment of hypertension are similar between genders, except for women of childbearing potential or during pregnancy. The 2023 ESC Guidelines for the management of cardiovascular disease in patients with diabetes emphasize how during these periods, certain drugs, such as RAS blockers, can have adverse effects on the fetus, particularly in early gestation [6].

These distinct risk factors are not isolated pathologies but rather interact with each other. When compared to women and men without DM, women typically exhibit more notable differences in BP and higher rates of hypertension than men at the time of DM diagnosis [10]. Additionally, women tend to have poorer BP control following diagnosis. Furthermore, sex-specific hypertension-mediated organ damage is associated with a significantly elevated risk of HF with preserved ejection fraction (HFpEF) in women, especially in the presence of DM [6]. Ventura-Clapier et al. demonstrated that women with hypertension have a 3-fold higher risk of HF or stroke than men and have higher rates of recurring myocardial infarction (MI) after an initial MI [11].

Evidence indicates that sex hormones and sex-specific molecular mechanisms play a role in influencing glucose and lipid metabolism, as well as cardiac energy metabolism and function. Males tend to have a more pro-atherogenic lipid profile, characterized by lower high-density lipoprotein and higher low-density lipoprotein and triglycerides [12].

Dyslipidemia emerges as a significant contributor to gender-based variations observed in HF. As shown by Meloni A. et al., the impact of abnormal lipid profiles, including elevated levels of cholesterol and triglycerides, varies between men and women, influencing the development and progression of HF differently [13]. Recognizing these gender-specific aspects of dyslipidemia is crucial for tailoring effective preventive and therapeutic strategies for HF in both male and female populations.

Cigarette smoking accounts for 50% of all preventable deaths in smokers, with half of these attributable to atherosclerotic cardiovascular disease. Notably, prolonged smoking poses a greater risk for women than men [5]; however, a meta-analysis of over three million individuals demonstrated that except for women aged 30–44 years, female smokers had a 25% greater risk of CVD than male smokers [14].

Young women who smoke face an elevated risk of sudden death due to MI, the pathology most strongly associated with smoking. The risk of myocardial infarction in male smokers is approximately five times higher than in women, with an increase corresponding to the number of cigarettes smoked. This difference is believed to be linked to the protective role of female hormones in the cardiovascular system [15].

In summary, given the under-representation of women in clinical trials and the absence of evidence for sex-specific recommendations regarding CVD management, the implementation of sex-balanced recruitment strategies is recommended for future cardiovascular outcome trials. Most importantly, concerted efforts should be made to ensure that women receive equal healthcare opportunities in the management of CVD.

3. Gender Differences in Pathophysiology

As remarked by Lam et al., microvascular dysfunction is attributed to endothelial inflammation, often stemming from cardiometabolic comorbidities such as obesity, which is more prevalent in females, and diabetes, disrupting the nitric oxide (NO) pathway [1].

In women, many sex-related conditions can lead to microvascular disease, such as postmenopausal estrogen loss and a higher tendency of autoimmune diseases, consequently leading to the increased production of pro-inflammatory cytokines. This, coupled with diastolic dysfunctions often caused by autoimmune diseases, adds to the complexity of the cardiovascular scenario [1].

Ischemic cardiopathy is the primary cause of HF with reduced ejection fraction (HFrEF) in both genders, while among the non-ischemic causes, hypertensive heart disease emerges as the predominant cause of HF with preserved ejection fraction (HFpEF). Long-standing hypertensive heart disease can progress to HF through cardiomyocyte dysfunction, fibrosis due to increased extracellular matrix, and the rarefaction of intramyocardial microvasculature. Diastolic dysfunction commonly presents early in HFpEF caused by hypertensive heart disease, induced by persistent pressure overload, and it results in concentric left ventricular hypertrophy [16].

An acute and transient HF presentation is frequently observed in Takotsubo cardiomyopathy, being more prevalent in females and triggered by impaired neurohormonal regulation during acute emotional or psychological stress. Women experiencing higher psychological distress are more prone to developing cardiovascular events than men [1]. As described in Circulation by Pelliccia et al., about 90% of patients with Takotsubo syndrome are postmenopausal women; women are also more predisposed to experience Takotsubo major adverse events, including cardiogenic shock, cardiac arrest, and mortality [17].

Breast cancer, the most prevalent cancer in females, presents an additional risk of HF due to cardiotoxicity from modern anti-cancer treatments, including chemotherapy and radiotherapy. Cadeddu Dessalvi et al., reported in their review that anthracyclines, which are a cornerstone for breast cancer and many other oncologic treatments, have a higher cardiotoxicity in the female sex, and this may be explained by gender differences in metabolic pathways which represent an intriguing ongoing research field to obtain more tailored therapies [18,19]. Radiotherapy, on the other hand, is associated with a heightened risk of major coronary events, such as myocardial infarction and coronary revascularization. This risk increases linearly with the mean dose to the heart, starting within the first 5 years post-radiation and continuing for at least 20 years. While cardiomyocytes are resistant to radiation, radiotherapy induces microvascular endothelial damage, leading to coronary microvascular artery rarefaction, oxidative stress, and fibrosis. Breast cancer and CVD share common risk factors, including age, obesity, and tobacco use, which may contribute to HF development [20,21].

4. Gender Differences in Diagnostic and Clinical Presentation

Diagnostic and clinical approaches at the onset of HF may vary based on the HF phenotype, clinical presentation, and gender. In terms of clinical presentation, reduced ejection fraction (EF) is more often associated with the male sex, whereas HFpEF is more prevalent in females and is linked to worse clinical outcomes [22,23]. At the time of diagnosis, women tend to present symptoms of chronic HF, such as exertional dyspnea, jugular vein distention, and peripheral edema, more frequently than men [22–24].

HF is primarily diagnosed clinically, stemming from structural and/or functional cardiac abnormalities. While the diagnosis is mainly clinical, confirmation and phenotype classification require an echocardiographic study; alternative diagnostic tools may be advantageous in specific scenarios [25]. Diagnostic tools that expose patients to radiation, such as computed tomography and nuclear imaging, are less frequently requested in females [25].

Biomarker plasma concentrations play a pivotal role in HF diagnosis, and the difference between men and women can only be partially explained by hormone status. Given the higher prevalence of HFpEF in women, natriuretic peptides are lower compared to men, as men are more affected by HFrEF, which typically carries higher natriuretic peptide levels. There is substantial evidence that most biomarkers, regardless of gender, exhibit similar diagnostic and prognostic effectiveness [26].

When an ischemic etiology is suspected, patients undergo coronary angiography without gender differences, but women are less likely to undergo percutaneous coronary intervention (PCI) in one-vessel disease. They are more likely to undergo PCI in multi-vessel disease and less likely to undergo coronary artery bypass graft (CABG) [27]. Diagnostic imaging is crucial in detecting ischemic etiology, particularly in women who frequently present ischemia and vascular dysfunction without obstructive coronary artery disease or due to spontaneous coronary artery dissection [28]. Despite the proven efficacy of pharmacological therapy, intracoronary imaging, and revascularization, women undergo invasive and non-invasive interventional strategies less frequently than men [29].

Regarding dilated cardiomyopathy, no significant gender differences exist in diagnosis, and the relationship between gender and the expression of pathogenic gene mutations remains unclear. Therefore, the role of genetic testing is similar between genders. However, a gender difference is noted in alcoholic cardiomyopathy, more common in men due to higher alcohol consumption [30]. Among secondary dilated cardiomyopathies, peripartum cardiomyopathy affects females and should be considered in the differential diagnosis for female patients presenting with dyspnea during pregnancy or postpartum [31].

Stress cardiomyopathy is more frequent in the female sex, with men commonly presenting with a physical trigger and being more prone to developing cardiogenic shock with worse clinical outcomes [32]. Myocarditis incidence is not significantly dissimilar between genders, but some registries indicate that men are hospitalized more frequently than women, despite there being higher mortality rates in women [33].

5. Gender Differences in Medical Treatment and Relationship with Invasive Cardiological Care or General Medicine Care

5.1. Medical Treatment

Current guidelines do not differentiate HF therapies between women and men, despite evidence pointing to gender differences. Primarily, variations in pharmacokinetics and pharmacodynamics contribute to differences in drug absorption, distribution, metabolism, excretion, and, consequently, drug effects [34,35].

Moreover, adverse drug effects vary between genders, with women experiencing 1.5 times higher rates than men. For instance, women with HF receiving diuretic therapy are more prone to ion imbalance and subsequent severe arrhythmias or ACE inhibitor cough [36].

The benefits of beta-blocker treatment in the context of HF with reduced ejection fraction are well-established for both males and females, as demonstrated by the "COPERNICUS" and "CIBIS II" trials [37,38]. Although the "MERIT-HF" trial did not find a beneficial effect on mortality in small subgroups of women [39,40], a post hoc analysis revealed a reduction in all-cause death or hospitalization in both women and men, with a more marked difference in the reduction in the risk of HF hospitalization in women [41].

In all the mentioned trials, females have been notably underrepresented, including in the evaluation of the efficacy of ACE inhibitors and angiotensin receptor blockers (ARBs) in HF patients. A post hoc analysis of the "CONSENSUS" study did not show a significant reduction in the primary endpoint of death with the use of Enalapril in women, as observed in men [37,42,43]. Meanwhile, the ATLAS and HEAAL trials suggested that lower doses of Lisinopril and Losartan may be effective in women, while men may require higher doses [44,45].

ARBs may have a more significant treatment effect in females than males in HFpEF. In the I-PRESERVE trial, Irbesartan showed a lower rate of all-cause mortality or first cardiovascular hospitalization in women compared to the male subgroup [46].

One of the new milestones in HFrEF treatment is the angiotensin receptor neprilysin inhibitors (ARNi). The PARADIGM-HF trial significantly favored sacubitril/valsartan over Enalapril in both males and females for the composite endpoint of cardiovascular mortality and HF hospitalization, with no significant sex differences [47].

In HFpEF patients, ARNi showed a significant effect on the composite endpoint only in the female subgroup (RR 0.73 vs. 1.03 in males), with females appearing more responsive to treatment at higher LVEF ranges than men [48,49]. In a subgroup analysis of the PROVE-HF trial, the initiation of sacubitril/valsartan in women demonstrated more rapid reductions in NT-proBNP and earlier reverse left ventricular remodeling [50].

As the RALES and EMPHASIS-HF trials reveal, using mineralocorticoid receptor antagonists is associated with reducing all-cause death in both males and females in the NYHA III-IV class, with no sex differences [51,52]. However, there is a sex disparity among HFpEF patients, as the TOPCAT trial demonstrates that spironolactone reduces the risk of all-cause death in females but not in males (HR 0.66 vs. 1.06) [53].

The last pillar in the treatment of HFrEF is represented by sodium–glucose cotransporter-2 inhibitors such as Dapagliflozin and Empagliflozin. Both drugs appear to provide benefits, such as a reduction in cardiovascular death and HF hospitalization, in both genders without significant gender disparity, as revealed in the DAPA-HF and EMPEROR-Reduced trials [54,55]. The newest EMPEROR-Preserved trial describes similar effects of Empagliflozin treatment in patients with HFpEF [56]. At the same time, a systematic review and meta-analysis of the five most essential trials about SGLT-2i, including DELIVER and SOLOIST, define that the reduction in worsening HF and death from cardiovascular causes was less pronounced in women [57].

In HFrEF patients, the use of digoxin determines the reduction in HF-related hospitalizations, as shown by the DIG trial, but a post hoc analysis defined a higher risk of all-cause mortality in women compared to men [58].

5.2. Invasive Cardiological Care

In the context of ischemic cardiomyopathy, there is a sex-specific disparity in access to coronary artery bypass grafting (CABG) [59]. However, over ten years, women exhibited lower all-cause mortality and cardiovascular mortality than men, emphasizing the critical importance of avoiding any delays in surgery based on gender [60].

Furthermore, gender differences come into play in the management of secondary mitral regurgitation (SMR) resulting from left ventricular remodeling in HFrEF patients. Women experience delayed referral for surgical intervention, leading to a less favorable scenario at presentation, fewer opportunities for valve repair, and a worse postoperative prognosis [61,62]. The quantitative cutoff values for effective regurgitant orifice area (EROA) and regurgitant volume are not adjusted for gender, potentially contributing to an overestimation of SMR severity in women [63,64].

A sub-analysis of the COAPT trial revealed that women undergoing transcatheter mitral valve repair with the MitraClip had a worse quality of life and functional capacity compared to men. Although transcatheter edge-to-edge repair (TEER) resulted in improved outcomes for both genders, the benefits were less pronounced in females (HR 0.78 vs. 0.43 in men) [65].

6. Gender Differences in Non-Medical Treatment: Devices and Surgery

6.1. Cardiac Resynchronization Therapy

Cardiac resynchronization therapy (CRT-P and -D) is now well established as a therapeutic option for selected patients with HFrEF and a prolonged QRS interval or when a high threshold of right ventricle pacing is expected [66]. CRT significantly improves HF symptoms, reduces hospitalizations, and lowers mortality [67–71].

It is essential to note that women are underrepresented in CRT trials, comprising only about 20% of enrollees, which complicates the assessment of sex differences. However, females tend to derive more significant benefits from CRT, particularly in terms of reductions in mortality, compared to males. Despite this, women undergo device implantation less frequently [72]. Furthermore, females exhibit a high response rate irrespective of QRS duration, experiencing a decrease in mortality and HF hospitalization for QRS durations between 130 and 149 ms in CRT-D recipients. This highlights that a 150 ms duration threshold for CRT implantation might be a limiting factor in accessing therapy [12].

Fewer women than men undergo CRT implantation [68,69], and a relatively higher percentage of these patients receive CRT-P instead of CRT-D in Europe [73], with reasons for this choice remaining unclear. The net clinical benefit from CRT seems similar between genders, although some evidence suggests that response rates in women may be superior to those in men [68,69,74,75]. This is possibly linked to a lower rate of ischemic etiology and fewer scarred segments at baseline compared to men [76]. In a meta-analysis by Zusterzeel et al. [77], it was found that women exhibit up to a 76% risk reduction compared to men, suggesting the need for a sex-specific definition of left bundle branch block for patient selection in CRT, with a potentially lower QRS duration cut-off value for women and men [1]. Conversely, a recent study revealed that this sex difference may not be a sex-specific result but may rather be because the smaller height and heart size of women are the actual predictors of being a responder to CRT [78].

6.2. Implantable Cardioverter Defibrillator

The implantable cardioverter defibrillator has demonstrated efficacy in reducing sudden cardiac death in both primary and secondary prevention. However, a notable challenge is the underrepresentation of women in randomized control trials evaluating ICD therapy, constituting only 10–32% of enrolled patients [79]. This insufficient representation hampers the ability of trials to adequately assess sex-specific outcomes. Despite this, findings from CRT trials indicate that there is not a significant interaction by sex regarding the benefits of ICD therapy, irrespective of whether the cardiomyopathy is ischemic or non-ischemic [74,80–82].

Aggregate registry data reveal that woman receiving an ICD experience lower mortality and a reduced incidence of proper therapies for life-threatening arrhythmias. However, it is important to note that they also face higher rates of complications, including infection and pneumothorax [83]. Additionally, women inherently exhibit a lower lifetime risk of ventricular arrhythmias and sudden cardiac death compared to men.

While various devices such as Cardiac Contractility Modulation and Cardio-MEM are now available, there is currently no robust evidence indicating significant gender differences in their effectiveness. Further research is needed to elucidate the potential nuances in outcomes across genders associated with these emerging technologies.

6.3. Heart Transplantation

Heart transplantation (HT) remains the gold standard for treating advanced HF, yet a significant gender disparity exists, with women constituting only approximately 25% of heart transplant recipients annually. This is in contrast to real-world population studies, which suggest that women make up to 45% of individuals with advanced HF [84]. Research by DeFilippis et al. highlights that women are less likely to be referred for HT and left ventricular assist devices (LVADs), despite their higher incidence of HF [85]. Moreover, women face higher waitlist mortality during the HT evaluation process and encounter more allo-sensitization disadvantages compared to men. It is noteworthy that women listed for HT are generally younger than their male counterparts and exhibit a distinct distribution of HF etiology [86].

Despite these disparities, early and late mortality outcomes after HT do not show significant differences between genders [87] (Table 1). However, during the follow-up period, women experience higher rates and a greater severity of rejection but demonstrate a lower prevalence of cardiac allograft vasculopathy and lower rates of malignancies compared to men [85]. These nuances highlight the need for a more comprehensive understanding of gender-specific factors influencing the entire heart transplantation process, from referral to post-transplant outcomes.

Table 1. Gender differences in CABG, MitraClip, heart transplant, and LVAD according to reported outcomes. CABG: coronary-artery bypass grafting. CAV: cardiac allograft vasculopathy. LVAD: left ventricular assist device.

Therapy	Endpoint	Male	Female
CABG	Mortality	↑	↓
MitraClip	Survival	↑	↓
	Quality of life	↑	↓
Heart Transplant	% of patients	≈75%	≈25%
	Possibility of referral	↑	↓
	Waiting list mortality	↓	↑
	Early and late mortality	=	=
	Rejection	↓	↑
	CAV	↑	↓
	Malignancies	↓	↓↑=
LVAD	% of patients	≈78%	≈22%
	Mortality	↓	↑
	Bridge to transplant	↑	↓
	Adverse events	↓	↑

6.4. Left Ventricular Assist Devices and Surgery

Recent data derived from INTERMACS reveal that females constitute approximately 21.4–22.7% of total LVAD implantations [88]. The Momentum-3 trial, however, did not observe a significant interaction between gender groups in their prespecified subgroup analysis [89]. Conversely, an observational study focusing on LVAD recipients suggests that women face a higher risk of mortality, reduced likelihood of heart transplantation, and an increased rate of adverse events [90]. These disparities in clinical outcomes persist even when stratified by race, device strategy, or implantation center (Table 1).

In the realm of surgical interventions for patients with HFrEF, CABG is a common procedure. This may be performed alone or combined with surgical ventricular reconstruction and mitral valve surgery for regurgitation. Limited data from randomized trials indicate that sex is not a significant factor associated with the effects of CABG plus medical therapy compared to medical therapy alone, specifically concerning all-cause mortality and cardiovascular mortality. Consequently, treatment decisions about CABG in these patients should not be influenced by gender considerations [91].

7. Overall Prognosis and Therapy Limitations in Both Genders

The prognostic stratification of HF poses a clinical challenge, particularly in women. HF in women exhibits specific characteristics in clinical presentation, response to therapy, and adherence to guidelines, leading to disparities between men and women [92–94] (Figure 1). Moreover, the underrepresentation of women in randomized clinical trials contributes to a lack of sex-oriented assessment in current prognostic scores [92].

Numerous studies indicate that women with HF generally experience better survival rates and lower hospitalization rates than their male counterparts. In the Olmsted County study, age-adjusted all-cause mortality rates were comparable between genders, while cardiovascular death rates were higher in men, and hospitalization rates were lower in women [95,96]. This pattern could be attributed to a lower prevalence of ischemic myocardial disease and a later onset of symptoms in older women [46,92]. Notably, the most common phenotype of HF in women is non-ischemic HFpEF [1]. In the acute HF setting, the ARIC study reported similar 28-day and 1-year case fatality rates between men and women (10% and 30%, respectively) [97].

Furthermore, the impact of chronic HF on quality of life appears to be more pronounced in women than in men [98]. Women affected by HF report more significant physical limitations and higher rates of anxiety and depression than their male counterparts, potentially influencing the effectiveness of therapy [24,99]. Additionally, as women are more frequently affected by HFpEF and often present with comorbidities such as chronic kidney disease, their ability to receive a complete prescription of optimal medical therapy may be limited, impacting prognosis [100].

8. Future Perspectives

Heart failure represents one of the most critical challenges for cardiology. While the development of highly effective diagnostic and therapeutic strategies has improved the survival and quality of life of patients with cardiovascular pathologies, it has concurrently expanded the population affected by heart failure.

In this context, there is a pressing need for an increased focus on gender-specific characteristics in pathophysiology, pharmacokinetics, and pharmacodynamics. The ongoing efforts of researchers in the realm of personalized medicine must systematically incorporate gender as a pivotal factor amidst biological, environmental, behavioral, and psychological considerations.

Moreover, given the current scarcity of robust gender-oriented data in the scientific literature, substantial attention should be directed toward the design of basic research and randomized clinical trials. These endeavors aim to elucidate gender-related distinctions in both disease manifestation and therapeutic responses, contributing to a more comprehensive understanding of heart failure and paving the way for tailored and effective interventions.

9. Conclusions

In this review, we have highlighted notable gender differences in the context of HF, emphasizing that men are more susceptible to HFrEF, while women are predisposed to HFpEF due to distinct comorbidities. We have delved into the variations in risk factors, pathophysiology, and clinical presentation, noting that women with HF generally exhibit better survival rates. However, the impact of the disease on their quality of life can be more substantial.

A significant concern that persists is the underrepresentation of women in clinical trials related to HF. This disparity raises questions about the applicability of research findings to women, highlighting the need for a more inclusive approach in clinical studies. Additionally, there is an urgent requirement for healthcare professionals to integrate sex-specific considerations into the diagnosis, treatment, and hospital care of individuals with HF, ensuring that both men and women receive optimal and tailored interventions. This ongoing issue underscores the importance of addressing gender disparities to enhance overall management and outcomes in HF.

Funding: This research received no external funding.

Conflicts of Interest: The authors declare no conflicts of interest.

References

1. Lam, C.S.P.; Arnott, C.; Beale, A.L.; Chandramouli, C.; Hilfiker-Kleiner, D.; Kaye, D.M.; Ky, B.; Santema, B.T.; Sliwa, K.; Voors, A.A. Sex differences in heart failure. *Eur. Heart J.* **2019**, *40*, 3859–3868c. [CrossRef]
2. Kaur, G.; Lau, E. Sex differences in heart failure with preserved ejection fraction: From traditional risk factors to sex-specific risk factors. *Women's Health* **2022**, *18*, 17455057221140209. [CrossRef] [PubMed]
3. Tibrewala, A.; Yancy, C.W. Heart Failure with Preserved Ejection Fraction in Women. *Heart Fail. Clin.* **2019**, *15*, 9–18. [CrossRef] [PubMed]
4. Maffei, S.; Guiducci, L.; Cugusi, L.; Cadeddu, C.; Deidda, M.; Gallina, S.; Sciomer, S.; Gastaldelli, A.; Kaski, J.C. Women-specific predictors of cardiovascular disease risk—New paradigms. *Int. J. Cardiol.* **2019**, *286*, 190–197. [CrossRef] [PubMed]
5. Salerni, S.; Di Francescomarino, S.; Cadeddu, C.; Acquistapace, F.; Maffei, S.; Gallina, S. The different role of sex hormones on female cardiovascular physiology and function: Not only oestrogens. *Eur. J. Clin. Investig.* **2015**, *45*, 634–645. [CrossRef]
6. Marx, N.; Federici, M.; Schütt, K.; Müller-Wieland, D.; Ajjan, R.A.; Antunes, M.J.; Christodorescu, R.M.; Crawford, C.; Di Angelantonio, E.; Eliasson, B.; et al. 2023 ESC Guidelines for the management of cardiovascular disease in patients with diabetes: Developed by the task force on the management of cardiovascular disease in patients with diabetes of the European Society of Cardiology (ESC). *Eur. Heart J.* **2023**, *44*, 4043–4140. [CrossRef] [PubMed]
7. Kautzky-Willer, A.; Harreiter, J.; Pacini, G. Sex and Gender Differences in Risk, Pathophysiology and Complications of Type 2 Diabetes Mellitus. *Endocr. Rev.* **2016**, *37*, 278–316. [CrossRef] [PubMed]
8. Wilson, P.W.; D'Agostino, R.B.; Sullivan, L.; Parise, H.; Kannel, W.B. Overweight and obesity as determinants of cardiovascular risk: The Framingham experience. *Arch. Intern. Med.* **2002**, *162*, 1867–1872. [CrossRef] [PubMed]
9. Yusuf, S.; Hawken, S.; Ôunpuu, S.; Dans, T.; Avezum, A.; Lanas, F.; McQueen, M.; Budaj, A.; Pais, P.; Varigos, J.; et al. Effect of potentially modifiable risk factors associated with myocardial infarction in 52 countries (the INTERHEART study): Case-control study. *Lancet* **2004**, *364*, 937–952. [CrossRef]
10. Cadeddu, C.; Franconi, F.; Cassisa, L.; Campesi, I.; Pepe, A.; Cugusi, L.; Maffei, S.; Gallina, S.; Sciomer, S.; Mercuro, G.; et al. Arterial hypertension in the female world: Pathophysiology and therapy. *J. Cardiovasc. Med.* **2016**, *17*, 229–236. [CrossRef]
11. Ventura-Clapier, R.; Piquereau, J.; Garnier, A.; Mericskay, M.; Lemaire, C.; Crozatier, B. Gender issues in cardiovascular diseases. Focus on energy metabolism. *Biochim. Biophys. Acta Mol. Basis Dis.* **2020**, *1866*, 165722. [CrossRef]
12. Connelly, P.J.; Azizi, Z.; Alipour, P.; Delles, C.; Pilote, L.; Raparelli, V. The Importance of Gender to Understand Sex Differences in Cardiovascular Disease. *Can. J. Cardiol.* **2021**, *37*, 699–710. [CrossRef]
13. Meloni, A.; Cadeddu, C.; Cugusi, L.; Donataccio, M.P.; Deidda, M.; Sciomer, S.; Gallina, S.; Vassalle, C.; Moscucci, F.; Mercuro, G.; et al. Gender Differences and Cardiometabolic Risk: The Importance of the Risk Factors. *Int. J. Mol. Sci.* **2023**, *24*, 1588. [CrossRef]
14. Huxley, R.R.; Woodward, M. Cigarette smoking as a risk factor for coronary heart disease in women compared with men: A systematic review and meta-analysis of prospective cohort studies. *Lancet* **2011**, *378*, 1297–1305. [CrossRef]
15. Kaplan, A.; Abidi, E.; Diab, R.; Ghali, R.; Al-Awassi, H.; Booz, G.W.; Zouein, F.A. Sex differences in cardiac remodeling post myocardial infarction with acute cigarette smoking. *Biol. Sex Differ.* **2022**, *13*, 36. [CrossRef]
16. Ballard-Hernandez, J.; Itchhaporia, D. Heart Failure in Women Due to Hypertensive Heart Disease. *Heart Fail. Clin.* **2019**, *15*, 497–507. [CrossRef] [PubMed]
17. Pelliccia, F.; Kaski, J.C.; Crea, F.; Camici, P.G. Pathophysiology of Takotsubo Syndrome. *Circulation* **2019**, *135*, 2426–2441. [CrossRef] [PubMed]

18. Cadeddu Dessalvi, C.; Pepe, A.; Penna, C.; Gimelli, A.; Madonna, R.; Mele, D.; Monte, I.; Novo, G.; Nugara, C.; Zito, C.; et al. Sex differences in anthracycline-induced cardiotoxicity: The benefits of estrogens. *Heart Fail. Rev.* **2019**, *24*, 915–925. [CrossRef] [PubMed]
19. Fazzini, L.; Caggiari, L.; Deidda, M.; Onnis, C.; Saba, L.; Mercuro, G.; Cadeddu Dessalvi, C. Metabolomic Profiles on Antiblastic Cardiotoxicity: New Perspectives for Early Diagnosis and Cardioprotection. *J. Clin. Med.* **2022**, *11*, 6745. [CrossRef] [PubMed]
20. Saiki, H.; Petersen, I.A.; Scott, C.G.; Bailey, K.R.; Dunlay, S.M.; Finley, R.R.; Ruddy, K.J.; Yan, E.; Redfield, M.M. Risk of Heart Failure with Preserved Ejection Fraction in Older Women after Contemporary Radiotherapy for Breast Cancer. *Circulation* **2017**, *135*, 1388–1396. [CrossRef] [PubMed]
21. Darby, S.C.; Ewertz, M.; McGale, P.; Bennet, A.M.; Blom-Goldman, U.; Brønnum, D.; Correa, C.; Cutter, D.; Gagliardi, G.; Gigante, B.; et al. Risk of ischemic heart disease in women after radiotherapy for breast cancer. *N. Engl. J. Med.* **2013**, *368*, 987–998. [CrossRef] [PubMed]
22. Sotomi, Y.; Hikoso, S.; Nakatani, D.; Mizuno, H.; Okada, K.; Dohi, T.; Kitamura, T.; Sunaga, A.; Kida, H.; Oeun, B.; et al. PURSUIT-HFpEF Investigators. Sex Differences in Heart Failure with Preserved Ejection Fraction. *J. Am. Heart Assoc.* **2021**, *10*, e018574. [CrossRef]
23. Stolfo, D.; Uijl, A.; Vedin, O.; Strömberg, A.; Faxén, U.L.; Rosano, G.M.C.; Sinagra, G.; Dahlström, U.; Savarese, G. Sex-Based Differences in Heart Failure Across the Ejection Fraction Spectrum. *J. Am. Coll. Cardiol. Heart Fail.* **2019**, *7*, 505–515. [CrossRef] [PubMed]
24. Dewan, P.; Rørth, R.; Raparelli, V.; Campbell, R.T.; Shen, L.; Jhund, P.S.; Petrie, M.C.; Anand, I.S.; Carson, P.E.; Desai, A.S.; et al. Sex-related differences in heart failure with preserved ejection fraction. *Circ. Heart Fail.* **2019**, *12*, e006539. [CrossRef] [PubMed]
25. Kozor, R.; Abiodun, A.; Kott, K.; Manisty, C. Non-invasive Imaging in Women with Heart Failure—Diagnosis and Insights Into Disease Mechanisms. *Curr. Heart Fail. Rep.* **2022**, *19*, 114–125. [CrossRef] [PubMed]
26. Lala, A.; Tayal, U.; Hamo, C.E.; Youmans, Q.; Al-Khatib, S.M.; Bozkurt, B.; Davis, M.B.; Januzzi, J.; Mentz, R.; Sauer, A.; et al. Sex Differences in Heart Failure. *J. Card. Fail.* **2022**, *28*, 477–498. [CrossRef]
27. Gudnadottir, G.S.; Andersen, K.; Thrainsdottir, I.S.; James, S.K.; Lagerqvist, B.; Gudnason, T. Gender differences in coronary angiography, subsequent interventions, and outcomes among patients with acute coronary syndromes. *Am. Heart J.* **2017**, *191*, 65–74. [CrossRef]
28. Hayes, S.N.; Tweet, M.S.; Adlam, D.; Kim, E.S.H.; Gulati, R.; Price, J.E.; Rose, C.H. Spontaneous Coronary Artery Dissection: JACC State-of-the-Art Review. *J. Am. Coll. Cardiol.* **2020**, *76*, 961–984. [CrossRef]
29. Arata, A.; Ricci, F.; Khanji, M.Y.; Mantini, C.; Angeli, F.; Aquilani, R.; Di Baldassarre, A.; Renda, G.; Mattioli, A.V.; Nodari, S.; et al. Sex Differences in Heart Failure: What Do We Know? *J. Cardiovasc. Dev. Dis.* **2023**, *10*, 277. [CrossRef]
30. Piano, M. Effects of Alcohol on the Cardiovascular System in Women. *ARCR* **2020**, *40*, 12. [CrossRef]
31. De Filippis, E.M.; Haythe, J.H.; Walsh, M.N.; Kittleson, M.M. Intersection of Heart Failure and Pregnancy: Beyond Peripartum Cardiomyopathy. *Circ. Heart Fail.* **2021**, *14*, e008223. [CrossRef]
32. Arcari, L.; Núñez Gil, I.J.; Stiermaier, T.; El-Battrawy, I.; Guerra, F.; Novo, G.; Musumeci, B.; Cacciotti, L.; Mariano, E.; Caldarola, P.; et al. Gender Differences in Takotsubo Syndrome. *J. Am. Coll. Cardiol.* **2022**, *79*, 2085–2093. [CrossRef]
33. Shah, Z.; Mohammed, M.; Vuddanda, V.; Ansari, M.W.; Masoomi, R.; Gupta, K. National Trends, Gender, Management, and Outcomes of Patients Hospitalized for Myocarditis. *Am. J. Cardiol.* **2019**, *124*, 131–136. [CrossRef]
34. Jochmann, N.; Stangl, K.; Garbe, E.; Baumann, G.; Stangl, V. Female-specific aspects in the pharmacotherapy of chronic cardiovascular diseases. *Eur. Heart J.* **2005**, *26*, 1585–1595. [CrossRef]
35. Soldin, O.P.; Mattison, D.R. Sex differences in pharmacokinetics and pharmacodynamics. *Clin. Pharmacokinet.* **2009**, *48*, 143–157. [CrossRef]
36. Rosano, G.M.; Lewis, B.; Agewall, S.; Wassmann, S.; Vitale, C.; Schmidt, H.; Drexel, H.; Patak, A.; Torp-Pedersen, C.; Kjeldsen, K.P.; et al. Gender differences in the effect of cardiovascular drugs: A position document of the Working Group on Pharmacology and Drug Therapy of the ESC. *Eur. Heart J.* **2015**, *36*, 2677–2680. [CrossRef]
37. Shekelle, P.G.; Rich, M.W.; Morton, S.C.; Atkinson, C.S.; Tu, W.; Maglione, M.; Rhodes, M.; Barrett, M.; Fonarow, G.C.; Greenberg, B.; et al. Efficacy of angiotensin converting enzyme inhibitors and beta-blockers in the management of left ventricular systolic dysfunction according to race, gender, and diabetic status. *J. Am. Coll. Cardiol.* **2003**, *41*, 1529–1538. [CrossRef] [PubMed]
38. Simon, T.; Mary-Krause, M.; Funck-Brentano, C.; Jaillon, P. Sex differences in the prognosis of congestive heart failure: Results from the Cardiac Insufficiency Bisoprolol Study (CIBIS II). *Circulation* **2001**, *103*, 375–380. [CrossRef] [PubMed]
39. MERIT-HF Study Group. Effect of metoprolol CR/XL in chronic heart failure: Metoprolol CR/XL randomised intervention trial in congestive heart failure (MERIT-HF). *Lancet* **1999**, *353*, 2001–2007. [CrossRef]
40. Packer, M.; Bristow, M.R.; Cohn, J.N.; Colucci, W.S.; Fowler, M.B.; Gilbert, E.M.; Shusterman, N.H.; U.S. Carvedilol Heart Failure Study Group. The effect of carvedilol on morbidity and mortality in patients with chronic heart failure. *N. Engl. J. Med.* **1996**, *334*, 1349–1355. [CrossRef] [PubMed]
41. Ghali, J.K.; Piña, I.L.; Gottlieb, S.S.; Deedwania, P.C.; Wikstrand, J.C.; MERIT-HF Study Group. Metoprolol CR/XL in female patients with heart failure: Analysis of the experience in Metoprolol Extended-Release Randomized Intervention Trial in Heart Failure (MERIT-HF). *Circulation* **2002**, *105*, 1585–1591. [CrossRef]

42. Kostis, J.B.; Shelton, B.; Gosselin, G.; Goulet, C.; Hood, W.B., Jr.; Kohn, R.M.; Kubo, S.H.; Schron, E.; Weiss, M.B.; Willis, P.W., 3rd; et al. Adverse effects of enalapril in the Studies of Left Ventricular Dysfunction (SOLVD). *Am. Heart J.* **1996**, *131*, 350–355. [CrossRef]
43. CONSENSUS Trial Study Group. Effects of enalapril on mortality in severe congestive heart failure. Results of the Cooperative North Scandinavian Enalapril Survival Study (CONSENSUS). *N. Engl. J. Med.* **1987**, *316*, 1429–1435. [CrossRef] [PubMed]
44. Packer, M.; Poole-Wilson, P.A.; Armstrong, P.W.; Cleland, J.G.; Horowitz, J.D.; Massie, B.M.; Rydén, L.; Thygesen, K.; Uretsky, B.F.; ATLAS Study Group. Comparative effects of low and high doses of the angiotensin-converting enzyme inhibitor, lisinopril, on morbidity and mortality in chronic heart failure. *Circulation* **1999**, *100*, 2312–2318. [CrossRef] [PubMed]
45. Konstam, M.A.; Neaton, J.D.; Dickstein, K.; Drexler, H.; Komajda, M.; Martinez, F.A.; Riegger, G.A.; Malbecq, W.; Smith, R.D.; Guptha, S.; et al. Effects of high-dose versus low-dose losartan on clinical outcomes in patients with heart failure (HEAAL study): A randomised, double-blind trial. *Lancet* **2009**, *374*, 1840–1848. [CrossRef] [PubMed]
46. Lam, C.S.; Carson, P.E.; Anand, I.S.; Rector, T.S.; Kuskowski, M.; Komajda, M.; McKelvie, R.S.; McMurray, J.J.; Zile, M.R.; Massie, B.M.; et al. Sex differences in clinical characteristics and outcomes in elderly patients with heart failure and preserved ejection fraction: The Irbesartan in Heart Failure with Preserved Ejection Fraction (I-PRESERVE) trial. *Circ. Heart Fail.* **2012**, *5*, 571–578. [CrossRef] [PubMed]
47. McMurray, J.J.; Packer, M.; Desai, A.S.; Gong, J.; Lefkowitz, M.P.; Rizkala, A.R.; Rouleau, J.L.; Shi, V.C.; Solomon, S.D.; Swedberg, K.; et al. Angiotensin-neprilysin inhibition versus enalapril in heart failure. *N. Engl. J. Med.* **2014**, *371*, 993–1004. [CrossRef] [PubMed]
48. Solomon, S.D.; Rizkala, A.R.; Gong, J.; Wang, W.; Anand, I.S.; Ge, J.; Lam, C.S.P.; Maggioni, A.P.; Martinez, F.; Packer, M.; et al. Angiotensin Receptor Neprilysin Inhibition in Heart Failure with Preserved Ejection Fraction: Rationale and Design of the PARAGON-HF Trial. *JACC Heart Fail.* **2017**, *5*, 471–482. [CrossRef] [PubMed]
49. Solomon, S.D.; Vaduganathan, M.; LClaggett, B.; Packer, M.; Zile, M.; Swedberg, K.; Rouleau, J.; APfeffer, M.; Desai, A.; Lund, L.H.; et al. Sacubitril/Valsartan Across the Spectrum of Ejection Fraction in Heart Failure. *Circulation* **2020**, *141*, 352–361. [CrossRef] [PubMed]
50. Ibrahim, N.E.; Piña, I.L.; Camacho, A.; Bapat, D.; Felker, G.M.; Maisel, A.S.; Butler, J.; Prescott, M.F.; Abbas, C.A.; Solomon, S.D.; et al. Sex-based differences in biomarkers, health status, and reverse cardiac remodelling in patients with heart failure with reduced ejection fraction treated with sacubitril/valsartan. *Eur. J. Heart Fail.* **2020**, *22*, 2018–2025. [CrossRef]
51. Zannad, F.; McMurray, J.J.; Krum, H.; van Veldhuisen, D.J.; Swedberg, K.; Shi, H.; Vincent, J.; Pocock, S.J.; Pitt, B.; EMPHASIS-HF Study Group. Eplerenone in patients with systolic heart failure and mild symptoms. *N. Engl. J. Med.* **2011**, *364*, 11–21. [CrossRef]
52. Pitt, B.; Pfeffer, M.A.; Assmann, S.F.; Boineau, R.; Anand, I.S.; Claggett, B.; Clausell, N.; Desai, A.S.; Diaz, R.; Fleg, J.L.; et al. Spironolactone for heart failure with preserved ejection fraction. *N. Engl. J. Med.* **2014**, *370*, 1383–1392. [CrossRef]
53. Merrill, M.; Sweitzer, N.; Lindenfeld, J.; Kao, D.P. Sex differences in outcomes and response to spironolactone in HFpEF: A secondary analysis of TOPCAT. *JACC Heart Fail.* **2019**, *7*, 228–238. [CrossRef]
54. McMurray, J.J.V.; Solomon, S.D.; Inzucchi, S.E.; Køber, L.; Kosiborod, M.N.; Martinez, F.A.; Ponikowski, P.; Sabatine, M.S.; Anand, I.S.; Bělohlávek, J.; et al. Dapagliflozin in patients with heart failure and reduced ejection fraction. *N. Engl. J. Med.* **2019**, *381*, 1995–2008. [CrossRef] [PubMed]
55. Packer, M.; Anker, S.D.; Butler, J.; Filippatos, G.; Pocock, S.J.; Carson, P.; Januzzi, J.; Verma, S.; Tsutsui, H.; Brueckmann, M.; et al. Cardiovascular and renal outcomes with empagliflozin in heart failure. *N. Engl. J. Med.* **2020**, *383*, 1413–1424. [CrossRef] [PubMed]
56. Anker, S.D.; Butler, J.; Filippatos, G.; Ferreira, J.P.; Bocchi, E.; Böhm, M.; Brunner-La Rocca, H.P.; Choi, D.J.; Chopra, V.; Chuquiure-Valenzuela, E.; et al. Empagliflozin in heart failure with a preserved ejection fraction. *N. Engl. J. Med.* **2021**, *385*, 1451–1461. [CrossRef] [PubMed]
57. Rivera, F.B.; Tang, V.A.S.; De Luna, D.V.; Lerma, E.V.; Vijayaraghavan, K.; Kazory, A.; Shah, N.S.; Volgman, A.S. Sex differences in cardiovascular outcomes of SGLT-2 inhibitors in heart failure randomized controlled trials: A systematic review and meta-analysis. *Am. Heart J. Plus* **2023**, *26*, 100261. [CrossRef] [PubMed]
58. Rathore, S.S.; Wang, Y.; Krumholz, H.M. Sex-based differences in the effect of digoxin for the treatment of heart failure. *N. Engl. J. Med.* **2002**, *347*, 1403–1411. [CrossRef] [PubMed]
59. Sun, L.Y.; Tu, J.V.; Bader Eddeen, A.; Liu, P.P. Prevalence and long-term survival after coronary artery bypass grafting in women and men with heart failure and preserved versus reduced ejection fraction. *J. Am. Heart Assoc.* **2018**, *7*, e008902. [CrossRef] [PubMed]
60. Velazquez, E.J.; Lee, K.L.; Jones, R.H.; Al-Khalidi, H.R.; Hill, J.A.; Panza, J.A.; Michler, R.E.; Bonow, R.O.; Doenst, T.; Petrie, M.C.; et al. STICHES Investigators. Coronary-Artery Bypass Surgery in Patients with Ischemic Cardiomyopathy. *N. Engl. J. Med.* **2016**, *374*, 1511–1520. [CrossRef]
61. Chan, V.; Chen, L.; Messika-Zeitoun, D.; Elmistekawy, E.; Ruel, M.; Mesana, T. Is late left ventricle remodeling after repair of degenerative mitral regurgitation worse in women? *Ann. Thorac. Surg.* **2019**, *108*, 1189–1193. [CrossRef] [PubMed]
62. Vassileva, C.M.; Stelle, L.M.; Markwell, S.; Boley, T.; Hazelrigg, S. Sex differences in procedure selection and outcomes of patients undergoing mitral valve surgery. *Heart Surg. Forum* **2011**, *14*, E276–E282. [CrossRef] [PubMed]

63. Nishimura, R.A.; Otto, C.M.; Bonow, R.O.; Carabello, B.A.; Erwin, J.P., 3rd; Fleisher, L.A.; Jneid, H.; Mack, M.J.; McLeod, C.J.; O'Gara, P.T.; et al. 2017 AHA/ACC Focused Update of the 2014 AHA/ACC Guideline for the Management of Patients with Valvular Heart Disease: A Report of the American College of Cardiology/American Heart Association Task Force on Clinical Practice Guidelines. *Circulation* **2017**, *135*, e1159–e1195. [CrossRef] [PubMed]
64. Lindenfeld, J.; Abraham, W.T.; Grayburn, P.A.; Kar, S.; Asch, F.M.; Lim, D.S.; Nie, H.; Singhal, P.; Sundareswaran, K.S.; Weissman, N.J.; et al. Association of Effective Regurgitation Orifice Area to Left Ventricular End-Diastolic Volume Ratio with Transcatheter Mitral Valve Repair Outcomes: A Secondary Analysis of the COAPT Trial. *JAMA Cardiol.* **2021**, *6*, 427–436. [CrossRef] [PubMed]
65. Kosmidou, I.; Lindenfeld, J.; Abraham, W.T.; Rinaldi, M.J.; Kapadia, S.R.; Rajagopal, V.; Sarembock, I.J.; Brieke, A.; Gaba, P.; Rogers, J.H.; et al. Sex specific outcomes of transcatheter mitral-valve repair and medical therapy for mitral regurgitation in heart failure. *JACC Heart Fail.* **2021**, *9*, 674–683. [CrossRef] [PubMed]
66. McDonagh, T.A.; Metra, M.; Adamo, M.; Gardner, R.S.; Baumbach, A.; Böhm, M.; Burri, H.; Butler, J.; Čelutkienė, J.; Chioncel, O.; et al. 2021 ESC Guidelines for the diagnosis and treatment of acute and chronic heart failure. *Eur. Heart J.* **2021**, *42*, 3599–3726. [CrossRef] [PubMed]
67. Abraham, W.T.; Fisher, W.G.; Smith, A.L.; Delurgio, D.B.; Leon, A.R.; Loh, E.; Kocovic, D.Z.; Packer, M.; Clavell, A.L.; Hayes, D.L.; et al. Cardiac resynchronization in chronic heart failure. *N. Engl. J. Med.* **2002**, *346*, 1845–1853. [CrossRef]
68. Cleland, J.G.; Daubert, J.C.; Erdmann, E.; Freemantle, N.; Gras, D.; Kappenberger, L.; Tavazzi, L.; Cardiac Resynchronization-Heart Failure (CARE-HF) Study Investigators. The effect of cardiac resynchronization on morbidity and mortality in heart failure. *N. Engl. J. Med.* **2005**, *352*, 1539–1549. [CrossRef]
69. Bristow, M.R.; Saxon, L.A.; Boehmer, J.; Krueger, S.; Kass, D.A.; De Marco, T.; Carson, P.; DiCarlo, L.; DeMets, D.; White, B.G.; et al. Cardiac-resynchronization therapy with or without an impantable defibrillator in advanced chronic heart failure. *N. Engl. J. Med.* **2004**, *350*, 2140–2150. [CrossRef]
70. Ruschitzka, F.; Abraham, W.T.; Singh, J.P.; Bax, J.J.; Borer, J.S.; Brugada, J.; Dickstein, K.; Ford, I.; Gorcsan, J., 3rd; Gras, D.; et al. Cardiac-resynchronization therapy in heart failure with a narrow QRS complex. *N. Eng. J. Med.* **2013**, *369*, 1395–1405. [CrossRef]
71. Amuthan, R.; Curtis, A.B. Sex-specific considerations in drug and device therapy of cardiac arrhythmias: JACC Focus Seminar 6/7. *J. Am. Coll. Cardiol.* **2022**, *79*, 1519–1529. [CrossRef]
72. Randolph, T.C.; Hellkamp, A.S.; Zeitler, E.P.; Fonarow, G.C.; Hernandez, A.F.; Thomas, K.L.; Peterson, E.D.; Yancy, C.W.; Al-Khatib, S.M. Utilization of cardiac resynchronization therapy in eligible patients hospitalized for heart failure and its association with patient outcomes. *Am. Heart J.* **2017**, *189*, 48–58. [CrossRef]
73. Alaeddini, J.; Wood, M.A.; Amin, M.S.; Ellenbogen, K.A. Gender disparity in the use of cardiac resynchronization therapy in the United States. *Pacing Clin. Electrophysiol.* **2008**, *31*, 468–472. [CrossRef]
74. Moss, A.J.; Hall, W.J.; Cannom, D.S. Cardiac-resynchronization therapy for the prevention of heart failure events. *N. Engl. J. Med.* **2009**, *361*, 1329–1338. [CrossRef]
75. Arshad, A.; Moss, A.J.; Foster, E.; Padeletti, L.; Barsheshet, A.; Goldenberg, I.; Greenberg, H.; Hall, W.J.; McNitt, S.; Zareba, W.; et al. MADIT-CRT Executive Committee Cardiac resynchronization therapy is more effective in women than in men: The MADIT-CRT (Multicenter Automatic Defibrillator Implantation Trial with Cardiac Resynchronization Therapy) trial. *J. Am. Coll. Cardiol.* **2011**, *57*, 813–820. [CrossRef] [PubMed]
76. Beela, A.S.; Duchenne, J.; Petrescu, A.; Unlu, S.; Penicka, M.; Aakhus, S.; Winter, S.; Aarones, M.; Stefanidis, E.; Fehske, W.; et al. Sex-specific difference in outcome after cardiac resynchronization therapy. *Eur. Heart J. Cardiovasc. Imaging* **2019**, *20*, 504–5119. [CrossRef] [PubMed]
77. Zusterzeel, R.; Curtis, J.P.; Canos, D.A.; Sanders, W.E.; Selzman, K.A.; Pina, I.L.; Spatz, E.S.; Bao, H.; Ponirakis, A.; Varosy, P.D.; et al. Sex-specific mortality risk by QRS morphology and duration in patients receiving CRT: Results from the NCDR. *J. Am. Coll. Cardiol.* **2014**, *64*, 887–894. [CrossRef] [PubMed]
78. Linde, C.; Cleland, J.G.F.; Gold, M.R.; Claude Daubert, J.; Tang, A.S.L.; Young JBSherfesee, L.; Abraham, W.T. The interaction of sex, height, and QRS duration on the effects of cardiac resynchronization therapy on morbidity and mortality: An individual patient data meta-analysis. *Eur. J. Heart Fail.* **2018**, *20*, 780–791. [CrossRef] [PubMed]
79. Linde, C.; Bongiorni, M.G.; Birgersdotter-Green, U.; Curtis, A.B.; Deisenhofer, I.; Furokawa, T.; Gillis, A.M.; Haugaa, K.H.; Lip, G.Y.H.; Van Gelder, I.; et al. Sex differences in cardiac arrhythmia: A consensus document of the European Heart Rhythm Association, endorsed by the Heart Rhythm Society and Asia Pacific Heart Rhythm Society. *EP Eur.* **2018**, *20*, 1565–1565ao. [CrossRef]
80. Tompkins, C.M.; Kutyifa, V.; Arshad, A.; McNitt, S.; Polonsky, B.; Wang, P.J.; Moss, A.J.; Zareba, W. Sex Differences in Device Therapies for Ventricular Arrhythmias or Death in the Multicenter Automatic Defibrillator Implantation Trial with Cardiac Resynchronization Therapy (MADIT-CRT) Trial. *J. Cardiovasc. Electrophysiol.* **2015**, *26*, 862–871. [CrossRef]
81. Bardy, G.H.; Lee, K.L.; Mark, D.B.; Poole, J.E.; Packer, D.L.; Boineau, R.; Domanski, M.; Troutman, C.; Anderson, J.; Johnson, G.; et al. Amiodarone or an implantable cardioverter-defibrillator for congestive heart failure. *N. Engl. J. Med.* **2005**, *352*, 225–237. [CrossRef]
82. Russo, A.M.; Poole, J.E.; Mark, D.B.; Anderson, J.; Hellkamp, A.S.; Lee, K.L.; Johnson, G.W.; Domanski, M.; Bardy, G.H. Primary prevention with defibrillator therapy in women: Results from the Sudden Cardiac Death in Heart Failure Trial. *J. Cardiovasc. Electrophysiol.* **2008**, *19*, 720–724. [CrossRef]

83. Sticherling, C.; Arendacka, B.; Svendsen, J.H.; Wijers, S.; Friede, T.; Stockinger, J.; Dommasch, M.; Merkely, B.; Willems, R.; Lubinski, A.; et al. Sex differences in outcomes of primary prevention implantable cardioverter-defibrillator therapy: Combined registry data from eleven European countries. *EP Eur.* **2018**, *20*, 963–970. [CrossRef]
84. Dunlay, S.M.; Roger, V.L.; Killian, J.M.; Weston, S.A.; Schulte, P.J.; Subramaniam, A.V.; Blecker, S.B.; Redfield, M.M. Advanced Heart Failure Epidemiology and Outcomes: A Population-Based Study. *JACC Heart Fail.* **2021**, *9*, 722–732. [CrossRef]
85. DeFilippis, E.M.; Nikolova, A.; Holzhauser, L.; Khush, K.K. Understanding and Investigating Sex-Based Differences in Heart Transplantation: A Call to Action. *JACC Heart Fail.* **2023**, *11*, 1181–1188. [CrossRef] [PubMed]
86. Moayedi, Y.; Fan, C.P.S.; Cherikh, W.S.; Stehlik, J.; Teuteberg, J.J.; Ross, H.J.; Khush, K.K. Survival Outcomes after Heart Transplantation: Does Recipient Sex Matter? *Circ. Heart Fail.* **2019**, *12*, e006218. [CrossRef] [PubMed]
87. Hsich, E.; Singh, T.P.; Cherikh, W.S.; Harhay, M.O.; Hayes, D., Jr.; Perch, M.; Potena, L.; Sadavarte, A.; Lindblad, K.; Zuckermann, A.; et al. The International thoracic organ transplant registry of the international society for heart and lung transplantation: Thirty-ninth adult heart transplantation report-2022; focus on transplant for restrictive heart disease. *J. Heart Lung Transplant.* **2022**, *41*, 1366–1375. [CrossRef] [PubMed]
88. Yuzefpolskaya, M.; Schroeder, S.E.; Houston, B.A.; Robinson, M.R.; Gosev, I.; Reyentovich, A.; Koehl, D.; Cantor, R.; Jorde, U.P.; Kirklin, J.K.; et al. The Society of Thoracic Surgeons Intermacs 2022 Annual Report: Focus on the 2018 Heart Transplant Allocation System. *Ann. Thorac. Surg.* **2023**, *115*, 311–327. [CrossRef] [PubMed]
89. Mehra, M.R.; Goldstein, D.J.; Cleveland, J.C.; Cowger, J.A.; Hall, S.; Salerno, C.T.; Naka, Y.; Horstmanshof, D.; Chuang, J.; Wang, A.; et al. Five-Year Outcomes in Patients with Fully Magnetically Levitated vs. Axial-Flow Left Ventricular Assist Devices in the MOMENTUM 3 Randomized Trial. *JAMA* **2022**, *328*, 1233–1242. [CrossRef] [PubMed]
90. Shetty, N.S.; Parcha, V.; Abdelmessih, P.; Patel, N.; Hasnie, A.A.; Kalra, R.; Pandey, A.; Breathett, K.; Morris, A.A.; Arora, G.; et al. Sex-Associated Differences in the Clinical Outcomes of Left Ventricular Assist Device Recipients: Insights from Interagency Registry for Mechanically Assisted Circulatory Support. *Circ. Heart Fail.* **2023**, *16*, e010189. [CrossRef] [PubMed]
91. Piña, I.L.; Zheng, Q.; She, L.; Szwed, H.; Lang, I.M.; Farsky, P.S.; Castelvecchio, S.; Biernat, J.; Paraforos, A.; Kosevic, D.; et al. Sex Difference in Patients with Ischemic Heart Failure Undergoing Surgical Revascularization: Results from the STICH Trial (Surgical Treatment for Ischemic Heart Failure). *Circulation* **2018**, *137*, 771–780. [CrossRef]
92. Sciomer, S.; Moscucci, F.; Salvioni, E.; Marchese, G.; Bussotti, M.; Corrà, U.; Piepoli, M.F. Role of gender, age and BMI in prognosis of heart failure. *Eur. J. Prev. Cardiol.* **2020**, *27* (Suppl. 2), 46–51. [CrossRef] [PubMed]
93. Lainščak, M.; Milinković, I.; Polovina, M.; Crespo-Leiro, M.G.; Lund, L.H.; Anker, S.D.; Laroche, C.; Ferrari, R.; Coats, A.J.S.; McDonagh, T. Sex- and age-related differences in the management and outcomes of chronic heart failure: An analysis of patients from the ESC HFA EORP Heart Failure Long-Term Registry. *Eur. J. Heart Fail.* **2020**, *22*, 92–102. [CrossRef]
94. Garcia, M.; Mulvagh, S.L.; Merz, C.N.; Buring, J.E.; Manson, J.E. Cardiovascular Disease in Women: Clinical Perspectives. *Circ. Res.* **2016**, *118*, 1273–1293. [CrossRef]
95. Wang, X.; Vaduganathan, M.; Claggett, B.L.; Hegde, S.M.; Pabon, M.; Kulac, I.J.; Vardeny, O.; O'Meara, E.; Zieroth, S.; Katova, T.; et al. Sex Differences in Characteristics, Outcomes, and Treatment Response with Dapagliflozin Across the Range of Ejection Fraction in Patients with Heart Failure: Insights from DAPA-HF and DELIVER. *Circulation* **2023**, *147*, 624–634. [CrossRef] [PubMed]
96. Gerber, Y.; Weston, S.A.; Redfield, M.M.; Chamberlain, A.M.; Manemann, S.M.; Jiang, R.; Killian, J.M.; Roger, V.L. A contemporary appraisal of the heart failure epidemic in Olmsted County, Minnesota, 2000 to 2010. *JAMA Intern. Med.* **2015**, *175*, 996–1004. [CrossRef]
97. Chang, P.P.; Wruck, L.M.; Shahar, E.; Rossi, J.S.; Loehr, L.R.; Russell, S.D.; Agarwal, S.K.; Konety, S.H.; Rodriguez, C.J.; Rosamond, W.D. Trends in hospitalizations and survival of acute decompensated heart failure in four US Communities (2005–2014): ARIC Study Community Surveillance. *Circulation* **2018**, *138*, 12–24. [CrossRef] [PubMed]
98. Passino, C.; Aimo, A.; Emdin, M.; Vergaro, G. Quality of life and outcome in heart failure with preserved ejection fraction: When sex matters. *Int. J. Cardiol.* **2018**, *267*, 141–142. [CrossRef]
99. Lewis, E.F.; Lamas, G.A.; O'Meara, E.; Granger, C.B.; Dunlap, M.E.; McKelvie, R.S.; Probstfield, J.L.; Young, J.B.; Michelson, E.L.; Halling, K.; et al. Characterization of health-related quality of life in heart failure patients with preserved versus low ejection fraction in CHARM. *Eur. J. Heart Fail.* **2007**, *9*, 83–91. [CrossRef]
100. Janse, R.J.; Fu, E.L.; Dahlström, U.; Benson, L.; Lindholm, B.; van Diepen, M.; Dekker, F.W.; Lund, L.H.; Carrero, J.J.; Savarese, G. Use of guideline-recommended medical therapy in patients with heart failure and chronic kidney disease: From physician's prescriptions to patient's dispensations, medication adherence and persistence. *Eur. J. Heart Fail.* **2022**, *24*, 2185–2195. [CrossRef]

Disclaimer/Publisher's Note: The statements, opinions and data contained in all publications are solely those of the individual author(s) and contributor(s) and not of MDPI and/or the editor(s). MDPI and/or the editor(s) disclaim responsibility for any injury to people or property resulting from any ideas, methods, instructions or products referred to in the content.

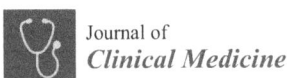

Article

Cardiovascular Risk Perception and Knowledge among Italian Women: Lessons from IGENDA Protocol

Silvia Maffei [1,*], Antonella Meloni [2], Martino Deidda [3], Susanna Sciomer [4], Lucia Cugusi [5], Christian Cadeddu [3], Sabina Gallina [6], Michela Franchini [7], Giovanni Scambia [8], Anna Vittoria Mattioli [9], Nicola Surico [10], Giuseppe Mercuro [3] and IGENDA Study Group [†] on behalf of the Italian Society of Cardiology (SIC) and the Italian Society of Obstetrics and Gynecology (SIGO)

1. Cardiovascular and Gynaecological Endocrinology Unit, Fondazione G Monasterio CNR-Regione Toscana, 56124 Pisa, Italy
2. Department of Radiology, Fondazione G Monasterio CNR-Regione Toscana, 56124 Pisa, Italy; antonella.meloni@ftgm.it
3. Department of Medical Sciences and Public Health, University of Cagliari, 09042 Cagliari, Italy; martino.deidda@tiscali.it (M.D.); cadedduc@unica.it (C.C.); giuseppemercuro@gmail.com (G.M.)
4. Department of Cardiovascular, Respiratory Nephrological, Anesthesiological and Geriatric Sciences, Sapienza University, 00186 Roma, Italy; susanna.sciomer@uniroma1.it
5. Department of Biomedical Sciences, University of Sassari, 07100 Sassari, Italy; lucia.cugusi@uniss.it
6. Department of Neuroscience, Imaging and Clinical Sciences, University of Chieti-Pescara, 66100 Chieti, Italy; sgallina@unich.it
7. Epidemiology and Health Research Lab, Institute of Clinical Physiology, National Research Council, 56124 Pisa, Italy; michela.franchini@ifc.cnr.it
8. Gynecologic Oncology, Department of Woman and Child Health and Public Health, Fondazione Policlinico Universitario A. Gemelli, IRCCS, 00168 Roma, Italy; giovanni.scambia@policlinicogemelli.it
9. Surgical, Medical and Dental Department of Morphological Sciences Related to Transplant, Oncology and Regenerative Medicine, University of Modena and Reggio Emilia, 41124 Modena, Italy; vittoria@unimore.it
10. Department of Translational Medicine, Università Piemonte Orientale, 28100 Novara, Italy; nicola.surico@med.unipmn.it
* Correspondence: silvia.maffei@ftgm.it; Tel.: +39-050-315-2216
† IGENDA study group (in alphabetical order): Maria Gabriella Aiello (Studio Ginecologico "Le Pleiadi", Scandicci, Italy); Antonio Alfeo (Struttura complessa Ginecologia ed Ostetricia, Azienda sanitaria locale TO4 di Ciriè, Chivasso e Ivrea, Italy); Antonio Amorosi (UOC Ginecologia Ostetricia Territoriale, ASP Regione Basilicata, Potenza, Italy); Rita Argentieri (Ambulatorio di ginecologia, S. Pietro Vernotico ASL Brindisi, Italy); Sonia Baldi (Consultorio, ASL 10, Firenze, Italy); Lorella Battini (UO Ostetricia e Ginecologia 2, Università di Pisa—Ospedale Santa Chiara, Pisa, Italy); Angelamaria Becorpi (Ambulatorio Menopausa Oncologica, AOU Careggi, Firenze, Italy); Pierluigi Benedetti Panici (Dipartimento Assistenziale Integrato Ostetricia e Ginecologia, Policlinico Umberto I—Università "La Sapienza", Roma, Italy); Chiara Benedetto (SCDU Ginecologia e Ostetricia C, Ospedale S. Anna, Torino, Italy); Ilaria Betella (Clinica Ginecologica, AOU Maggiore della Carità, Novara, Italy); Anna Biasoli (Clinica Ostetrica e Ginecologica, AOU Santa Maria della Misericordia, Udine, Italy); Maria Sandra Bucciantini (Clinica Ostetrica e Ginecologica, AOU Careggi, Firenze, Italy); Angelo Cagnacci (Clinica Ostetrica e Ginecologica, Università di Modena, Modena, Italy); Federica Campolo (SCDU Ginecologia e Ostetricia C, Ospedale S. Anna, Torino, Italy); Antonio Canino (UOC Ginecologia e Ostetricia, Ospedale Niguarda Ca' Granda, Milano, Italy); Gianpiero Capobianco (Dipartimento di Scienze Clinica Ostetrica e Ginecologica, Università degli Studi di Sassari, Sassari, Italy); Pia Cassinelli (Struttura complessa Ginecologia ed Ostetricia, Azienda sanitaria locale TO4 di Ciriè, Chivasso e Ivrea, Italy); Antonina Cermigliaro (Struttura complessa Ginecologia ed Ostetricia, Azienda sanitaria locale TO4 di Ciriè, Chivasso e Ivrea, Italy); Ettore Cicinelli (Ginecologia e Ostetricia, Azienda Ospedaliero-Universitaria Consorziale Policlinico di Bari, Bari, Italy); Nicola Colacurci (Dipartimento Scienze Ginecologiche, Ostetriche e della Riproduzione, Seconda Università di Napoli, Napoli, Italy); Giuseppe D'Amato (Procreazione Medica Assistita, Presidio Ospedaliero Jaia, Conversano, Italy); Rosaraio D'Anna (Clinica Ostetrica e Ginecologica, Università di Messina, Messina, Italy); Barbara Del Bravo (Unità Funzionale Consultoriale, Azienda Usl Toscana Nord Ovest, Pisa, Italy); Vincenzo De Leo (Clinica Ostetrica e Ginecologica, AOU Senese Policlinico Santa Maria alle Scotte, Siena, Italy); Monica Della Martina (Clinica Ostetrica e Ginecologica, AOU Santa Maria della Misericordia, Udine, Italy); Filippo De Luca (Clinica Ostetrica e Ginecologica, Università di Messina, Messina, Italy); Francesco De Seta (Clinica Ostetrica e Ginecologica, IRCCS B. Garofolo, Trieste, Italy); Maria Gabriella De Silvio (Unità materno infantile territoriale distretto 60, ASL Salerno, Salerno, Italy); Salvatore Dessole (Dipartimento di Scienze Clinica Ostetrica e Ginecologica, Università degli Studi di Sassari, Sassari, Italy); Costantino Di Carlo (Dipartimento di Ostetricia e Ginecologia, AOU Federico II, Napoli, Italy);

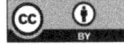

Citation: Maffei, S.; Meloni, A.; Deidda, M.; Sciomer, S.; Cugusi, L.; Cadeddu, C.; Gallina, S.; Franchini, M.; Scambia, G.; Mattioli, A.V.; et al. Cardiovascular Risk Perception and Knowledge among Italian Women: Lessons from IGENDA Protocol. *J. Clin. Med.* 2022, *11*, 1695. https://doi.org/10.3390/jcm11061695

Academic Editor: Jeffrey L. Anderson

Received: 8 February 2022
Accepted: 16 March 2022
Published: 18 March 2022

Copyright: © 2022 by the authors. Licensee MDPI, Basel, Switzerland. This article is an open access article distributed under the terms and conditions of the Creative Commons Attribution (CC BY) license (https://creativecommons.org/licenses/by/4.0/).

Giovanni Di Vagno (U.O.C. Ginecologia e Prevenzione Ginecologica, IRCCS-Ospedale Oncologico, Bari, Italy); Valeria Dubini (Consultorio, ASL 10, Firenze, Italy); Giovanni Fattorini (Poliambulatorio Mazzacurati, Bologna, Italy); Luigi Fedele (Dipartimento della donna, del bambino e del neonato, Fondazione IRCCS Ospedale Maggiore Policlinico, Milano, Italy); Simone Ferrero (Clinica Ostetrica e Ginecologica, AOU San Martino, Genova, Italy); Fabio Focardi (Azienda Sanitaria Firenze/Unità Funzionale Consultori, Prato, Italy); Angiolo Gadducci (UO Ostetricia e Ginecologia 1, Università di Pisa—Ospedale Santa Chiara, Pisa, Italy); Mario Gallo (Struttura complessa Ginecologia ed Ostetricia, Azienda sanitaria locale TO4 di Ciriè, Chivasso e Ivrea, Italy); Diana Giobbi (Ambulatori Ginecologia e Ostetricia, San Benedetto del Tronto, Italy); Barbara Giussy (Dipartimento della donna, del bambino e del neonato, Fondazione IRCCS Ospedale Maggiore Policlinico, Milano, Italy); Pantaleo Greco (Universitaria, Università degli Studi di Foggia, Foggia, Italy); Secondo Guaschino (Ambulatorio Menopausa Oncologica, AOU Careggi, Firenze, Italy); Maurizio Guida (UO Ginecologia e Ostetricia, Università degli Studi di Salerno, Salerno, Italy); Michele Lisco (Consultorio Familiare, ASL Brindisi 1, Brindisi, Italy); Stefano Luisi (Clinica Ostetrica e Ginecologica, AOU Senese Policlinico Santa Maria alle Scotte, Siena, Italy); Laura Manzan (Azienda Sanitaria Firenze/Unità Funzionale Consultori, Prato, Italy); Carlo Mapelli (UOC Ginecologia e Ostetricia, Ospedale Niguarda Ca'Granda, Milano, Italy); Diego Marchesoni (Clinica Ostetrica e Ginecologica, AOU Santa Maria della Misericordia, Udine, Italy); Enrico Marseglia (Consultorio familiare, Ostuni, Azienda sanitaria Locale, Brindisi, Italy); Patrizia Masi (Poliambulatorio Mazzacurati, Bologna, Italy); Gian Benedetto Melis (Dipartimento di scienze chirurgiche, Università di Cagliari, Clinica Ostetrica e Ginecologica AOU di Cagliari, Cagliari, Italy); Guido Menato (SCDU Ginecologia e Ostetricia, A.O. Ordine Mauriziano, Torino, Italy); Angelo Multinu (Ginecologia e Ostetricia, Ospedale S. Francesco, Nuoro, ATS Sardegna, Italy); Carmine Nappi (Dipartimento di Ostetricia e Ginecologia, AOU Federico II, Napoli, Italy); Luigi Nappi (U.O. di Ginecologia ed Ostetricia Universitaria, Università degli Studi di Foggia, Foggia, Italy); Francesca Nocera (Ginecologia ed Ostetricia, Azienda Ospedaliera per l'Emergenza Cannizzaro, Catania, Italy); Silvia Ottanelli (Studi medici, Firenze, Italy); Maria Carmela Pandolfo (U.O.C. di Ginecologia ed Ostetricia, Ospedale Buccheri La Ferla FBF, Palermo, Italy); Anna Maria Paoletti (Dipartimento di scienze chirurgiche, Università di Cagliari, Clinica Ostetrica e Ginecologica AOU di Cagliari, Cagliari, Italy); Anna Pasi (Centro Medico Donna Si Cura, Ravenna, Italy); Felice Petraglia (Clinica Ostetrica e Ginecologica, AOU Senese Policlinico Santa Maria alle Scotte, Siena, Italy); Monica Pilloni (Dipartimento di scienze chirurgiche, Università di Cagliari, Clinica Ostetrica e Ginecologica AOU di Cagliari, Cagliari, Italy); Elena Rosa Potì (ASL Brindisi, Presidio di Brindisi "Di Summa—Perrino", Brindisi, Italy); Maria Cristina Pozzi (Centro Medico Donna Si Cura, Ravenna, Italy); Carmela Ruscello (Consultorio, ASP Caltanissetta, Caltanissetta, Italy); Maria Giovanna Salerno (UO Ostetricia e Ginecologia 2, Università di Pisa—Ospedale Santa Chiara, Pisa, Italy); Stefania Sanna (Ginecologia ed Ostetricia, Ospedale S. Martino, Oristano, ATS Sardegna, Italy); Vincenzo Sanzarello (Consultorio, ASP Messina, Messina, Italy); Giovanni Scalabrino (Consultorio Canicattì e Castrofilippo, ASP Agrigento, Agrigento, Italy); Silvano Scarponi (Divisione Ostetrica e Ginecologica, USL Umbria 1, Perugia, Italy); Paolo Scollo (Ginecologia ed Ostetricia, Azienda Ospedaliera per l'Emergenza Cannizzaro, Catania, Italy); Claudia Scumace (Clinica Ginecologica, AOU Maggiore della Carità, Novara, Italy); Ettore Simoncini (Consultori, Azienda Usl Toscana Nord Ovest, Livorno, Italy); Massimo Stomati (Unità operativa di Ostetricia e Ginecologia, ASL Brindisi, Presidio di Francavilla Fontana, Italy); Onorato Succu (Ginecologia ed Ostetricia, Ospedale S. Martino, Oristano, ATS Sardegna, Italy); Daniela Surico (Clinica Ginecologica, AOU Maggiore della Carità, Novara, Italy); Giuseppina Trimarchi (Unità Funzionale Consultoriale, Azienda Usl Toscana Nord Ovest, Pisa, Italy); Riccarda Triolo (Centro della Salute, Azienda Usl Toscana Centro, Pistoia, Italy); Giuseppe Trojano (UO Ostetricia e Ginecologia 2, Università di Pisa—Ospedale Santa Chiara, Pisa, Italy); Vito Trojano (U.O.C. Ginecologia e Prevenzione Ginecologica, IRCCS-Ospedale Oncologico, Bari, Italy); Valerio Vallerino (Dipartimento di scienze chirurgiche, Università di Cagliari, Clinica Ostetrica e Ginecologica AOU di Cagliari, Cagliari, Italy); Pier Luigi Venturini (Clinica Ostetrica e Ginecologica, AOU San Martino, Genova, Italy); Paola Villa (Dipartimento per la tutela della salute della donna, Policlinico Universitario Agostino Gemelli, Roma, Italy); Flora Vota (Struttura complessa Ginecologia ed Ostetricia, Azienda sanitaria locale TO4 di Ciriè, Chivasso e Ivrea, Italy); Maurizio Zaza (UOC Ginecologia e Ostetricia, Ospedale Sant'Eugenio, Roma, Italy).

Abstract: A multicenter, cross-sectional observational study (Italian GENder Differences in Awareness of Cardiovascular risk, IGENDA study) was carried out to evaluate the perception and knowledge of cardiovascular risk among Italian women. An anonymous questionnaire was completed by 4454 women (44.3 ± 14.1 years). The 70% of respondents correctly identified cardiovascular disease (CVD) as the leading cause of death. More than half of respondents quoted cancer as the greatest current and future health problem of women of same age. Sixty percent of interviewed women considered CVD as an almost exclusively male condition. Although respondents showed a good knowledge of the major cardiovascular risk factors, the presence of cardiovascular risk factors was not associated with higher odds of identifying CVD as the biggest cause of death. Less than 10% of respondents perceived themselves as being at high CVD risk, and the increased CVD risk perception was associated with ageing, higher frequency of cardiovascular risk factors and disease, and a poorer self-rated health status. The findings of this study highlight the low perception of cardiovascular risk in Italian women and suggest an urgent need to enhance knowledge and perception of CVD risk in women as a real health problem and not just as a as a life-threatening threat.

Keywords: awareness; cardiovascular disease; cardiovascular risk factors; knowledge; perception; women

1. Introduction

The cardiovascular (CV) risk involves anthropometric, metabolic, biological, and behavioral factors, which, in turn, interact with sex and are modulated by aging [1–3]. CV risk is not uniformly distributed across the world, as it is also influenced by genetics, lifestyle, environment, and the culture of each population. Countries, therefore, can be divided into two main groups, based on the high or low risk of CV disease (CVD) of their populations. In Europe, Italy is a low-CV-risk country [4], although CVD is also in this country the leading cause of disability and death.

Objective CV risk assessment (e.g., Framingham score) does not include the individual knowledge of CV risk or CVD prevalence [5–7]. This lack has a strong impact on the problem and its correction, because to adopt a healthy lifestyle, a correct perception of personal risk is necessary: its deficiency is to be considered almost as an additional risk factor [8]. The problem is even more significant among women, due to the wrong and settled belief that CVD is primarily, if not exclusively, a male disease. In turn, this misunderstanding is generated by the differences in the clinical presentation of CVD in the two sexes and by the increased prevalence of CVD in women of advanced postmenopausal age [8,9]. Moreover, several female-specific risk factors for CVD, such as polycystic ovary syndrome, premature ovarian failure, hypertensive disorders of pregnancy, gestational diabetes, and preterm birth, are underappreciated clinically and not receive adequate attention in CVD risk prediction [10–12].

A lack of knowledge of CV risk factors (CVRF) among women has been demonstrated by the majority of published studies [13–21]. The knowledge that CVD is the leading cause of death proved to be suboptimal among Australian and US women [19,21,22]. A nationwide survey conducted by the Women's Heart Alliance in 2014 to determine barriers and opportunities for women and physicians with regard to CVD showed that almost half of 1011 interviewed women did not recognize CVD as the number one killer of women in the US [23]. Conversely, in a survey conducted in Austria, 75.3% of women correctly defined CVD as the leading cause of death [18].

Instead, with regard to the assessment of the impact of the CVD on their personal health status, several studies revealed a wrong perception even amongst women with CVRF [14,22,24]. For example, Mosca et al., in their survey of 2010, found that only 16% of women recognized the CVD as their biggest health problem, while 46% perceived cancer as the leading cause of illness in the female gender and the greatest threat to their future health [22].

It should be recognized that 90% of the published studies investigated US and Australian women [14,19,21,22,24], while the European situation in terms of knowledge and perception of CVD remains almost totally unexplored.

To the best of our knowledge, only one population-based study was conducted in Italy [25], which showed that only 26.5% of respondents correctly identified the main CVRF, with the exception for smoking (89.4%) and high cholesterol level (74.7%). Unfortunately, this study involved only 830 women recruited at random in five public schools (mothers of children aged 3 to 18 years), who lived in a single, limited urban area (Naples and Salerno). Therefore, this cohort cannot be considered representative of the entire Italian female population.

On the basis of these inadequate premises, we conducted a national CV health survey on a large sample of 5000 women attending one of the 80 outpatient gynecological centers throughout the Italian Society of Obstetrics and Gynecology (SIGO) network [26]. Indeed, all the project phases were conducted in strict collaboration with the Italian Society of Cardiology (SIC) and SIGO. In this representative female population, we investigated the degree of knowledge of CVD and CVRF and the perception of CV health status.

2. Materials and Methods

2.1. Study Design and Participants

The Italian GENder Differences in Awareness of CV risk (IGENDA) is a cross-sectional, observational, multicenter study whose protocol has already been described [26]. As part of this study, an anonymous, self-administered questionnaire was distributed to 5000 consecutive Italian women aged 18 to 70 years, who attended one of the 80 outpatient gynecological centers through the SIGO network. Exclusion criteria were a diagnosis of malignancy in the last 5 years and/or an ongoing chemotherapy treatment.

The study was conducted in accordance with the Declaration of Helsinki [27] and the GCP guidelines of the European Commission. Ethical approval was obtained from the Ethical Committee of Pisa (Comitato Etico Area Vasta Nord Ovest) on 13 March 2014 (Protocol Number 17857). All participants gave their signed informed consent to the project and received a brief description of the study's aims and how to complete the questionnaire.

2.2. Structure of the Questionnaire

The questionnaire for the participants included the following three main parts.

Part 1, baseline assessment, collected general information on survey participants as well as their knowledge of CVD as the greatest health problem or risk.

Part 2, on CVDs, investigated the knowledge of traditional CVRF: women were asked if they were aware on the fact that a given condition/behavior represented a CVRF.

Part 3, on individual health status and perceived CVD risk. Participants were asked on their individual CVD history, such as pre-existing coronary artery disease, myocardial infarction, or stroke. The perception of subjective health status and personal CVD risk profile was assessed by a Self-Rating of Health (SRH), using the single-items "How would you rate your current health status on a scale from 0 to 10?" and "Which is your personal risk of developing a CVD in the future on a scale from 0 (very low) to 10 (very high)?". Ratings for SRH were poor <4, acceptable 5–7, and good 8–10. Similarly, ratings for perceived risk were low <4, intermediate 5–7, and high 8–10.

The completion of the questionnaire required at least 20 min.

Data on the educational level of the participants were included in a general health questionnaire compiled by their physicians.

2.3. Statistical Analysis

Data analyses were conducted with the IBM SPSS Statistics 20 statistical package. Continuous variables were described as mean ± standard deviation (SD) and categorical variables as frequencies and percentages. The normality of distribution of the parameters was assessed by using the Kolmogorov–Smirnov test. For continuous values with normal distribution, comparisons between groups were made by independent-samples t-test (for two groups) or one-way ANOVA (for more than two groups). Wilcoxon's signed rank test and Kruskal–Wallis test were applied for continuous values with non-normal distribution. The Bonferroni correction test was used in all pairwise comparisons. The χ^2 testing was performed for non-continuous variables. The odds ratios (ORs) and 95% confidence intervals (CIs) were calculated using logistic regression analysis.

A two-tailed probability $p < 0.05$ was considered statistically significant.

3. Results

3.1. Characteristics of Respondents

A total of 4454 respondents filled out the questionnaire. Their demographic and health characteristics are summarized in Table 1. The mean age was 44.3 ± 14.1 years, with 62% of participants over 40 years old. Three quarters of the women had a medium to high education level.

Table 1. Demographics and health characteristics of respondents.

Age Group	n (%)
<30 years	820 (18.4)
30–39 years	851 (19.1)
40–49 years	1011 (22.7)
50–59 years	1149 (25.8)
≥60 years	623 (14.0)
Cardiovascular risk factors	n (%)
Yes	2592 (58.2)
Cardiovascular disease	n (%)
Yes	125 (2.8)
Highest educational level	n (%)
Lower secondary school or less	1114 (25.0)
High school	1897 (42.6)
University	1443 (32.4)

The 58.2% of women had one or more CVRF; in detail, 44.5% had a single CVRF, 25.4% reported two CVRF, and the remaining 30.1% reported three or more CVRF. Among the CVRF, the following frequencies were detected: menopause 27.7%, obesity/overweight 19.2%, smoking habit 17.9%, hypertension 17.5%, family CVD history 17.1%, dyslipidemia 13.0%, and diabetes mellitus 6.7%.

The 2.8% of respondents reported to suffer from a diagnosed CVD. Women with CVD were significantly older than those without CVD (54.9 ± 14.9 vs. 42.1 ± 13.4; $p < 0.0001$).

3.2. Knowledge of CVD

The 69.8% of women correctly identified CVD as the leading cause of death in the Italian population (Figure 1a). Those who gave the correct answer were older (45.1 ± 14.1 vs. 42.2 ± 14.1 years; $p < 0.0001$) and had the highest level of education (university vs. secondary school 74.0% vs. 65.8%; $p < 0.0001$, and university vs. high school, 74.0% vs. 68.5%; $p = 0.006$). The percentage of women who answered this question correctly was similar in subjects with and without CVD (76.0% vs. 69.0%; $p = 0.134$). Furthermore, this percentage was significantly higher among women with at least one CVRF compared to those who reported none (70.5% vs. 65.7%; $p = 0.005$).

The 60.8% of women believed that CVD is an almost exclusively male condition (Figure 1b).

In the multiple choice questions, more than half of women identified cancer as the biggest health problem for people of the same age and gender (74%) and as the greatest danger to their health in the future (64%) (Figure 2). Only 20.7% and 24.6% of women, respectively, selected CVD in the two aforementioned questions. Noteworthily, these women most often suffered from CVD (4.6% vs. 2.2%, $p = 0.002$; OR 2.1, 95% CI: 1.4–3.4; $p = 0.001$) and were older (46.6 ± 14.3 vs. 43.3 ± 14.1 years; $p < 0.0001$).

3.3. Knowledge of the Main CVRF

Table 2 shows respondents' degree of knowledge of CVRF and how age and level of education, as well as the presence of CVRF or CVD, influences this knowledge. Greater recognition of all CVRF was found in progressively older age groups and among women with the highest level of education. Women affected by CVRF correctly identified only family history of CVD, high cholesterol, and menopause as CVRF. The presence of CVD did not correlate with a higher level of knowledge of the individual CVRF.

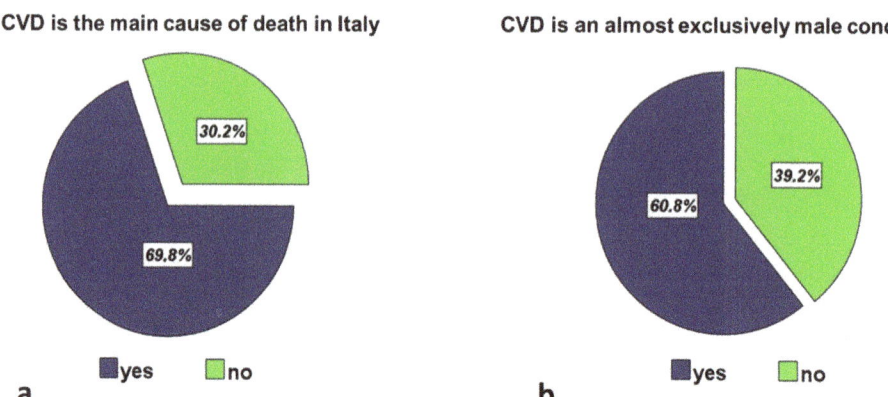

Figure 1. (**a**) Percentages of women who identified/did not identify CVD as the leading cause of death in Italy. (**b**) Percentage distribution of women who stated or excluded that CVD is an almost exclusively male condition.

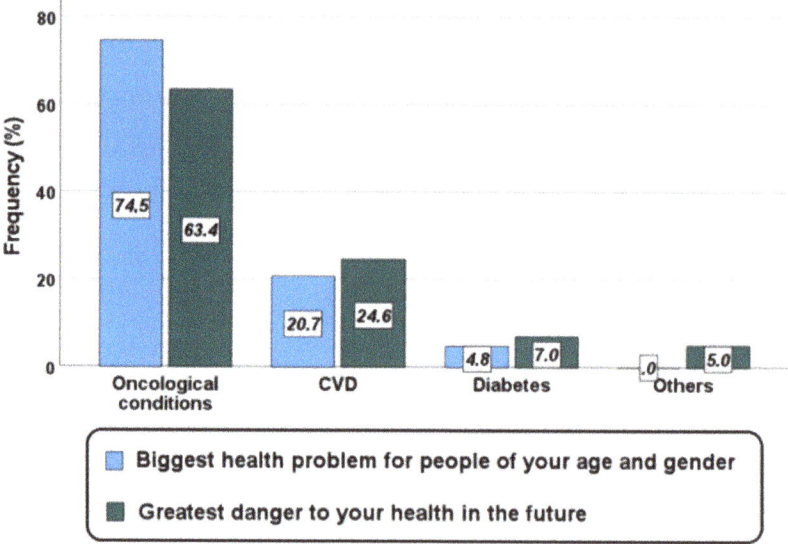

Figure 2. Percent response to the multiple choice questions "What is the biggest health problem for people of your age and gender and what is the greatest danger to your health in the future?".

3.4. Self-Rating of Health

The characteristics of the three groups based on SRH status are presented in Table 3. The 10.4% of women rated their health as bad, 47.6% as acceptable, and 42.0% as good. Age was significantly higher in the poor SRH group than in both the acceptable and good SHR groups ($p < 0.0001$), as well as in the acceptable SRH group in comparison with good SRH ($p = 0.003$). Women who reported good SRH had significantly lower prevalence of both CVRF and CVD than respondents with acceptable and poor SRH ($p < 0.0001$; Table 3).

Table 2. Logistic regression for awareness of CVRF.

| CVRF | Correctly Identified n (%) | Age (Years) | | | | Level of Schooling | | CVRF [c] | CVD [d] |
| | | 30–40 [a] | 40–50 [a] | 50–60 [a] | ≥60 [a] | High School [b] | University [b] | | |
		OR (95%CI) p-Value	OR (95%CI) p-Value	OR (95%CI) p-Value	OR (95%CI) p-Value	OR (95%CI) p-Value	OR (95%CI) p-Value	OR (95%CI) p-Value	OR (95%CI) p-Value
Family CVD history	3804 (85.4)	1.02 (0.78–1.35) p = 0.844	1.12 (0.86–1.46) p = 0.416	0.95 (0.74–1.22) p = 0.668	1.51 (1.09–2.09) p = 0.014	1.64 (1.33–2.02) p < 0.0001	2.68 (2.09–3.43) p < 0.0001	1.31 (1.08–1.60) p = 0.007	1.11 (0.63–1.96) p = 0.725
Smoke	4343 (97.5)	1.34 (0.76–2.36) p = 0.312	1.20 (0.71–2.04) p = 0.491	3.09 (1.59–6.01) p = 0.001	1.54 (0.80–2.95) p = 0.194	1.75 (1.09–2.81) p = 0.021	1.72 (1.03–2.86) p = 0.037	1.44 (0.93–2.24) p = 0.107	2.77 (0.38–20.08) p = 0.313
High blood pressure	4316 (96.9)	1.42 (0.89–2.27) p = 0.141	1.88 (1.16–3.04) p = 0.010	3.72 (2.10–6.57) p < 0.0001	2.84 (1.48–5.43) p = 0.002	1.94 (1.31–2.88) p = 0.001	3.19 (1.94–5.24) p < 0.0001	1.32 (0.90–1.93) p = 0.150	3.58 (0.49–25.88) p = 0.206
High cholesterol	4271 (95.9)	0.97 (0.63–1.49) p = 0.875	1.24 (0.80–1.92) p = 0.335	2.34 (1.37–3.66) p = 0.001	1.72 (0.99–2.99) p = 0.053	1.92 (1.35–2.74) p < 0.0001	3.32 (2.12–5.19) p < 0.0001	1.70 (1.19–2.44) p = 0.004	2.16 (0.53–8.86) p = 0.283
Overweight	4360 (97.9)	1.62 (0.80–3.29) p = 0.178	1.47 (0.76–2.82) p = 0.251	1.57 (0.82–2.98) p = 0.172	0.88 (0.45–1.70) p = 0.884	2.23 (1.37–3.62) p = 0.001	3.94 (2.09–7.43) p < 0.0001	0.54 (0.52–1.40) p = 0.536	0.86 (0.52–1.40) p = 0.536
Physical inactivity	4258 (95.6)	1.55 (1.00–2.42) p = 0.050	1.86 (1.19–2.88) p = 0.006	1.83 (1.19–2.80) p = 0.005	1.44 (0.89–2.33) p = 0.133	1.44 (1.02–2.03) p = 0.039	2.35 (1.55–3.58) p < 0.0001	0.97 (0.69–1.37) p = 0.874	2.30 (0.56–9.43) p = 0.246
Diabetes	3910 (87.8)	1.51 (1.13–2.02) p = 0.005	1.12 (0.86–1.45) p = 0.400	1.61 (1.23–2.11) p = 0.001	2.15 (1.51–3.07) p < 0.0001	1.13 (0.89–1.42) p = 0.321	1.71 (1.31–2.24) p < 0.0001	0.97 (0.78–1.21) p = 0.776	1.68 (0.81–3.49) p = 0.162
Menopause	3692 (82.9)	0.87 (0.68–1.11) p = 0.266	0.91 (0.72–1.15) p = 0.437	1.99 (1.53–2.58) p < 0.0001	2.09 (1.52–2.87) p < 0.0001	1.39 (1.13–1.69) p = 0.002	1.96 (1.56–2.47) p < 0.0001	1.33 (1.11–1.61) p = 0.003	1.23 (0.71–2.14) p = 0.468

CVRF = cardiovascular risk factors; CVD = cardiovascular disease; OR = odds ratio. [a] Compared to 18–30 years old age group. [b] Compared to women with lower educational level (lower secondary school or less). [c] Compared to women without CVRF. [d] Compared to women without CVD.

Table 3. Characteristics of the three groups identified on the basis of the by SRH status.

| | SRH Status | | | p-Value |
	Poor	Acceptable	Good	
Age (years)	49.10 ± 15.16	46.54 ± 13.64	40.10 ± 12.93	<0.0001
CVRF %	64.4	65.4	47.7	<0.0001
CVD %	5.5	3.9	1.2	<0.0001

SRH = self-rated health; CVRF = cardiovascular risk factor; CVD = cardiovascular disease.

3.5. Perception of CVD Risk

The 44.5% of the women considered themselves to be at low CVD risk and 46.7% at intermediate risk, although the prevalence rates of CVRF in the two groups were 50.2% and 64.6%, respectively. Only the remaining 8.8% of the respondents reported to perceive a high CVD risk, commensurated with a 70.0% CVRF prevalence (Table 4). A direct correlation between perceived risk increase and age increase was detected: the group with a low perceived CVD risk was significantly younger than the groups of women with both intermediate and high perceived CVD risk ($p < 0.0001$). Finally, a good SRH status was associated with a low perceived CVD risk (Table 4).

Table 4. Perceived CVD risk compared to demographics and clinical conditions.

| | Perceived CVD Risk | | | p-Value |
	Low	Intermediate	High	
Age (years)	41.27 ± 13.79	46.08 ± 13.49	50.14 ± 14.56	<0.0001
CVRF %	50.2	64.6	70	<0.0001
CVD %	1.7	2.9	10.2	<0.0001
SRH status %				
Poor	9.9	9.8	19.5	<0.0001
Acceptable	40	55.9	51.4	
Good	50.1	34.4	29.1	

CVD = cardiovascular disease; CVRF = cardiovascular risk factor; SRH = self-rated health.

4. Discussion

This national survey documented several important findings. In Italy, women's knowledge of CVD as the main cause of death is higher (69.8%) than those reported by the US (56%) [28] and Australian (32%) [19] women and comparable to that found among Austrian women (75.3%) [18]. In Italy, the knowledge of CVD as the main cause of death was more associated with older age than with the presence of CVD, thereby suggesting that such consciousness may be influenced by life experiences (e.g., number of CVD deaths among friends and relatives).

On the other hand, most of the interviewed women, although correctly identifying the CVD as the main cause of death in Italy, considered themselves at risk of oncological diseases rather than CVD. This misperception was even more evident in younger women, in whom a further misunderstanding of CV risk could be due to the poor attention to their health status and lack of life experience of CVD. The apparent contradiction between the knowledge of CVD as a leading cause of mortality and the expectation of cancer in future life could be largely explained by the erroneous but widespread opinion that CVD is more common in males. Consistently, our data showed that over 60% of the respondents considered CVD as an almost exclusively male condition.

Italian women showed in our study a good knowledge of the main CVRF, unlike the US and Australian female populations [13–17,19,20]. Actually, in contrast to our data, the only previous population study conducted in Italy also showed a very poor knowledge of the main CVRF among women (26.5%) [25]. The discrepancy in the results could be largely explained by the small sample interviewed in that study, the survey area limited to two cities in southern Italy, and the low percentage of people over 60 years old. Moreover, the study by Tedesco was performed years ago and before the national campaign of information on CV risk [25]. Being overweight was the most commonly recognized CVRF by women with no differences between age groups. It is reasonable to assume that the widespread attention to the aesthetic aspect typical of our era contributes to this awareness. Conversely, menopause was the less frequently identified CVRF. This finding corresponds and could be explained by the underestimation of menopause as an individual CVRF also by the scientific community. Furthermore, younger women were less aware of this relevant problem than the postmenopausal respondents. Diabetes was one of the most underestimated CVRF in our survey, despite the recognized importance of diabetes as a CVD equivalent [1]. These data are in accordance with previous surveys [16,18], where diabetes was the less known CVRF, identified by less than half of the women surveyed. The knowledge of CVRF was strongly influenced by age and educational level, confirming the positive effect of schooling, in accordance with data reported by other studies [25,29]. Inexplicably, the presence of a known CVD did not improve the knowledge of the CVRF among women. This feature proved controversial in previous surveys. While some studies showed that women with CVRF or CVD have greater knowledge of CV risk [14,15,30], Hoare et al. [19] revealed only negligible differences in the knowledge of clinical CVRF among women with CVD or diabetes compared to healthy women. It has consistently been shown that women with diabetes and hypertension did not identify these conditions as CVRF [17] and that less than 50% of them had an exact knowledge of the normal cholesterol, blood pressure, or blood glucose [14,21,31]. Besides menopause, the knowledge of women-specific CVRF was not evaluated, but we are planning to explore this issue in our population. Two studies conducted in the USA showed that women with pre-eclampsia or gestational diabetes mellitus were unfamiliar with the relationship between these conditions and increased future CVD risk [32,33].

In this study, we assessed the female perception of health status and personal CVD risk profile by means of the SRH status assessment. This is a subjective reflection of one's general personal health condition, called "perceived" or "subjective" health, that integrates biological, mental, social, and functional aspects of a person, including individual and cultural beliefs and health behaviors [34]. As expected and in agreement with previous studies [35,36], we found that age was negatively correlated with the SRH status (younger women feel better than middle-aged and older women) and that a worse SRH status was associated with a more frequent reporting of CVRF and CVD [37].

In spite of these findings and their good knowledge of CVRF, our interviewees did not translate this information into a correct perception of their personal risk of developing CVD: although this insight would increase with age, higher CVRF and CVD reporting, and poorer SRH status, less than 10% of all women perceived the high possibility of CVD in their future life. Certainly, this lack of awareness is more concerning in women who reported having at least one CVRF, as more than one-third of them perceived their future CVD risk as low. These results confirm previous investigations. A Canadian study found that a significant percentage of participants were unaware of their CVD risk status [16]. Furthermore, a survey conducted on a smaller sample of elderly women (>70 years) confirmed that those with CVRF or CVD had a misperception of their health status, so that only 24.5% of the high-risk group—based on BMI, high blood pressure, cholesterol levels, and smoking habits—failed to recognize their actual risk of CVD [31]. These findings highlight a misperception of present and future health status in relation to the actual presence of CVRF, a mechanism for removing one's own risk of disease that has cultural and social roots. Women continue to be the reference for the whole family and are the family caregiver. They see and recognize the risk of illness in their family members but do not recognize their own risk, an attitude that can be traced back to the theory known in health psychology as "comparative optimism". The "comparative optimism" is the belief that negative events are more likely to happen to others, while positive events are more likely to happen to themselves [38]. It has been shown that people are likely to retrieve the information on the general perception of risk through social influence; however, when considering self-reported risk, positive prejudices are likely much more influential, with the consequence that people underestimate their personal risk [39].

5. Conclusions

Our data highlight the need to strengthen the knowledge of CVD, as well as CVRF, as a real health problem for both the sexes, removing the still widespread misunderstanding of a "male-limited" condition. For this purpose, a global campaign to improve knowledge and perception of CVD is of paramount importance. This campaign should be conducted within the health system, during patient visits, and by organizing specific seminars or conferences directed to the general population, and, above all, through various digital communication channels, including mass media (TV and radio advertisements and articles on newspapers and magazines), social media (blogs, micro-blogs, wikis, social networking sites, photo-sharing sites, instant messaging, video-sharing sites, and podcasts), and text messages or phone calls. The digital communication campaign can reach audiences in a low-cost, impactful, and effective way. Younger women should be the main focus of this educational project. Indeed, this is the key to providing a more prevention-oriented approach, a powerful and decisive contribution to reducing CVD risk among women.

Author Contributions: S.M.: conceptualization, methodology, funding acquisition, and writing—original draft preparation. A.M.: formal analysis and writing—original draft preparation. M.D.: data curation and writing—review and editing. S.S.: supervision. L.C.: data curation and writing—original draft preparation. C.C.: supervision. S.G.: supervision. M.F.: software, validation, and formal analysis. G.S.: supervision. A.V.M.: supervision and writing—review and editing. N.S.: project administration. G.M.: supervision and writing—review and editing. The members of the IGENDA Study group recruited the women, administrated the questionaries to the women, and compiled a general questionnaire on the educational level and general health status of the participants. All authors have read and agreed to the published version of the manuscript.

Funding: This cross-sectional observational multicenter study was supported by an unrestricted medical grant from Pfizer and Fondazione Banca Unicredit. The funders had no role in study design, data collection and analysis, decision to publish, or preparation of the manuscript.

Institutional Review Board Statement: The study was conducted in accordance with the Declaration of Helsinki (1964) and the GCP guidelines of the European Commission. Ethical approval was obtained from the Ethical Committee of Pisa (Comitato Etico Area Vasta Nord Ovest) on 13 March 2014 (Protocol Number 17857).

Informed Consent Statement: Informed consent was obtained from all subjects involved in the study.

Data Availability Statement: The data presented in this study are available on request from the corresponding author. The data are not publicly available due to privacy.

Acknowledgments: The authors would like to thank Roberto Marchioli for the important contribution in the drafting of the study protocol and the SIC secretaries Alessandra Bazzani and Antonella Amiconi and the SIGO secretaries Paola Ferri and Laura Montemagno for the precious technical support throughout the study period. Finally, we would like to thank all the women for their participation in our study.

Conflicts of Interest: The authors declare no conflict of interest.

References

1. Cannon, C.P. Cardiovascular disease and modifiable cardiometabolic risk factors. *Clin. Cornerstone* **2007**, *8*, 11–28. [CrossRef]
2. Mattioli, A.V.; Sciomer, S.; Moscucci, F.; Maiello, M.; Cugusi, L.; Gallina, S.; Dei Cas, A.; Lombardi, C.; Pengo, M.; Parati, G.; et al. Cardiovascular prevention in women: A narrative review from the Italian Society of Cardiology working groups on 'Cardiovascular Prevention, Hypertension and peripheral circulation' and on 'Women Disease'. *J. Cardiovasc. Med. (Hagerstown)* **2019**, *20*, 575–583. [CrossRef]
3. Song, P.S.; Kim, M.J.; Seong, S.-W.; Choi, S.W.; Gwon, H.-C.; Hur, S.-H.; Rha, S.-W.; Yoon, C.-H.; Jeong, M.H.; Jeong, J.-O.; et al. Gender Differences in All-Cause Mortality after Acute Myocardial Infarction: Evidence for a Gender–Age Interaction. *J. Clin. Med.* **2022**, *11*, 541. [CrossRef]
4. Conroy, R.M.; Pyorala, K.; Fitzgerald, A.P.; Sans, S.; Menotti, A.; De Backer, G.; De Bacquer, D.; Ducimetiere, P.; Jousilahti, P.; Keil, U.; et al. Estimation of ten-year risk of fatal cardiovascular disease in Europe: The SCORE project. *Eur. Heart J.* **2003**, *24*, 987–1003. [CrossRef]
5. Wilson, P.W.; Castelli, W.P.; Kannel, W.B. Coronary risk prediction in adults (the Framingham Heart Study). *Am. J. Cardiol.* **1987**, *59*, G91–G94. [CrossRef]
6. Alm-Roijer, C.; Fridlund, B.; Stagmo, M.; Erhardt, L. Knowing your risk factors for coronary heart disease improves adherence to advice on lifestyle changes and medication. *J. Cardiovasc. Nurs.* **2006**, *21*, E24–E31. [CrossRef]
7. Mosca, L.; Jones, W.K.; King, K.B.; Ouyang, P.; Redberg, R.F.; Hill, M.N. Awareness, perception, and knowledge of heart disease risk and prevention among women in the United States. American Heart Association Women's Heart Disease and Stroke Campaign Task Force. *Arch. Fam. Med.* **2000**, *9*, 506–515. [CrossRef] [PubMed]
8. Alm-Roijer, C.; Stagmo, M.; Udén, G.; Erhardt, L. Better knowledge improves adherence to lifestyle changes and medication in patients with coronary heart disease. *Eur. J. Cardiovasc. Nurs.* **2004**, *3*, 321–330. [CrossRef] [PubMed]
9. Ciambrone, G.; Kaski, J.C. The importance of gender differences in the diagnosis and management of cardiovascular disease. *Curr. Pharm. Des.* **2011**, *17*, 1079–1081. [CrossRef] [PubMed]
10. Maffei, S.; Guiducci, L.; Cugusi, L.; Cadeddu, C.; Deidda, M.; Gallina, S.; Sciomer, S.; Gastaldelli, A.; Kaski, J.C. Working Group on "Gender difference in cardiovascular disease" of the Italian Society of, C. Women-specific predictors of cardiovascular disease risk-New paradigms. *Int. J. Cardiol.* **2019**, *286*, 190–197. [CrossRef] [PubMed]
11. Arnott, C.; Patel, S.; Hyett, J.; Jennings, G.; Woodward, M.; Celermajer, D.S. Women and Cardiovascular Disease: Pregnancy, the Forgotten Risk Factor. *Heart Lung Circ.* **2020**, *29*, 662–667. [CrossRef]
12. Arnott, C.; Nelson, M.; Alfaro Ramirez, M.; Hyett, J.; Gale, M.; Henry, A.; Celermajer, D.S.; Taylor, L.; Woodward, M. Maternal cardiovascular risk after hypertensive disorder of pregnancy. *Heart* **2020**, *106*, 1927–1933. [CrossRef]
13. Mosca, L.; Ferris, A.; Fabunmi, R.; Robertson, R.M.; American Heart, A. Tracking women's awareness of heart disease: An American Heart Association national study. *Circulation* **2004**, *109*, 573–579. [CrossRef]
14. Mosca, L.; Mochari, H.; Christian, A.; Berra, K.; Taubert, K.; Mills, T.; Burdick, K.A.; Simpson, S.L. National study of women's awareness, preventive action, and barriers to cardiovascular health. *Circulation* **2006**, *113*, 525–534. [CrossRef]
15. Lynch, E.B.; Liu, K.; Kiefe, C.I.; Greenland, P. Cardiovascular disease risk factor knowledge in young adults and 10-year change in risk factors: The Coronary Artery Risk Development in Young Adults (CARDIA) Study. *Am. J. Epidemiol.* **2006**, *164*, 1171–1179. [CrossRef]
16. McDonnell, L.A.; Pipe, A.L.; Westcott, C.; Perron, S.; Younger-Lewis, D.; Elias, N.; Nooyen, J.; Reid, R.D. Perceived vs. actual knowledge and risk of heart disease in women: Findings from a Canadian survey on heart health awareness, attitudes, and lifestyle. *Can. J. Cardiol.* **2014**, *30*, 827–834. [CrossRef]
17. McKenzie, C.; Skelly, A.H. Perceptions of coronary heart disease risk in African American women with type 2 diabetes: A qualitative study. *Diabetes Educ.* **2010**, *36*, 766–773. [CrossRef]

18. Haidinger, T.; Zweimüller, M.; Stütz, L.; Demir, D.; Kaider, A.; Strametz-Juranek, J. Effect of gender on awareness of cardiovascular risk factors, preventive action taken, and barriers to cardiovascular health in a group of Austrian subjects. *Gend. Med.* **2012**, *9*, 94–102. [CrossRef]
19. Hoare, E.; Stavreski, B.; Kingwell, B.A.; Jennings, G.L. Australian adults' behaviours, knowledge and perceptions of risk factors for heart disease: A cross-sectional study. *Prev. Med. Rep.* **2017**, *8*, 204–209. [CrossRef]
20. Lange, J.; Evans-Benard, S.; Cooper, J.; Fahey, E.; Kalapos, M.; Tice, D.; Wang-D'Amato, N.; Watsky, N. Puerto Rican Women's Perceptions of Heart Disease Risk. *Clin. Nurs. Res.* **2009**, *18*, 291–306. [CrossRef]
21. Mochari, H.; Ferris, A.; Adigopula, S.; Henry, G.; Mosca, L. Cardiovascular disease knowledge, medication adherence, and barriers to preventive action in a minority population. *Prev. Cardiol.* **2007**, *10*, 190–195. [CrossRef] [PubMed]
22. Mosca, L.; Mochari-Greenberger, H.; Dolor, R.J.; Newby, L.K.; Robb, K.J. Twelve-year follow-up of American women's awareness of cardiovascular disease risk and barriers to heart health. *Circ. Cardiovasc. Qual. Outcomes* **2010**, *3*, 120–127. [CrossRef] [PubMed]
23. Bairey Merz, C.N.; Andersen, H.; Sprague, E.; Burns, A.; Keida, M.; Walsh, M.N.; Greenberger, P.; Campbell, S.; Pollin, I.; McCullough, C.; et al. Knowledge, Attitudes, and Beliefs Regarding Cardiovascular Disease in Women: The Women's Heart Alliance. *J. Am. Coll. Cardiol.* **2017**, *70*, 123–132. [CrossRef] [PubMed]
24. Christian, A.H.; Rosamond, W.; White, A.R.; Mosca, L. Nine-year trends and racial and ethnic disparities in women's awareness of heart disease and stroke: An American Heart Association national study. *J. Womens Health (Larchmt)* **2007**, *16*, 68–81. [CrossRef] [PubMed]
25. Tedesco, L.M.; Di Giuseppe, G.; Napolitano, F.; Angelillo, I.F. Cardiovascular diseases and women: Knowledge, attitudes, and behavior in the general population in Italy. *BioMed Res. Int.* **2015**, *2015*, 324692. [CrossRef] [PubMed]
26. Maffei, S.; Cugusi, L.; Meloni, A.; Deidda, M.; Colasante, E.; Marchioli, R.; Surico, N.; Mercuro, G. IGENDA protocol: Gender differences in awareness, knowledge and perception of cardiovascular risk: An Italian multicenter study. *J. Cardiovasc. Med. (Hagerstown)* **2019**, *20*, 278–283. [CrossRef] [PubMed]
27. World Medical Association Declaration of Helsinki: Ethical principles for medical research involving human subjects. *JAMA* **2013**, *310*, 2191–2194. [CrossRef] [PubMed]
28. Mosca, L.; Hammond, G.; Mochari-Greenberger, H.; Towfighi, A.; Albert, M.A. Fifteen-year trends in awareness of heart disease in women: Results of a 2012 American Heart Association national survey. *Circulation* **2013**, *127*, 1254–1263. [CrossRef] [PubMed]
29. Winham, D.M.; Jones, K.M. Knowledge of young African American adults about heart disease: A cross-sectional survey. *BMC Public Health* **2011**, *11*, 248. [CrossRef]
30. Crouch, R.; Wilson, A. An exploration of rural women's knowledge of heart disease and the association with lifestyle behaviours. *Int. J. Nurs. Pract.* **2011**, *17*, 238–245. [CrossRef] [PubMed]
31. Mazalin Protulipac, J.; Sonicki, Z.; Reiner, Ž. Cardiovascular disease (CVD) risk factors in older adults-Perception and reality. *Arch. Gerontol. Geriatr.* **2015**, *61*, 88–92. [CrossRef]
32. Nicklas, J.M.; Zera, C.A.; Seely, E.W.; Abdul-Rahim, Z.S.; Rudloff, N.D.; Levkoff, S.E. Identifying postpartum intervention approaches to prevent type 2 diabetes in women with a history of gestational diabetes. *BMC Pregnancy Childbirth* **2011**, *11*, 23. [CrossRef]
33. Seely, E.W.; Rich-Edwards, J.; Lui, J.; Nicklas, J.M.; Saxena, A.; Tsigas, E.; Levkoff, S.E. Risk of future cardiovascular disease in women with prior preeclampsia: A focus group study. *BMC Pregnancy Childbirth* **2013**, *13*, 240. [CrossRef] [PubMed]
34. Stanojevic Jerkovic, O.; Sauliune, S.; Sumskas, L.; Birt, C.A.; Kersnik, J. Determinants of self-rated health in elderly populations in urban areas in Slovenia, Lithuania and UK: Findings of the EURO-URHIS 2 survey. *Eur. J. Public Health* **2017**, *27*, 74–79. [CrossRef]
35. Andersen, F.K.; Christensen, K.; Frederiksen, H. Self-rated health and age: A cross-sectional and longitudinal study of 11,000 Danes aged 45—102. *Scand. J. Public Health* **2007**, *35*, 164–171. [CrossRef]
36. Berdahl, T.A.; McQuillan, J. Self-Rated Health Trajectories among Married Americans: Do Disparities Persist over 20 Years? *J. Aging Res.* **2018**, *2018*, 1208598. [CrossRef] [PubMed]
37. Veromaa, V.; Kautiainen, H.; Juonala, M.; Rantanen, A.; Korhonen, P.E. Self-rated health as an indicator of ideal cardiovascular health among working-aged women. *Scand. J. Prim. Health Care* **2017**, *35*, 322–328. [CrossRef]
38. Lichtenstein, S.; Slovic, P.; Fischhoff, B.; Layman, M.; Combs, B. Judged frequency of lethal events. *J. Exp.Psychol. Hum. Learn. Mem.* **1978**, *4*, 551–578. [CrossRef]
39. van der Pligt, J. Risk appraisal and health behaviour. In *Social Psychology and Health: European Perspectives*; Avebury/Ashgate Publishing Co.: Brookfield, VT, USA, 1994; pp. 131–151.

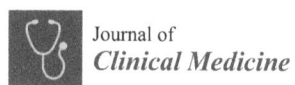 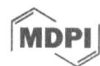

Article

Sex-Specific Risk Factors for Short- and Long-Term Outcomes after Surgery in Patients with Infective Endocarditis

Christine Friedrich [1,*], Mohamed Salem [1], Thomas Puehler [1], Bernd Panholzer [1], Lea Herbers [1], Julia Reimers [1], Lars Hummitzsch [2], Jochen Cremer [1] and Assad Haneya [1]

1 Department of Cardiovascular Surgery, University Hospital Schleswig-Holstein, Campus Kiel, 24105 Kiel, Germany; mohamed.salem@uksh.de (M.S.); thomas.puehler@uksh.de (T.P.); bernd.panholzer@uksh.de (B.P.); lea.herbers@uksh.de (L.H.); julia.reimers@uksh.de (J.R.); jochen.cremer@uksh.de (J.C.); assad.haneya@uksh.de (A.H.)
2 Department of Anaesthesiology and Intensive Care Medicine, University Medical Center Schleswig-Holstein, Campus Kiel, 24105 Kiel, Germany; lars.hummitzsch@uksh.de
* Correspondence: christine.friedrich@uksh.de; Tel.: +49-431-5002-2176

Abstract: (1) Background: Surgery for infective endocarditis (IE) is associated with considerable mortality and it is controversial whether the female gender is predictive for a worse outcome. This large single-center study investigated the impact of sex on outcomes after surgery for IE. (2) Methods: 413 patients (25.4% female) were included into this retrospective observational study. Univariate and multivariable analyses identified sex-specific risk factors for 30 day and late mortality. Survival was estimated by the Kaplan-Meier-method. (3) Results: Women presented more often with mitral valve infection ($p = 0.039$). Men presented more frequently with previous endocarditis ($p = 0.045$), coronary heart disease ($p = 0.033$), and aortic valve infection ($p = 0.005$). Blood transfusion occurred more frequently intraoperatively in women ($p < 0.001$), but postoperatively in men ($p = 0.015$) and men had a longer postoperative stay ($p = 0.046$). Women showed a higher 30 day mortality than men ($p = 0.007$) and female gender was predictive for 30 day mortality (OR 2.090). Late survival showed no sex-specific difference ($p = 0.853$), and the female gender was not an independent predictor for late mortality ($p = 0.718$). Risk factors for early and late mortality showed distinct sex-specific differences such as increased preoperative CRP level in women and culture-negative IE in men.

Keywords: infective endocarditis; sex-specific; gender; risk factors; survival

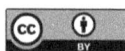

1. Introduction

Infective endocarditis (IE) is a rare but severe disease with a higher incidence in men and a male/female ratio ranging mostly from 1.3:1 to 3:1 in hospital-based studies [1–5]. Though the causes for this sex-specific difference are not fully understood, a higher rate of pre-disposing heart conditions in men [5,6] may contribute to a lower incidence of IE in women.

Early diagnosis and therapy are essential to reduce morbidity and mortality in patients suffering from IE [7]. Surgical treatment was carried out in about 50% of cases in the European infective endocarditis registry [3], but women underwent cardiac surgery for IE less frequently than men in several studies [4,8,9].

Despite major medical advances in diagnostics and therapy, IE is still associated with severe morbidity and a high early mortality of around 20% [3,10,11]. In cases of IE, female gender shows no protective effect, since several studies demonstrate a similar or higher early mortality when compared to men [8,12–15]. The persistently poor overall prognosis regarding hospital mortality is, besides the female gender, attributed to several possible causative factors such as the increase of elderly and more severely ill patients, previous cardiac surgery, an increasing rate of IE in prosthetic heart valves and devices, cerebral complications, renal failure, preoperative ventilation, New York Heart Association heart failure (NYHA) stage, paravalvular abscess, *S. aureus* infection, and withholding of indicated surgery [3,10,12,16]. However, there are controversial implications if the female gender is an independent predictor for mortality after surgery for IE [4,13,16,17]. Older age, a different spectrum of comorbidities, and a lower rate of surgical treatment are discussed as risk factors for a poorer outcome in women [8,9,12]. Sex-specific analysis revealed older age, preoperative dialysis, identification of the endocarditis focus [12], and a poor response to antibiotics [2] as independent risk factors in female patients. Likewise, studies on mid- or long-term outcome provide conflicting results. While some studies revealed a lower survival rate in women [9,12], others found a similar survival rate [18], and in several studies the female gender was no independent predictor for late mortality [8,9,17,19].

Sex-specific subgroup analyses on adjusted risk factors for early and late mortality after surgery for IE are scarce, therefore we analyzed predictors for early and late mortality for women and men separately to detect underlying causes for their different outcomes.

2. Materials and Methods

2.1. Patients and Study Design

This retrospective observational single-center study included 413 consecutive patients ≥ 18 years, 105 (25.4%) women and 308 (74.6%) men, who were operated on for IE between January 2002 and February 2020 in our department.

Pre-, intra-, and post-operative findings of women and men and their risk factors for mortality were analyzed and compared. Data were collected from the institution's database and patient records. The primary endpoints were 30-day mortality and survival during follow-up; secondary endpoints were pre- and peri-operative details, post-operative outcome, and sex-specific risk factors for early and late mortality. All-cause survival during follow-up was obtained by inquiries at the registry offices. The number of patients in the intraoperative course and during the follow-up is shown in Supplementary Figure S1. Active IE was defined as patients receiving antibiotic therapy at the time of admission. The study protocol was approved by the local Ethics Committee and informed patient consent was obtained at primary hospital stay.

Preliminary sub-results of this study without sex-specific risk factor analysis were published in German [20].

2.2. Patient Management

A transthoracic echocardiogram (Vivid E9, General Electric Company, Boston, MA, USA) was performed on every patient, recording the location and size of vegetations, the presence of valve destruction or abscess, as well as left ventricular ejection fraction (LVEF). The antibiotic treatment started immediately after diagnosis of IE and an intravenous treatment regimen was initiated for at least 4–6 weeks independently of the time of surgery. Blood cultures were obtained from all patients to identify the pathogenic organisms and their sensitivities to medical treatment. All patients admitted with stroke underwent brain scan computer tomography to exclude any risk of bleeding prior to surgery and also to get a prognosis for intubated patients and coma patients. A neurologist was consulted to evaluate the neurological findings. The indication for the operation was made after interdisciplinary discussion between cardiologists and cardiac surgeons on the basis of the currently valid guidelines.

2.3. Surgical Procedure

Women and men with IE underwent curative surgery performed exclusively by senior surgeons. Cardiopulmonary bypass was performed by direct cannulation of the ascending aorta. In cases of aortic valve endocarditis, venous drainage was carried out through direct cannulation of the right atrium, while double cannulation of the superior and inferior vena cava was performed in cases of mitral or tricuspid valve endocarditis, with subsequent cross-clamping of ascending aorta. The decision for biological or mechanical prosthesis or valve repair was made depending on the age of the patients, the intraoperative findings, and the extent of valve destruction, as well as the patient's preference and their compliance with long-term anticoagulation. Transesophageal echocardiography (GE Vivid E95, General Electric Company, Boston, MA, USA) was performed for assessment after surgical repair and to control the presence of residual air in the left side of the heart during rewarming. The operative technique has been described in more detail in previous papers [21].

2.4. Statistical Analysis

Pre-, intra-, and post-operative findings of women and men and of 30 day survivors and non-survivors were compared by univariate statistics. Continuous variables were assessed for normal distribution by the Kolmogorov-Smirnov-Test and are presented as median with range or interquartile range as appropriate, and compared by the Mann-Whitney-U-Test. Categorical variables were shown as absolute frequencies (n) and simple percentages and were compared by the Chi-squared or Fisher's exact test as appropriate. Missing data were excluded pairwise and variables with missing data > 5% are indicated in the tables.

Preoperative variables with univariate association to 30 day mortality ($p \leq 0.1$) were assessed for their adjusted impact on early mortality by multivariable logistic regression for the overall group, as well as for women and men separately, with a goodness of fit, described by Cox and Snell R-Squared, of 0.214, 0.377, and 0.231, respectively. Age was categorized as sex-specific according to the highest impact on 30 day mortality. Although EuroSCORE I and II (The European System for Cardiac Operative Risk Evaluation) [22,23] showed a significant association with mortality, we excluded it from the multivariable analyses since it complicated the detection of single risk factors due to multicollinearity. Sex-specific interaction was assessed by logistic regression analysis.

Follow-up outcome was defined as all-cause mortality of patients who survived 30 days postoperatively. Survival was estimated by the Kaplan-Meier method for right censored data and analyzed for sex-specific differences by the log rank-test. Risk factors for mortality during follow-up were assessed by Cox proportional hazards regression with forward selection for the groups separately and then included into the final models. Age of the overall group was categorized to ≥ 65 years for multivariable analysis based on the median value of 64 years.

All tests were conducted as two-sided and a p-value of ≤ 0.05 was assumed to be statistically significant. Statistical analysis was performed using the IBM SPSS Statistics software (version 26.0 and 28.0).

3. Results

The number of patients per year with surgical treatment of infective endocarditis increased over the study period (Figure 1).

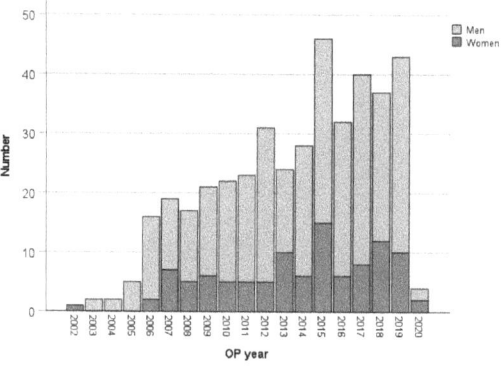

Figure 1. Number of patients during the study period.

3.1. Demographics and Clinical Details of the Study Population

Men were affected almost three times as often as women (74.6 vs. 25.4%, Table 1) and female patients with IE were only slightly older than male patients (65 vs. 64 years, $p = 0.082$). Men presented more often with coronary heart disease (46.3 vs. 34.3%, $p = 0.033$), with previous surgically treated IE (16.6 vs. 8.6%, $p = 0.045$) and with isolated infection of the aortic valve (34.7 vs. 20.0%, $p = 0.005$).

Table 1. Baseline patient characteristics stratified by gender.

Variable	Overall (n = 413)	Men (n = 308, 74.6%)	Women (n = 105, 25.4%)	p-Value
Age, years	64 (52;73)	64 (50;73)	65 (57;75)	0.082
Body mass index (kg/m^2)	25.9 (23.0;29.4)	25.7 (23.0;29.0)	26.1 (23.0;30.8)	0.223
Body mass index > 30 (kg/m^2)	92 (22.4%)	63 (20.6%)	29 (27.6%)	0.136
Logistic EuroSCORE	27.2 (12.5;49.1)	24.8 (11.7;45.6)	35.7 (14.6;53.6)	0.054
EuroSCORE II	12.1 (5.2;27.3)	11.6 (5.0;25.2)	16.3 (6.1;30.8)	0.127
Co-morbidity				
COPD	50 (12.1%)	37 (12.0%)	13 (12.4%)	0.920
Arterial hypertension	240 (58.1%)	177 (57.5%)	63 (60.0%)	0.650
Pulmonary hypertension (>25 mmHg)	86 (20.9%)	60 (19.5%)	26 (25.0%)	0.231
Atrial fibrillation	81 (19.6%)	61 (19.8%)	20 (19.0%)	0.866
Peripheral vascular disease	36 (8.7%)	28 (9.1%)	8 (7.6%)	0.644
Type 1 Diabetes mellitus	3 (0.7%)	2 (0.6%)	1 (1.0%)	1.000
Type 2 Diabetes mellitus	83 (20.1%)	58 (18.8%)	25 (23.8%)	0.272
IDDM	45 (10.9%)	30 (9.7%)	15 (14.3%)	0.197
Hyperlipoproteinemia	116 (28.1%)	82 (26.6%)	34 (32.4%)	0.257
Dialysis (acute and chronic)	45 (10.9%)	32 (10.4%)	13 (12.4%)	0.572
Acute renal insufficiency	53 (12.8%)	42 (13.6%)	11 (10.5%)	0.403
Chronic dialysis preoperative	18 (4.4%)	11 (3.6%)	7 (6.7%)	0.177
Chronic renal insufficiency	116 (28.1%)	92 (29.9%)	24 (22.9%)	0.167
NYHA IV	83 (20.2%)	65 (21.2%)	18 (17.3%)	0.388
Tumor	55 (13.3%)	40 (13.0%)	15 (14.3%)	0.735
Rheumatic disease	23 (5.6%)	16 (5.2%)	7 (6.7%)	0.570
History of liver disease	55 (13.3%)	42 (13.7%)	13 (12.4%)	0.735
Drug abuse	23 (5.6%)	16 (5.2%)	7 (6.7%)	0.570
Smoking [1]	103 (27.8%)	78 (28.4%)	25 (26.0%)	0.662
Immunosuppressive therapy	11 (2.7%)	6 (1.9%)	5 (4.8%)	0.156
Previous endocarditis	60 (14.5%)	51 (16.6%)	9 (8.6%)	**0.045**
LVEF poor (<30)	41 (10.5%)	35 (12.0%)	6 (6.1%)	0.096

Table 1. Cont.

Variable	Overall (n = 413)	Men (n = 308, 74.6%)	Women (n = 105, 25.4%)	p-Value
Coronary heart disease	178 (43.2%)	142 (46.3%)	36 (34.3%)	**0.033**
Single-vessel disease	76 (18.4%)	56 (18.2%)	20 (19.0%)	0.854
Two-vessel-disease	36 (8.7%)	29 (9.4%)	7 (6.7%)	0.384
Three-vessel disease	66 (16.0%)	57 (18.6%)	9 (8.6%)	**0.016**
Previous cardiac surgery	171 (41.4%)	125 (40.6%)	46 (43.8%)	0.562
Previous CABG	9 (2.2%)	7 (2.3%)	2 (1.9%)	1.000
Aortic valve replacement	69 (16.7%)	45 (14.6%)	24 (22.9%)	**0.050**
Mitral valve replacement/resection	6 (1.5%)	4 (1.3%)	2 (1.9%)	0.067
Combined valve surgery	79 (19.1%)	63 (20.5%)	16 (15.2%)	0.241
TAVI	2 (0.5%)	2 (0.6%)	0 (0%)	1.000
Clinical presentation				
Acute myocardial infarction (≤48 h)	14 (3.4%)	11 (3.6%)	3 (2.9%)	1.000
Cardiogenic shock	21 (5.1%)	18 (5.8%)	3 (2.9%)	0.229
CPR (≤48 h)	9 (2.2%)	8 (2.6%)	1 (1.0%)	0.449
Emergency	90 (21.8%)	72 (23.4%)	18 (17.1%)	0.181
Transfer from intensive care unit	109 (26.5%)	80 (26.1%)	29 (27.6%)	0.754
Intubated at admission	38 (9.2%)	29 (9.4%)	9 (8.6%)	0.796
Neurological deficits (TIA or stroke)	81 (19.6%)	55 (17.9%)	26 (24.8%)	0.124
Stroke	76 (18.4%)	53 (17.2%)	23 (21.9%)	0.283
Preoperative embolization	114 (27.6%)	81 (26.3%)	33 (31.4%)	0.310
Embolization of several organs	28 (6.8%)	17 (5.5%)	11 (10.5%)	0.081
Fever (≥38 °C)	270 (66.5%)	206 (68.0%)	64 (62.1%)	0.277
Fever until surgery	63 (15.5%)	48 (15.8%)	15 (14.6%)	0.757
Time from diagnosis to surgery > 7 days	243 (59.3%)	180 (58.8%)	63 (60.6%)	0.753
Time from antibiotic start to surgery				
≤1 day	59 (14.5%)	49 (16.1%)	10 (9.6%)	0.104
2–3 days	38 (9.3%)	23 (7.6%)	15 (14.4%)	**0.038**
4–7 days	47 (11.5%)	39 (12.8%)	8 (7.7%)	0.157
>7 days	264 (64.7%)	193 (63.5%)	71 (68.3%)	0.378
Pathogens				
Staphylococcus aureus	82 (20.0%)	59 (19.3%)	23 (21.9%)	0.562
Enterococcus	61 (14.8%)	48 (15.7%)	13 (12.4%)	0.411
Streptococcus viridans	43 (10.5%)	35 (11.4%)	8 (7.6%)	0.270
Gram-positive streptococcus	37 (9.0%)	26 (8.5%)	11 (10.5%)	0.541

Table 1. Cont.

Variable	Overall (n = 413)	Men (n = 308, 74.6%)	Women (n = 105, 25.4%)	p-Value
HACEK group	1 (0.2%)	1 (0.3%)	0 (0%)	1.000
Mycosis	6 (1.5%)	3 (1.0%)	3 (2.9%)	0.177
Culture negative IE	113 (27.5%)	85 (27.8%)	28 (26.7%)	0.826
Staphylococcus epidermidis	28 (6.8%)	18 (5.9%)	10 (9.5%)	0.201
MRSA	14 (3.4%)	10 (3.3%)	4 (3.8%)	0.760
Affected valves				
Aortic valve endocarditis	168 (40.7%)	137 (44.5%)	31 (29.5%)	**0.007**
Isolated Aortic valve endocarditis	128 (31.0%)	107 (34.7%)	21 (20.0%)	**0.005**
Mitral valve endocarditis	129 (31.2%)	90 (29.2%)	39 (37.1%)	0.130
Isolated Mitral valve endocarditis	92 (22.3%)	61 (19.8%)	31 (29.5%)	**0.039**
Tricuspid valve endocarditis	16 (3.9%)	8 (2.6%)	8 (7.6%)	**0.036**
Isolated Tricuspid valve endocarditis	7 (1.7%)	4 (1.3%)	3 (2.9%)	0.377
Isolated Prosthetic endocarditis	143 (34.6%)	104 (33.8%)	39 (37.1%)	0.530
Paravalvular leak	17 (4.1%)	13 (4.2%)	4 (3.8%)	1.000
Valve insufficiency (at least grade 2)	359 (87.3%)	267 (87.3%)	92 (87.6%)	0.923
Aortic valve	108 (26.3%)	87 (28.4%)	21 (20.0%)	0.090
Mitral valve	78 (19.0%)	55 (18.0%)	23 (21.9%)	0.375
Tricuspid valve	8 (1.9%)	3 (1.0%)	5 (4.8%)	**0.029**
Peri-annular abscess	113 (27.8%)	81 (26.6%)	32 (31.1%)	0.386
Vegetation	285 (70.4%)	209 (69.2%)	76 (73.8%)	0.309
Preoperative laboratory results				
C-reactive protein (mg/L)	42.7 (16.4;90.5)	43.5 (19.3;91.1)	41.2 (13.6;88.2)	0.565

Significant p-values are indicated in bold. Quantitative data are presented as median with 25th and 75th percentiles, while categorical data are presented as number of patients (n) with percentage (%). Missing values > 5%: [1] 10.2% missing. European System for Cardiac Operative Risk Evaluation is abbreviated to EuroSCORE, chronic obstructive pulmonary disease to COPD, insulin dependent diabetes mellitus to IDDM, New York Heart Association heart failure stage to NYHA, left ventricular ejection fraction to LVEF, Coronary artery bypass grafting to CABG, transcatheter aortic valve implantation to TAVI, cardiopulmonary resuscitation to CPR, transient ischemic attack to TIA, *Haemophilus, Aggregatibacter, Cardiobacterium, Eikenella, Kingella* to HACEK, methicillin-resistant *Staphylococcus aureus* to MRSA.

Women presented more often with previous aortic valve replacement (22.9 vs. 14.6%, $p = 0.050$), isolated infection of the mitral valve (29.5 vs. 19.8%, $p = 0.039$), and of the tricuspid valve combined with infection of other valves (7.6 vs. 2.6%, $p = 0.036$). A significant association was shown between preoperative embolization and neurological complications preoperative for both women and men (Chi^2 $p < 0.001$).

Intraoperatively, no significant sex-specific differences regarding procedural times were observed, but women received more blood transfusions (red blood cell concentrates, 4 (0–14) vs. 2 (0–27), $p < 0.001$). Men more often underwent aortic valve surgery (78.1 vs. 62.9%, $p = 0.002$), had a higher need for blood transfusion postoperatively (2 (0–27) vs. 2 (0–17), $p = 0.015$), and a longer postoperative stay (10 vs. 9 days, $p = 0.046$; Tables 2 and 3). In-hospital mortality tended to be higher in women (22.3 vs. 14.7%, $p = 0.070$), while 30 day mortality was significantly higher when compared to mortality in men (26.7 vs. 14.9%, $p = 0.007$).

Table 2. Operative data stratified by gender.

Variable	Overall (n = 413)	Men (n = 308, 74.6%)	Women (n = 105, 25.4%)	p-Value
Length of surgery (min)	273 (220;355)	274 (224;357)	271 (216;337)	0.411
Cardiopulmonary bypass time (min)	166 (125;215)	166 (126;214)	166 (121;219)	0.879
Cross-clamp time (min)	116 (86;156)	115 (86;157)	116 (83;144)	0.433
Circulatory arrest (min)	0 (0–36)	0 (0–36)	0 (0–32)	0.520
Number of packed red blood cells (unit)	3 (0–27)	2 (0–27)	4 (0–14)	**<0.001**
Number of fresh frozen plasma (unit)	0 (0–13)	0 (0–13)	0 (0–12)	0.900
Number of platelet concentrate (unit)	1 (0–6)	1 (0–6)	1 (0–4)	0.143
Aortic valve surgery	305 (74.2%)	239 (78.1%)	66 (62.9%)	**0.002**
Mitral valve surgery	155 (37.7%)	110 (35.9%)	45 (42.9%)	0.207
Tricuspid valve surgery	15 (3.6%)	8 (2.6%)	7 (6.7%)	0.070
Thoracic aortic surgery	55 (13.4%)	43 (14.1%)	12 (11.5%)	0.509
CABG	49 (11.9%)	37 (12.1%)	12 (11.4%)	0.856

Significant p-values are indicated in bold. Quantitative data are presented as median with 25th and 75th percentiles, while categorical data are presented as number of patients (n) with percentage (%).

Table 3. Postoperative data and outcomes stratified by gender.

Variable	Overall (n = 413)	Men (n = 308, 74.6%)	Women (n = 105, 25.4%)	p-Value
AKI KDIGO stages	115 (29.3%)	85 (29.2%)	30 (29.4%)	0.969
New–onset of hemodialysis	61 (15.6%)	46 (15.8%)	15 (14.9%)	0.819
24 h-drainage loss (mL)	600 (300;1100)	650 (388;1150)	510 (250;1060)	0.123
Rethoracotomy (bleeding/tamponade)	50 (12.4%)	40 (13.3%)	10 (9.7%)	0.341
Number of packed red blood cells (unit) [1]	2 (0–27)	2 (0–27)	2 (0–17)	**0.015**
Number of fresh frozen plasma, (unit) [1]	0 (0–35)	0 (0–35)	0 (0–32)	0.269
Number of platelet concentrate, (unit) [1]	0 (0–9)	0 (0–8)	0 (0–9)	0.357
Ventilation time (h)	16 (9;45)	16 (9;44)	16 (9;55)	0.801
Reintubation	49 (12.3%)	33 (11.1%)	16 (15.7%)	0.220
Tracheotomy	57 (14.5%)	47 (16.2%)	10 (9.9%)	0.125
ICU time (d)	3 (1;7)	3 (1;7)	3 (1;6)	0.245
Postoperative days (d)	10 (7;16)	10 (7;17)	9 (5;15)	**0.046**
Postoperative delirium	64 (16.1%)	54 (18.2%)	10 (10.0%)	0.054
Stroke	18 (4.5%)	11 (3.7%)	7 (6.9%)	0.265
CPR	22 (5.5%)	17 (5.7%)	5 (4.9%)	0.759

Table 3. Cont.

Variable	Overall (n = 413)	Men (n = 308, 74.6%)	Women (n = 105, 25.4%)	p-Value
Pacemaker patient	47 (11.6%)	37 (12.2%)	10 (9.8%)	0.511
Postoperative myocardial infarction	5 (1.3%)	4 (1.3%)	1 (1.0%)	1.000
Bronchopulmonary infection	45 (11.1%)	36 (11.8%)	9 (8.9%)	0.422
Sepsis	54 (13.3%)	40 (13.1%)	14 (13.9%)	0.839
Sternal wound infection [2]	9 (2.5%)	8 (2.9%)	1 (1.1%)	0.694
Hospital mortality	68 (16.6%)	45 (14.7%)	23 (22.3%)	0.070
Cardiac death	10 (14.3%)	6 (13.3%)	4 (16.0%)	0.737
Cerebral death	1 (1.4%)	1 (2.2%)	0 (0%)	1.000
Sepsis	9 (12.9%)	5 (11.1%)	4 (16.0%)	0.712
MOF	50 (71.4%)	33 (73.3%)	17 (68.0%)	0.636
30 day mortality	74 (17.9%)	46 (14.9%)	28 (26.7%)	**0.007**
Survival/follow-up time (years)	3.9 (1.2;7.7)	3.7 (1.1;7.8)	4.6 (1.4;7.8)	0.535

Significant p-values are indicated in bold. Quantitative data are presented as median with 25th and 75th percentiles, while categorical data are presented as number of patients (n) with percentage (%). Missing values > 5%: [1] Number of blood products given within 48 hr postoperatively, 5.8% missing, [2] 11.1% missing. AKI is abbreviated to acute kidney injury, Kidney Disease: Improving Global Outcomes to KDIGO, intensive care unit to ICU, cardiopulmonary resuscitation to CPR, multiple organ failure to MOF.

3.2. Univariate Association to 30-Day Mortality

Though being without significance in the total group, sex-specific analyses revealed a significant association for pulmonary hypertension, diabetes mellitus Type 1 and 2, embolization of several organs, time from antibiotic start to surgery < 7 days, culture negative IE, and combined surgery in the male group. Only in the female group did peripheral arterial disease (PAD) show a significant association to 30 day mortality, which was confirmed by interaction analysis (Supplementary Table S1). A univariate subgroup analysis based on the overall cohort revealed that culture-negative cases had an antibiotic treatment before surgery > 7 days (62 (55.9%) less frequently when compared to culture-positive cases (202 (68.2%), p = 0.020). Additional sex-specific association is shown in Table S1.

3.3. Independent Predictors for 30 Day Mortality

In the overall group, female gender was an independent predictor for 30 day mortality (Table 4). Acute or chronic dialysis was revealed as a risk factor for early mortality in women and men. In women only, age ≥ 65 years, preoperative transfer from the intensive care unit (ICU), and increased C-reactive protein (CRP) level were risk factors. In men, age ≥ 70 years, body mass index (BMI), pulmonary hypertension, NYHA IV, cardiogenic shock, fever until surgery, culture negative IE, abscess, and embolization of several organs were predictors for early mortality.

Table 4. Independent preoperative risk factors for 30 day mortality.

Risk Factors Group	Odds Ratio Overall	95% CI	p-Value	Odds Ratio Men	95% CI	p-Value	Odds Ratio Women	95% CI	p-Value
Age (years)	1.036	1.010–1.063	0.006						
Age ≥ 65 years							4.921	1.048–23.099	0.043
Age ≥ 70 years				2.836	1.265–6.357	0.011			
Female gender	2.090	1.077–4.053	0.029						
Body mass index				1.104	1.026–1.189	0.008			
PH				3.500	1.440–8.508	0.006			
Dialysis				5.943	2.019–17.494	0.001	6.974	1.133–42.922	0.036
NYHA IV	2.719	1.344–5.500	0.005	3.108	1.344–7.189	0.008			
Cardiogenic shock	3.415	1.027–11.350	0.045	9.083	2.418–34.112	0.001			
Stroke	2.664	1.281–5.543	0.009						
Transfer from ICU							10.086	1.791–56.806	0.009
AV insufficiency	0.341	0.133–0.879	0.026						
Fever until surgery				2.828	1.030–7.768	0.044			
Culture negative				2.661	1.161–6.100	0.021			
Abscess	2.513	1.332–4.742	0.004	2.570	1.075–6.142	0.034			
CRP (mg/L)	1.008	1.003–1.012	0.001				1.012	1.002–1.022	0.021
AV endocarditis							0.041	0.004–0.432	0.007
Embolization				4.678	1.032–21.194	0.045			

Pulmonary hypertension > 25 mm Hg is abbreviated to PH, New York heart association heart failure stage to NYHA, intensive care unit to ICU, Aortic valve to AV, C-reactive protein to CRP. Dialysis = Acute and chronic dialysis, Embolization = Embolization of several organs.

3.4. Survival Analysis

Median follow-up time was 3.9 (1.2; 7.7) years. Crude survival showed no sex-specific difference (p = 0.853, Figure 2) and women and men showed a cumulative survival of 82% vs. 72%. after 5 years and 61% in both groups after 8 years.

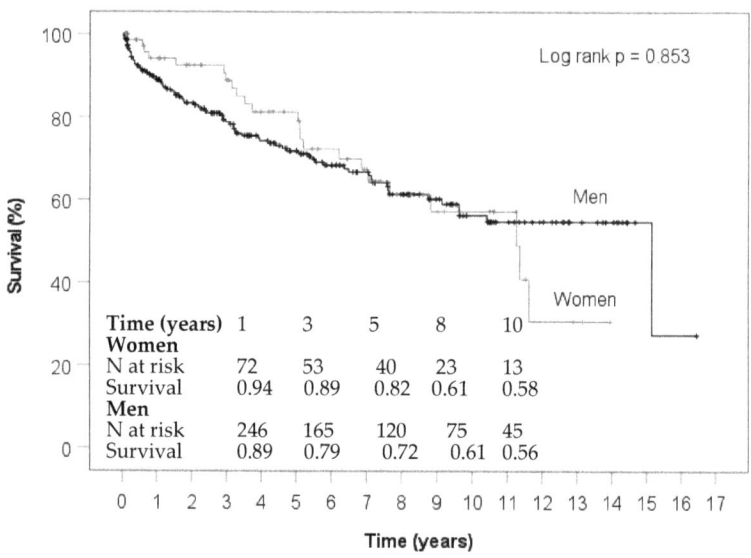

Figure 2. Survival of women and men during follow-up.

3.5. Risk Factors for Long-Term Survival

Female gender did not prove to be a risk factor for mortality during follow-up (p = 0.718, Table 5).

Table 5. Independent preoperative risk factors for mortality during follow-up.

Risk Factors Group	Hazard Ratio Overall	95% CI	p-Value	Hazard Ratio Men	95% CI	p-Value	Hazard Ratio Women	95% CI	p-Value
Age ≥ 65 years	2.198	1.385–3.488	<0.001	1.921 *	1.287–2.868	0.001	2.066	1.056–4.040	0.034
Female gender	1.097	0.662–1.820	0.718						
AHT				1.685	1.076–2.637	0.022			
NYHA IV							4.192	1.954–8.993	<0.001
Poor LVEF (<30%)	1.945	1.000–3.783	0.050	2.166	1.342–3.497	0.002			
PAD	2.515	1.291–4.900	0.007	1.795	1.023–3.152	0.041			
CAD stage 3							4.040	1.633–9.994	0.003
Dialysis	2.186	1.102–4.338	0.025	1.926	1.145–3.241	0.014	3.383	1.317–8.688	0.011
Combined surgery	2.223	1.236–3.998	0.008	1.709	1.054–2.770	0.030			
Cardiogenic shock				3.601	1.803–7.189	<0.001			
Emergency							5.850	2.439–14.032	<0.001
Diagnosis > 7 days							2.902	1.341–6.282	0.007
Stroke				2.165	1.334–3.516	0.002			
Tumor				1.687	1.014–2.808	0.044			
Liver disease	1.912	1.090–3.355	0.024	2.114	1.310–3.413	0.002			
S. viridans				0.336	0.123–0.924	0.035			
S. epidermidis							4.878	1.680–14.160	0.004
AV endocarditis							0.300	0.123–0.734	0.008
Abscess				1.561	1.038–2.348	0.032			
CRP (mg/L)							1.006	1.001–1.010	0.018

Peripheral arterial disease is abbreviated to PAD, Arterial hypertension to AHT, New York heart association heart failure stage to NYHA, Coronary heart disease to CAD, *Streptococcus viridans* to *S. viridans*, *Staphylococcus epidermidis* to *S. epidermidis*, Aortic valve to AV, C-reactive protein to CRP, Dialysis = Acute and chronic dialysis, Combined surgery = Combined valve surgery, Diagnosis > 7 days = Diagnosis until surgery > 7 days. * Age in the male group was categorized to ≥ 70 years.

The Cox regression revealed sex-specific risk factors for late mortality. Age ≥ 70 years, arterial hypertension, LVEF < 30%, PAD, combined valve surgery, cardiogenic shock, preoperative stroke, tumor, liver disease, and abscess were identified as risk factors in the male group. Risk factors in the female group were age ≥ 65 years, NYHA IV, coronary three-vessel disease, emergency admission, diagnosis until surgery > 7 days, Staphylococcus epidermidis as a pathogenic microorganism, and preoperatively increased CRP (mg/L) level, while preoperative acute or chronic dialysis was evident in both groups.

4. Discussion

In this study, women showed a considerably higher early mortality when compared to men and the female gender was an independent predictor for 30 day mortality, while no significant difference was observed regarding mortality during follow-up. Independent risk factors for early and late mortality showed substantial sex-specific differences and differed strikingly from the results of the overall group.

In contrast to the review of Slipczuk et al. 2013 [10], who found a proportional increase in male IE patients from the 1970s to the 2000s, we could not show a further temporal trend in the male/female ratio during our study period from 2002 to 2020. The proportion of our surgically treated female patients was 25.4%, which is lower than 31.1% in the European infective endocarditis registry, which also included non-surgically treated patients [3]. This points to an underlying lower rate of referral to cardiac surgery in our female patients, a finding already described in several recent studies [3,9,13,15].

In contrast to previous findings [8,9,12,14], female patients in our study were not distinctly older and did not present with more comorbid conditions when compared to men. As shown in previous studies [9,13,17], IE affected the aortic valve in men most frequently, while in female patients, a predominant affection of the mitral valve was found.

Risk stratification by logistic EuroSCORE and EuroSCORE II showed a tendency towards a higher postoperative risk in female patients. However, particularly EuroSCORE II did not adequately predict the considerably higher mortality in women when compared to men. The EuroSCORE includes female gender as a risk factor, but it is based on a mixed female and male population and therefore does not take into account the different weighting of risk factors in men and women identified in previous studies [2,12] and confirmed by our results.

Despite comparable intraoperative procedural times, women received more blood transfusions than men. Higher transfusion rates and lower preoperative hemoglobin levels in women were already described for cardiac surgery [24,25], and may explain the observed intraoperative discrepancy in our study. Men tended to develop a delirium more often than women, as we already observed at aortic surgery [26]. This is in line with the findings of Wang et al. that male gender is an important predictor for postoperative delirium following cardiac surgery [27]. Moreover, red blood cell transfusion, which was more frequent in our male patients postoperatively, was shown to be an important initiating risk factor for delirium after cardiac surgery in a review by Koster et al. [28], as well as the association with prolonged postoperative stay in our male patients [29].

The overall early mortality of 17.9% in our study was comparable to the 17% mortality reported in the European endocarditis registry [3] and 17.2% mortality after surgery for IE of the aortic valve [12]. Women in our study experienced a significantly higher early mortality when compared to men as demonstrated previously [12,13,17]. However, in contrast to these studies, we found no major sex-specific differences regarding baseline clinical presentation, comorbidities, or pathogenic organisms that could explain the poorer outcome in women, but rather a gender-specific impact of risk factors, as the univariate and multivariable analysis indicated.

Weber et al. [17] stated that the severity of presentation, but not female gender, accounts for a worse outcome after IE. Contrary to their results, which included also postoperative factors and EuroSCORE II, female sex proved to be an independent predictor for early mortality in our study on preoperative predictors, confirming previous results [4,12,16]. The multivariable analysis, moreover, revealed distinct sex-specific predictors for early mortality. In female patients, an age ≥ 65 years, dialysis, preoperative transfer from the ICU, and increased CRP level were predictive. Elevated baseline CRP levels were predictive for early mortality after IE in a prospective hospital-based analysis [30], however, it was a risk factor only in our female surgical patients. Dialysis was shown to be a risk factor in women [12], but was confirmed by our study as being a risk for both genders as demonstrated recently [2]. A predominant affection of the mitral valve as identified in our female patients may be associated with a lower referral to early valve surgery in women [19], whereas affection of the aortic valve was identified as predictor for early valve surgery [19]. The protective effect of aortic valve IE identified in our female patients may support this theory of a possible earlier referral of women with aortic valve IE in a less severe preoperative condition. However, this observation should be further clarified. Only in the male group, age ≥ 70 years, BMI, pulmonary hypertension, and factors related to severity of IE, namely, fever until surgery, embolization of several organs, and culture-negative IE, were risk factors for 30 day mortality. The frequency of culture-negative IE was similar in women and men in our study but was overall higher (27.5%) when compared to the findings of the European endocarditis registry, which reports a frequency of 21% [3]. A recent study by Salsano et al. [31] showed that culture-negative IE is associated with a significantly higher adjusted postoperative risk for early mortality. Culture-negative IE may complicate treatment and result in a worse outcome, as observed in our male patients.

Unadjusted all-cause survival was similar between genders. Once the critical early period is overcome, women and men therefore seemed to have a comparable prognosis, as also shown in a previous hospital-based study [18]. In contrast, Dohmen et al. [12] and Weber et al. [17] found a significantly worse survival after surgery for IE in women when compared to men during a 12 year and a 1.76 year follow-up, respectively. A higher age and more severe degree of IE may explain the worse outcome in in these studies.

Previous studies demonstrated that female gender was not an independent predictor for mid-term and long-term mortality [8,9,17,19], which was confirmed by our analysis. Our multivariable analysis revealed distinct gender-specific risk factors for mortality during follow-up, except for age and preoperative dialysis, which were identified as risk factors in both genders, confirming the results of Dohmen et al. [12]. The meta-analysis of Liang et al. [32] indicated that a surgical treatment within one week after diagnosis was associated with lower in-hospital mortality; however, a time interval > 7 days was an independent predictor for follow-up mortality in female patients in our study, but not for early mortality, and, moreover, it did not prove as a risk factor for male patients.

This study has several limitations. The retrospective single-center design carries a possible risk for unknown confounders due to unregistered variables. The limited sample size of the female cohort decreases the statistical power and may have impaired the detection of risk factors in the female group.

5. Conclusions

Female gender was an independent predictor for 30 day mortality but not for late mortality after surgical treatment of IE. Striking differences regarding sex-specific risk factors indicate that analyses of a mixed male and female cohort may overlook important risk factors. The higher risk for early postoperative mortality in women should not per se lead to avoidance of surgical therapy in women, as surgical treatment was shown to be a protective factor against early mortality in IE in previous studies. Consideration of sex-specific risk factors in prevention, interdisciplinary diagnosis, therapy, and an early postoperative course, such as preoperative elevated CRP level and interval from diagnosis to surgery in female patients, as well as the potential risk of culture-negative IE in male patients, may improve outcomes in women and men.

Supplementary Materials: The following supporting information can be downloaded at: https://www.mdpi.com/article/10.3390/jcm11071875/s1, Table S1: Pre- and intraoperative characteristics associated with 30-day mortality ($p \leq 0.1$), Figure S1: Flow chart of case numbers over the course of the study.

Author Contributions: Conceptualization, C.F., M.S. and A.H.; methodology, C.F., M.S., L.H. (Lea Herbers), J.R. and A.H.; software, not applicable; validation, M.S., T.P., B.P., L.H. (Lars Hummitzsch) and A.H.; formal analysis, C.F.; investigation, C.F. and A.H.; resources, A.H. and J.C.; data curation, C.F., M.S., L.H. (Lea Herbers) and J.R.; writing—original draft preparation, C.F.; writing—review and editing, all authors; visualization, C.F.; supervision, A.H. and J.C.; project administration, C.F. and A.H.; funding acquisition, C.F. All authors have read and agreed to the published version of the manuscript.

Funding: We acknowledge financial support by DFG within the funding programme Open Access-Publikationskosten.

Institutional Review Board Statement: This retrospective single-centre cohort study was conducted in accordance with the Declaration of Helsinki (as revised in 2013) and approved by the local ethics committee of Christian-Albrechts University of Kiel (No. D458/20).

Informed Consent Statement: Written informed consent was obtained from all subjects involved in the study.

Data Availability Statement: The data presented in this study are available on request from the corresponding author.

Conflicts of Interest: The authors declare no conflict of interest.

References

1. Cresti, A.; Chiavarelli, M.; Scalese, M.; Nencioni, C.; Valentini, S.; Guerrini, F.; D'Aiello, I.; Picchi, A.; De Sensi, F.; Habib, G. Epidemiological and mortality trends in infective endocarditis, a 17-year population-based prospective study. *Cardiovasc. Diagn. Ther.* **2017**, *7*, 27–35. [CrossRef] [PubMed]
2. Elamragy, A.A.; Meshaal, M.S.; El-Kholy, A.A.; Rizk, H.H. Gender differences in clinical features and complications of infective endocarditis: 11-year experience of a single institute in Egypt. *Egypt. Heart J.* **2020**, *72*, 5. [CrossRef] [PubMed]
3. Habib, G.; Erba, P.A.; Iung, B.; Donal, E.; Cosyns, B.; Laroche, C.; Popescu, B.A.; Prendergast, B.; Tornos, P.; Sadeghpour, A.; et al. Clinical presentation, aetiology and outcome of infective endocarditis. Results of the ESC-EORP EURO-ENDO (European infective endocarditis) registry: A prospective cohort study. *Eur. Heart J.* **2019**, *40*, 3222–3232. [CrossRef] [PubMed]

4. Sousa, C.; Nogueira, P.; Pinto, F.J. Insight into the epidemiology of infective endocarditis in Portugal: A contemporary nationwide study from 2010 to 2018. *BMC Cardiovasc. Disord.* **2021**, *21*, 138. [CrossRef] [PubMed]
5. Ahtela, E.; Oksi, J.; Porela, P.; Ekström, T.; Rautava, P.; Kytö, V. Trends in occurrence and 30-day mortality of infective endocarditis in adults: Population-based registry study in Finland. *BMJ Open* **2019**, *9*, e026811. [CrossRef]
6. Thornhill, M.H.; Jones, S.; Prendergast, B.; Baddour, L.M.; Chambers, J.B.; Lockhart, P.B.; Dayer, M.J. Quantifying infective endocarditis risk in patients with predisposing cardiac conditions. *Eur. Heart J.* **2018**, *39*, 586–595. [CrossRef]
7. Rajani, R.; Klein, J.L. Infective endocarditis: A contemporary update. *Clin. Med.* **2020**, *20*, 31–35. [CrossRef]
8. Aksoy, O.; Meyer, L.T.; Cabell, C.H.; Kourany, W.M.; Pappas, P.A.; Sexton, D.J. Gender differences in infective endocarditis: Pre- and co-morbid conditions lead to different management and outcomes in female patients. *Scand. J. Infect. Dis.* **2007**, *39*, 101–107. [CrossRef]
9. Sambola, A.; Fernández-Hidalgo, N.; Almirante, B.; Roca, I.; González-Alujas, T.; Serra, B.; Pahissa, A.; García-Dorado, D.; Tornos, P. Sex differences in native-valve infective endocarditis in a single tertiary-care hospital. *Am. J. Cardiol.* **2010**, *106*, 92–98. [CrossRef]
10. Slipczuk, L.; Codolosa, J.N.; Davila, C.D.; Romero-Corral, A.; Yun, J.; Pressman, G.S.; Figueredo, V.M. Infective endocarditis epidemiology over five decades: A systematic review. *PLoS ONE* **2013**, *8*, e82665. [CrossRef]
11. Vincent, L.L.; Otto, C.M. Infective Endocarditis: Update on Epidemiology, Outcomes, and Management. *Curr. Cardiol. Rep.* **2018**, *20*, 86. [CrossRef]
12. Dohmen, P.M.; Binner, C.; Mende, M.; Daviewala, P.; Etz, C.D.; Borger, M.A.; Misfeld, M.; Eifert, S.; Mohr, F.W. Gender-Based Long-Term Surgical Outcome in Patients with Active Infective Aortic Valve Endocarditis. *Med. Sci. Monit.* **2016**, *22*, 2520–2527. [CrossRef]
13. Varela Barca, L.; Vidal-Bonnet, L.; Fariñas, M.C.; Muñoz, P.; Valerio Minero, M.; de Alarcón, A.; Gutiérrez Carretero, E.; Gutiérrez Cuadra, M.; Moreno Camacho, A.; Kortajarena Urkola, X.; et al. Analysis of sex differences in the clinical presentation, management and prognosis of infective endocarditis in Spain. *Heart* **2021**, *107*, 1717–1724. [CrossRef]
14. Polishchuk, I.; Stavi, V.; Awesat, J.; Ben Baruch Golan, Y.; Bartal, C.; Sagy, I.; Jotkowitz, A.; Barski, L. Sex Differences in Infective Endocarditis. *Am. J. Med. Sci.* **2021**, *361*, 83–89. [CrossRef]
15. van den Brink, F.S.; Swaans, M.J.; Hoogendijk, M.G.; Alipour, A.; Kelder, J.C.; Jaarsma, W.; Eefting, F.D.; Groenmeijer, B.; Kupper, A.J.F.; Ten Berg, J.M. Increased incidence of infective endocarditis after the 2009 European Society of Cardiology guideline update: A nationwide study in the Netherlands. *Eur. Heart J. Qual. Care Clin. Outcomes* **2017**, *3*, 141–147. [CrossRef]
16. Varela Barca, L.; Navas Elorza, E.; Fernández-Hidalgo, N.; Moya Mur, J.L.; Muriel García, A.; Fernández-Felix, B.M.; Miguelena Hycka, J.; Rodríguez-Roda, J.; López-Menéndez, J. Prognostic factors of mortality after surgery in infective endocarditis: Systematic review and meta-analysis. *Infection* **2019**, *47*, 879–895. [CrossRef]
17. Weber, C.; Gassa, A.; Rokohl, A.; Sabashnikov, A.; Deppe, A.C.; Eghbalzadeh, K.; Merkle, J.; Hamacher, S.; Liakopoulos, O.J.; Wahlers, T. Severity of Presentation, Not Sex, Increases Risk of Surgery for Infective Endocarditis. *Ann. Thorac. Surg.* **2019**, *107*, 1111–1117. [CrossRef]
18. Castillo, J.C.; Anguita, M.P.; Delgado, M.; Ruiz, M.; Mesa, D.; Romo, E.; Crespín, M.; García, D.; Arizón, J.M.; Suárez de Lezo, J. Clinical characteristics and prognosis of infective endocarditis in women. *Rev. Esp. Cardiol.* **2008**, *61*, 36–40. [CrossRef]
19. Curlier, E.; Hoen, B.; Alla, F.; Selton-Suty, C.; Schubel, L.; Doco-Lecompte, T.; Minary, L.; Erpelding, M.L.; Duval, X.; Chirouze, C. Relationships between sex, early valve surgery and mortality in patients with left-sided infective endocarditis analysed in a population-based cohort study. *Heart* **2014**, *100*, 1173–1178. [CrossRef]
20. Friedrich, C.; Salem, M.; Panholzer, B.; Cremer, J.; Haneya, A. Geschlechtsspezifische Ergebnisse nach operativer Therapie bei infektiöser Endokarditis. *CHAZ* **2021**, *22*, 35–39.
21. Salem, M.; Friedrich, C.; Saad, M.; Frank, D.; Salem, M.; Puehler, T.; Schoettler, J.; Schoeneich, F.; Cremer, J.; Haneya, A. Active Infective Native and Prosthetic Valve Endocarditis: Short- and Long-Term Outcomes of Patients after Surgical Treatment. *J. Clin. Med.* **2021**, *10*, 1868. [CrossRef] [PubMed]
22. Roques, F.; Michel, P.; Goldstone, A.R.; Nashef, S.A. The logistic EuroSCORE. *Eur. Heart J.* **2003**, *24*, 881–882. [CrossRef]
23. Nashef, S.A.; Roques, F.; Sharples, L.D.; Nilsson, J.; Smith, C.; Goldstone, A.R.; Lockowandt, U. EuroSCORE II. *Eur. J. Cardiothorac. Surg.* **2012**, *41*, 734–744, discussion 744–745. [CrossRef] [PubMed]
24. Blaudszun, G.; Munting, K.E.; Butchart, A.; Gerrard, C.; Klein, A.A. The association between borderline pre-operative anaemia in women and outcomes after cardiac surgery: A cohort study. *Anaesthesia* **2018**, *73*, 572–578. [CrossRef]
25. Faerber, G.; Zacher, M.; Reents, W.; Boergermann, J.; Kappert, U.; Boening, A.; Diegeler, A.; Doenst, T. Female sex is not a risk factor for post procedural mortality in coronary bypass surgery in the elderly: A secondary analysis of the GOPCABE trial. *PLoS ONE* **2017**, *12*, e0184038. [CrossRef]
26. Friedrich, C.; Salem, M.A.; Puehler, T.; Hoffmann, G.; Lutter, G.; Cremer, J.; Haneya, A. Sex-specific risk factors for early mortality and survival after surgery of acute aortic dissection type a: A retrospective observational study. *J. Cardiothorac. Surg.* **2020**, *15*, 145. [CrossRef]
27. Wang, H.; Guo, X.; Zhu, X.; Li, Y.; Jia, Y.; Zhang, Z.; Yuan, S.; Yan, F. Gender Differences and Postoperative Delirium in Adult Patients Undergoing Cardiac Valve Surgery. *Front. Cardiovasc. Med.* **2021**, *8*, 751421. [CrossRef]
28. Koster, S.; Hensens, A.G.; Schuurmans, M.J.; van der Palen, J. Risk factors of delirium after cardiac surgery: A systematic review. *Eur. J. Cardiovasc. Nurs.* **2011**, *10*, 197–204. [CrossRef]
29. Kumar, A.K.; Jayant, A.; Arya, V.K.; Magoon, R.; Sharma, R. Delirium after cardiac surgery: A pilot study from a single tertiary referral center. *Ann. Card. Anaesth.* **2017**, *20*, 76–82.
30. Mohanan, S.; Gopalan Nair, R.; Vellani, H.; Sajeev, C.G.; George, B.; Krishnan, M.N. Baseline C-reactive protein levels and prognosis in patients with infective endocarditis: A prospective cohort study. *Indian Heart J.* **2018**, *70* (Suppl. 3), S43–S49. [CrossRef]

31. Salsano, A.; Giacobbe, D.R.; Del Puente, F.; Natali, R.; Miette, A.; Moscatelli, S.; Perocchio, G.; Scarano, F.; Porto, I.; Mariscalco, G.; et al. Culture-negative infective endocarditis (CNIE): Impact on postoperative mortality. *Open Med.* **2020**, *15*, 571–579. [CrossRef]
32. Liang, F.; Song, B.; Liu, R.; Yang, L.; Tang, H.; Li, Y. Optimal timing for early surgery in infective endocarditis: A meta-analysis. *Interact Cardiovasc Thorac. Surg.* **2016**, *22*, 336–345. [CrossRef]

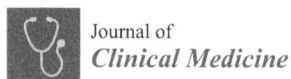

Article

Differences in Sex and the Incidence and In-Hospital Mortality among People Admitted for Infective Endocarditis in Spain, 2016–2020

Jose M. De Miguel-Yanes [1], Rodrigo Jimenez-Garcia [2,*], Javier De Miguel-Diez [3], Valentin Hernández-Barrera [4], David Carabantes-Alarcon [2], Jose J. Zamorano-Leon [2], Concepción Noriega [5] and Ana Lopez-de-Andres [2]

[1] Internal Medicine Department, Hospital General Universitario Gregorio Marañón, Universidad Complutense de Madrid, Instituto de Investigación Sanitaria Gregorio Marañón (IiSGM), 28007 Madrid, Spain
[2] Department of Public Health and Maternal & Child Health, Faculty of Medicine, Universidad Complutense de Madrid, 28040 Madrid, Spain
[3] Respiratory Care Department, Hospital General Universitario Gregorio Marañón, Universidad Complutense de Madrid, Instituto de Investigación Sanitaria Gregorio Marañón (IiSGM), 28007 Madrid, Spain
[4] Preventive Medicine and Public Health Teaching and Research Unit, Health Sciences Faculty, Universidad Rey Juan Carlos, 28922 Alcorcón, Spain
[5] Department of Nursery and Physiotherapy, Faculty of Medicine and Health Sciences, University of Alcalá, 28801 Alcalá de Henares, Spain
* Correspondence: rodrijim@ucm.es

Abstract: (1) Background: A description of the trends and outcomes during hospitalization for infective endocarditis (IE) according to sex. (2) Methods: Using Spanish national hospital discharge data (2016–2020), we built Poisson regression models to compare the age-adjusted time trends for the incidence rate. We used propensity score matching (PSM) to compare the clinical characteristics and the in-hospital mortality (IHM) between men and women hospitalized with IE. (3) Results: We identified 10,459 hospitalizations for IE (33.26% women). The incidence of IE remained stable during this five-year period. The age-adjusted incidence of IE was two-fold higher among men vs. women (IRR = 2.08; 95%CI 2.0–2.17). Before PSM, women with IE were significantly older than men (70.25 vs. 66.24 years; $p < 0.001$) and had lower comorbidity according to the Charlson comorbidity index (mean 1.38 vs. 1.43; $p = 0.019$). After PSM, the IHM among women admitted for IE remained >3 points higher than that among men (19.52% vs. 15.98%; $p < 0.001$). (4) Conclusions: The incidence of IE was two-fold higher among men than among women. IHM was significantly higher among women after accounting for the potential confounders.

Keywords: infective endocarditis; sex; heart valve surgery; comorbidities; in-hospital mortality

1. Introduction

Infective endocarditis (IE) has classically been associated with a grim prognosis, with an in-hospital mortality (IHM) ranging from 11% to 20% [1,2]. A deeper understanding of the factors that contribute to worsening the outcomes could inform clinical decisions to improve the management of the patients admitted to the hospital for IE.

Some authors have claimed that sex plays a role in the outcome of patients admitted for IE [3]. Beyond the distinct biological factors possibly underlying sex-related disparities in the host response to the infection, gender could influence patients' and doctors' behaviors and thus modify the clinical course of the disease [4]. For instance, lower rates of heart valve replacement surgery among women have been reported during hospitalization for IE [5].

Older research from our country found that the female sex is associated with IHM in IE [6]. However, this research work mainly focused on microbiological isolations and differences among treating hospitals and did not specifically address the effect exerted by

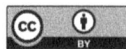

sex on mortality. Contrarily, other studies support a trend of a lower IHM among women [7]. Moreover, different researchers have published nonsignificant differences in IHM between both sexes, like the paper by Sevilla T et al. [8]. However, in this study, the IHM was 28% among men vs. 35% among women (p value = 0.1), conveying the idea that a lack of statistical power due to small study populations may add confusion. Residual confounding is an important issue concerning randomized clinical trials. Propensity score matching (PSM) might help reduce the impact of unaccounted factors in observational studies [9]. Recent research from our country using PSM has revealed higher mortality among women admitted for IE [10]. However, this work was not fully representative of national data because the registry used for this investigation is integrated by multidisciplinary groups from large academic centers that actively included new IE cases and specifically evaluated the role of surgery in people admitted for IE [10].

With this background, in this investigation, we aimed to describe the incidence of hospitalizations for IE among women and men in Spain for the period 2016–2020, assessing sex differences. We also compared the clinical characteristics, use of therapeutic procedures, and in-hospital outcomes according to sex using PSM.

2. Materials and Methods

2.1. Study Design, Study Population, and Data Assessment

We performed an observational, sex-stratified cohort study based on data from the Hospital Discharge Records of the Spanish National Health System (RAE-CMBD, *Registro de Actividad de Atención Especializada-Conjunto Mínimo Básico de Datos* [Register of Specialized Care–Basic Minimum Database]) for the period 1 January 2016 to 31 December 2020. The discharge records were coded based on the International Classification of Disease, Tenth Revision (ICD-10). Details on the RAE-CMBD are available online [11].

The study population comprised every person aged ≥ 18 years hospitalized with an ICD-10 diagnosis code for IE (I33.0; I33.9; I38) in the first or second diagnostic position in their discharge reports. This method to identify IE hospitalizations has been previously used for research purposes in our country [6].

We excluded patients with missing data for age (n = 4), sex (n = 6), and discharge destination (n = 10). If the same patient was admitted with a diagnosis of IE more than once during the 2016–2020 period, we only considered the first episode in this research.

The main variables were trends in the incidence of IE in men and women, IHM, and length of hospital stay (LOHS). We also analyzed comorbidities and therapeutic procedures in men and women with IE. Comorbidity was measured using the Charlson comorbidity index (CCI) calculated based on ICD-10 codes, as described elsewhere [12,13].

To calculate the incidence rates, we used the population data provided by the Spanish National Statistics Institute for the years 2016–2020, grouped by age and sex [14].

We reported, for each patient, the following diagnoses: prevalent heart valvulopathy, congenital malformation of the heart, prosthetic valve carrier status, drug abuse, COVID-19, atrial fibrillation, ischemic heart disease, periannular complications/atrioventricular block, septic arterial embolism and shock. As for pathogens, we sought bacteremia by *Staphylococcus*, *Streptococcus*, Gram-negative bacilli, and fungi.

We also collected data on procedures like dialysis, heart valve surgery, mechanical ventilation, and pacemaker implantation. The ICD10 codes used for these diagnoses and procedures are shown in Table S1.

Finally, the hospital department where the patients were admitted was analyzed.

2.2. Propensity Score Matching

The PSM method consisted of selecting (for each woman) a man with the same or closest propensity score (PS) obtained with multivariable logistic regression, so we could match the structure of the confounding factors for both sexes. We used year of hospitalization, age, and all the comorbidities present on admission as matching conditions to calculate the PS [15].

The matching method chosen was one-to-one using calipers of width equal to 0.2 of the standard deviation of the logit of the PS. Estimating the absolute standardized difference before and after matching allowed us to assess the quality of the PSM process. Populations are considered to be well balanced whenever the absolute standardized differences were <10% after PSM [15].

2.3. Statistical Analysis

We estimated the incidence of IE per man and woman hospitalized for each of the five years analyzed. Age-adjusted incidence rate ratios (IRRs) with their 95% confidence intervals (95% CIs) were calculated using Poisson regression models to compare the incidence of IE according to sex.

We show the mean and standard deviation (SD) or median and interquartile range (IQR) for the continuous variables and frequency and percentage for the categorical variables. We compared the continuous variables using the t test or the Mann–Whitney test, and categorical variables using the chi-square test.

To assess changes over time, we used Poisson regression for the incidence, Cochran-Armitage tests for categorical variables, and the Jonckheere-Terpstra test for the LOHS.

Multivariable trends in the incidence of IE adjusted by age were evaluated with Poisson regression. We provided the annual percentage change (APC) with 95% confidence interval.

The statistical analysis and the PSM were conducted using Stata version 14 (Stata, College Station, TX, USA), and significance was set at $p < 0.05$ (2-sided).

2.4. Ethics

The access to the RAE-CMBD is universal under request (to the Spanish Ministry of Health) [16]. Since this is an anonymous registry, it is not deemed necessary to ask for individual written consent from the patients or to apply for an ethics committee approval, following Spanish legislation.

3. Results

We identified a total of 10,459 patients aged ≥18 years with an admission diagnosis of IE in Spain during the period 2016–2020. Women represented 33.26% (n = 3479) of the study population.

3.1. Incidence of Patients Admitted to Hospitals with IE and Hospital Department of Admission According to Sex

The incidence of IE was significantly higher in men than in women for all the years analyzed ($p < 0.001$), with an age-adjusted IRR of 2.08 (95% CI 2.00–2.17) for men vs. women. As can be seen in Table 1, the crude incidence of IE remained stable from 2016 to 2020 among both men and women.

We could see no significant changes in the incidence of IE over time for women (APC −0.07%; 95% CI, −0.17% to 0.08%; p = 0.458) or men with IE (APC, 0.03%; 95% CI, −0.09% to 0.03%; p = 0.689) in the multivariable regression model.

Over time, the mean age increased only in men (65.53 ±17.31 years in 2016 vs. 67.45 ± 15.24 in 2020; $p < 0.001$). The presence of previous mitral, aortic, and tricuspid valve disease and the mean CCI increased significantly among both sexes. Congenital malformation of the heart remained constant over the study period for both sexes, with figures ranging from 2% to 4%.

Table 1. Incidence, clinical characteristics, and in-hospital outcomes of patients hospitalized with infective endocarditis in Spain from 2016 to 2020 according to sex.

		2016	2017	2018	2019	2020	p-Value *
N, (incidence per 100,000 people per year)	Both sexes	1975 (4.25)	2090 (4.49)	2242 (4.8)	2222 (4.72)	1930 (4.08)	0.656
N, (incidence per 100,000 people per year)	Women	646 (2.73)	704 (2.97)	772 (3.24)	715 (2.98)	642 (2.66)	0.672
	Men	1329 (5.83)	1386 (6.07)	1470 (6.42)	1507 (6.53)	1288 (5.55)	0.826
Age, mean (SD)	Women	70.21 (18.21)	69.00 (19.34)	69.88 (18.27)	70.53 (16.74)	71.78 (14.77)	0.064
	Men	65.53 (17.31)	64.62 (17.18)	67.23 (15.82)	66.36 (15.90)	67.45 (15.24)	<0.001
CCI index, mean (SD)	Women	1.27 (1.13)	1.35 (1.12)	1.30 (1.11)	1.46 (1.18)	1.50 (1.17)	<0.001
	Men	1.30 (1.19)	1.43 (1.21)	1.49 (1.25)	1.43 (1.25)	1.53 (1.27)	<0.001
Prosthetic valve carriers, n (%)	Women	69 (10.68)	68 (9.66)	65 (8.42)	55 (7.69)	65 (10.12)	0.287
	Men	121 (9.10)	117 (8.44)	136 (9.25)	121 (8.03)	103 (8.00)	0.647
Previous mitral valve disease, n (%)	Women	195 (30.19)	189 (26.85)	235 (30.44)	244 (34.13)	217 (33.80)	0.021
	Men	311 (23.40)	349 (25.18)	370 (25.17)	364 (24.15)	367 (28.49)	0.032
Previous aortic valve disease, n (%)	Women	128 (19.81)	163 (23.15)	174 (22.54)	206 (28.81)	177 (27.57)	<0.001
	Men	357 (26.86)	410 (29.58)	420 (28.57)	444 (29.46)	422 (32.76)	0.020
Previous tricuspid valve disease, n (%)	Women	43 (6.66)	54 (7.67)	90 (11.66)	82 (11.47)	74 (11.53)	0.001
	Men	66 (4.97)	80 (5.77)	101 (6.87)	111 (7.37)	112 (8.70)	0.002
Previous pulmonary valve disease, n (%)	Women	3 (0.46)	7 (0.99)	2 (0.26)	2 (0.28)	3 (0.47)	0.268
	Men	3 (0.23)	7 (0.51)	4 (0.27)	2 (0.13)	7 (0.54)	0.244
Congenital malformation of heart, n (%)	Women	13 (2.01)	25 (3.55)	28 (3.63)	20 (2.8)	19 (2.96)	0.403
	Men	44 (3.31)	51 (3.68)	57 (3.88)	55 (3.65)	40 (3.11)	0.820
Drug abuse, n (%)	Women	10 (1.55)	13 (1.85)	8 (1.04)	5 (0.70)	5 (0.78)	0.208
	Men	44 (3.31)	56 (4.04)	68 (4.63)	58 (3.85)	41 (3.18)	0.274
LOHS, median (IQR)	Women	16.5 (27)	17 (28)	18 (25)	19 (24)	18 (24)	0.681
	Men	20 (25)	19 (26)	19 (26)	19 (25)	19 (23)	0.897
IHM, n (%)	Women	125 (19.35)	128 (18.18)	142 (18.39)	144 (20.14)	140 (21.81)	0.441
	Men	191 (14.37)	183 (13.20)	232 (15.78)	233 (15.46)	200 (15.53)	0.275

* p value for time trend. SD: standard deviation; CCI: Charlson comorbidity index; LOHS: length of hospital stay; IQR: interquartile range; IHM: in-hospital mortality.

LOHS was around 18 days in women and 19 days in men. We found no significant differences in crude IHM among women (19.35% in 2016 vs. 21.81% in 2020; p = 0.441) or men (14.37% in 2016 vs. 15.53%; p = 0.275) over time (Table 1).

The distributions by hospital departments where patients with IE were admitted according to sex are shown in Table S2. For both sexes, the most common admission department was Internal Medicine, with a significantly higher proportion of women than men (43.32% vs. 38.94%; p < 0.001). However, Cardiology (17.98% vs. 16.21%; =0.025), Cardiovascular Surgery (14.15% vs. 9.89%; p < 0.01), and Infectious Diseases (10.33% vs. 7.85%; p < 0.001) were more frequent among men. No significant differences were found for the Intensive Care Unit (7.27% for women and 7.21% for men).

3.2. Clinical Characteristics and Hospital Outcomes for Women and Men Admitted to the Hospital for IE

Before PSM, when all patients hospitalized from 2016 to 2020 were grouped, women with IE were significantly older than men (70.25 vs. 66.24; p < 0.001) but had fewer comorbidities according to the CCI (1.38 vs. 1.43; p = 0.019) (Table 2). Men suffered from most of the comorbid conditions analyzed more frequently than women. Nonetheless, dementia and atrial fibrillation were more prevalent among women. After PSM, the differences seen between men and women before PSM became nonsignificant.

Table 2. Distribution of clinical characteristics of women and men with infective endocarditis in Spain (2016–20), before and after propensity score matching (PSM).

	BEFORE PSM				AFTER PSM			
	Women	Men	ASD	p-Value	Women	Men	ASD	p-Value
N	3479	6980	NA	NA	3479	3479	NA	NA
Age, mean (SD)	70.25 (17.59)	66.24 (16.33)	0.236	<0.001	70.25 (17.59)	70.11 (11.87)	0.07	0.697
CCI index, mean (SD)	1.38 (1.15)	1.43 (1.24)	0.049	0.019	1.38 (1.15)	1.42 (1.11)	0.047	0.140
Prosthetic valve carriers, n (%)	322 (9.26)	598 (8.57)	0.024	0.242	322 (9.26)	344 (9.89)	0.022	0.370
Previous mitral valve disease, n (%)	1080 (31.04)	1761 (25.23)	0.13	<0.001	1080 (31.04)	1069 (30.73)	0.065	0.781
Previous aortic valve disease, n (%)	848 (24.37)	2053 (29.41)	0.114	<0.001	848 (24.37)	789 (22.69)	0.09	0.097
Previous tricuspid valve disease, n (%)	343 (9.86)	470 (6.73)	0.113	<0.001	343 (9.86)	337 (9.69)	0.006	0.809
Previous pulmonary valve disease, n (%)	17 (0.49)	23 (0.33)	0.025	0.214	17 (0.49)	20 (0.57)	0.014	0.621
Congenital malformation of heart, n (%)	105 (3.02)	247 (3.54)	0.083	0.164	105 (3.02)	87 (2.52)	0.041	0.705
COVID-19, n (%)	20 (0.57)	31 (0.44)	0.028	0.366	20 (0.57)	27 (0.78)	0.018	0.306
Congestive heart failure, n (%)	392 (11.27)	717 (10.27)	0.032	0.119	392 (11.27)	382 (10.98)	0.009	0.703
Septic arterial embolism, n (%)	150 (4.31)	305 (4.37)	0.003	0.891	150 (4.31)	161 (4.63)	0.016	0.523
Dementia, n (%)	92 (2.64)	108 (1.55)	0.077	<0.001	92 (2.64)	82 (2.36)	0.02	0.443
Acute renal disease, n (%)	690 (19.83)	1500 (21.49)	0.041	0.050	690 (19.83)	676 (19.43)	0.01	0.673
Chronic renal disease, n (%)	640 (18.4)	1186 (16.99)	0.037	0.075	640 (18.40)	656 (18.86)	0.012	0.622
Ischemic heart disease, n (%)	343 (9.86)	1229 (17.61)	0.227	<0.001	343 (9.86)	379 (10.90)	0.081	0.156
COPD, n (%)	104 (2.99)	683 (9.79)	0.281	<0.001	104 (2.99)	131 (3.77)	0.097	0.072
Atrial fibrillation, n (%)	1167 (33.54)	1789 (25.63)	0.174	<0.001	1167 (33.54)	1223 (35.15)	0.035	0.157
Diabetes, n (%)	816 (23.46)	1792 (25.67)	0.052	0.013	816 (23.46)	793 (22.79)	0.015	0.513
Drug abuse, n (%)	41 (1.18)	267 (3.83)	0.17	<0.001	41 (1.18)	60 (1.73)	0.042	0.057
Shock, n (%)	65 (1.87)	163 (2.34)	0.033	0.123	65 (1.87)	63 (1.81)	0.004	0.858
Periannular complications/atrioventricular block, n (%)	142 (4.08)	425 (6.09)	0.191	<0.001	142 (4.08)	122 (3.51)	0.033	0.209

NA: not applicable; SD: standard deviation; CCI: Charlson comorbidity index; COPD: chronic obstructive pulmonary disease. ASD: absolute standardized differences.

Shown in Table 2 and Figure 1 are the absolute standardized differences before and after PSM. As can be seen in Figure 1, a significant imbalance could be ruled out since all the absolute standardized differences after PSM were below 10% [15].

In Table 3, we show the distribution of the isolated pathogens, therapeutic procedures, and hospital outcomes among women and men with IE, both before and after PSM. Streptococcus bacteremia was more incident in men, whereas Gram-negative bacilli were more incident in women, even after PSM. Women underwent heart valve surgery and pacemaker implantation less often than men, even after PSM (16.3% and 4.02% vs. 18.74% and 5.29%; $p = 0.007$ and $p = 0.012$, respectively). However, mechanical ventilation was more often coded among women than among men (10.32% vs. 8.88%; $p = 0.042$). IHM among women admitted for IE remained over 3% higher than among men (19.52% vs. 15.98%; $p < 0.001$).

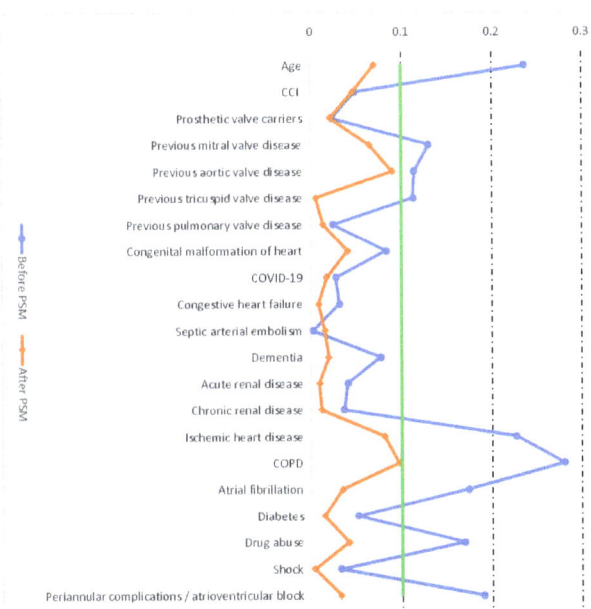

Figure 1. Love plot showing the comparison of covariate values for men and women: absolute standardized differences before and after propensity score matching (PSM). Green line shows the absolute standardized differences of 10%. Dotted lines show 20% and 30% standardized differences.

Table 3. Distribution of isolated pathogens, therapeutic procedures, and hospital outcomes among women and men with infective endocarditis in Spain (2016–2020), before and after propensity score matching (PSM).

	BEFORE PSM			AFTER PSM		
	Women	Men	p-Value	Women	Men	p-Value
Staphylococcus bacteremia, n (%)	992 (28.51)	2035 (29.15)	0.496	992 (28.51)	978 (28.11)	0.709
Streptococcus bacteremia, n (%)	705 (20.26)	1715 (24.57)	<0.001	705 (20.26)	848 (24.37)	<0.001
Gram-negative bacilli bacteremia, n (%)	353 (10.15)	459 (6.58)	<0.001	353 (10.15)	240 (6.90)	<0.001
Fungemia, n (%)	15 (0.43)	34 (0.49)	0.693	15 (0.43)	14 (0.40)	0.852
Heart valve surgery n (%)	567 (16.30)	1560 (22.35)	<0.001	567 (16.30)	652 (18.74)	0.007
Dialysis, n (%)	172 (4.94)	350 (5.01)	0.876	172 (4.94)	141 (4.05)	0.073
Pacemaker implantation, n (%)	140 (4.02)	385 (5.52)	0.001	140 (4.02)	184 (5.29)	0.012
Mechanical ventilation, n (%)	359 (10.32)	788 (11.29)	0.135	359 (10.32)	309 (8.88)	0.042
LOHS, median (IQR)	18 (25)	19 (25)	0.085	18 (25)	19 (25)	0.271
IHM, n (%)	679 (19.52)	1039 (14.89)	<0.001	679 (19.52)	556 (15.98)	<0.001

LOHS: length of hospital stay; IQR: interquartile range; IHM: in-hospital mortality. Heart valve surgery included aortic, mitral, tricuspid, and pulmonary.

3.3. Variables Associated with IHM for Women and Men Admitted to the Hospital with a Diagnosis of IE

We show IHM among women and men with IE before and after PSM according to the prespecified variables in Table 4. Older ages were associated with increased IHM among both sexes. Even after PSM, IHM among women was higher than among men for several conditions, such as previous mitral disease ($p < 0.001$), septic arterial embolism ($p = 0.032$), acute renal disease ($p = 0.005$), atrial fibrillation ($p = 0.036$), diabetes ($p = 0.004$), Gram-positive cocci bacteremia, and heart valve surgery ($p = 0.01$).

Table 4. In hospital mortality according to study variables of women and men with infective endocarditis in Spain (2016–2020), before and after propensity score matching (PSM).

	BEFORE PSM			AFTER PSM		
	Women	Men	p-Value	Women	Men	p-Value
N	679	1039	NA	679	556	NA
Age, mean (SD)	75.94 (11.72)	72.88 (12.03)	<0.001	75.94 (11.72)	75.97 (10.12)	0.966
<40 years old, n (%)	4 (1.71)	10 (2.28)	0.621	4 (1.71)	0 (0)	NA
40–66 years old, n (%)	121 (15.37)	273 (10.62)	<0.001	121 (15.37)	101 (10.58)	0.003
67–75 years old, n (%)	151 (18.48)	262 (15.35)	0.047	151 (18.48)	139 (14.32)	0.018
≥76 years old, n (%)	403 (24.56)	494 (21.82)	0.045	403 (24.56)	316 (20.80)	0.012
CCI index, mean (SD)	1.81 (1.16)	2.01 (1.25)	0.001	1.81 (1.16)	1.72 (1.15)	0.163
Prosthetic valve carriers, n (%)	61 (18.94)	79 (13.21)	0.022	61 (18.94)	48 (13.95)	0.083
Previous mitral valve disease, n (%)	227 (21.02)	260 (14.76)	<0.001	227 (21.02)	173 (14.65)	<0.001
Previous aortic valve disease, n (%)	175 (20.64)	342 (16.66)	0.011	175 (20.64)	142 (20.97)	0.872
Previous tricuspid valve disease, n (%)	73 (21.28)	67 (14.26)	0.009	73 (21.28)	52 (15.43)	0.050
Previous pulmonic valve disease, n (%)	2 (11.76)	1 (4.35)	0.397	2 (11.76)	1 (5.00)	0.465
Congenital malformation of heart, n (%)	7 (6.67)	4 (5.67)	0.718	7 (6.67)	4 (7.55)	0.832
COVID-19, n (%)	4 (20.00)	7 (22.58)	0.827	4 (20.00)	7 (25.93)	0.636
Congestive heart failure, n (%)	103 (26.28)	168 (23.43)	0.292	103 (26.28)	100 (26.18)	0.975
Septic arterial embolism, n (%)	52 (34.67)	58 (19.02)	<0.001	52 (34.67)	38 (23.60)	0.032
Dementia, n (%)	24 (26.09)	28 (25.93)	0.979	24 (26.09)	19 (23.17)	0.656
Acute renal disease, n (%)	256 (37.10)	442 (29.47)	<0.001	256 (37.10)	202 (29.88)	0.005
Chronic renal disease, n (%)	172 (26.88)	275 (23.19)	0.081	172 (26.88)	158 (24.09)	0.249
Ischemic heart disease, n (%)	89 (25.95)	230 (18.71)	0.003	89 (25.95)	25 (17.36)	0.042
COPD, n (%)	30 (28.85)	141 (20.64)	0.060	30 (28.85)	1 (20.00)	0.671
Atrial fibrillation, n (%)	269 (23.05)	368 (20.57)	0.109	269 (23.05)	239 (19.54)	0.036
Diabetes, n (%)	183 (22.43)	296 (16.52)	<0.001	183 (22.43)	133 (16.77)	0.004
Drug Abuse, n (%)	5 (12.20)	16 (5.99)	0.151	5 (12.20)	6 (9.38)	0.646
Shock, n (%)	45 (69.23)	89 (54.60)	0.044	45 (69.23)	33 (52.38)	0.052
Periannular complications/atrioventricular block, n (%)	30 (21.13)	83 (19.53)	0.680	30 (21.13)	39 (18.40)	0.525
Staphylococcus bacteremia, n (%)	274 (27.62)	420 (20.64)	<0.001	274 (27.62)	225 (23.01)	0.019
Streptococcus bacteremia, n (%)	75 (10.64)	118 (6.88)	0.002	75 (10.64)	65 (7.67)	0.042
Gram-negative bacteremia, n (%)	72 (20.40)	102 (22.22)	0.530	72 (20.40)	52 (21.67)	0.709
Fungemia, n (%)	6 (40.00)	15 (44.12)	0.788	6 (40.00)	9 (64.29)	0.196
Heart valve surgery, n (%)	130 (22.93)	253 (16.22)	<0.001	130 (22.93)	111 (17.02)	0.010
Dialysis, n (%)	81 (47.09)	131 (37.43)	0.035	81 (47.09)	54 (38.30)	0.119
Pacemaker implantation, n (%)	17 (12.14)	37 (9.61)	0.399	17 (12.14)	17 (9.24)	0.400
Mechanical ventilation, n (%)	152 (42.34)	278 (35.28)	0.022	152 (42.34)	111 (35.92)	0.091
LOHS, Median (IQR)	14 (21)	15 (21)	0.855	14 (21)	16 (21)	0.529

NA: not applicable; SD: standard deviation; CCI: Charlson comorbidity index; COPD: chronic obstructive pulmonary disease LOHS: length of hospital stay; IHM: in-hospital mortality. Heart valve surgery included aortic, mitral, tricuspid, and pulmonary.

4. Discussion

Here, we found that the incidence of IE among men doubled the incidence among women. Other studies have also reported higher incidence rates among men vs. women [5,17]. Two recent meta-analyses from one research group, which included European and North American studies, respectively, confirmed the preponderance of male sex among patients admitted for IE [18,19]. The reason for this consistent finding is not clear; it could perhaps be due to recognizable sex-specific predisposing conditions or, eventually, more frequent episodes of low-grade bacteremia among men [20]. It has been proposed that hormonal factors could diminish the incidence of IE among women by protecting them from endothelial damage [21].

In our population, the incidence of IE remained stable over time for both sexes. In this regard, we found conflicting results in the literature [17,19,22–26]. A systematic review by Talha et al. evaluated the population-based incidence of IE in Europe. The pooled regression estimate was a 4.1 ± 1.2% for yearly increments in IE incidence, which translated into a compound increase of 106% over 18 years (2000–2018) [18]. More years of follow-up will be needed to confirm the stabilization of the IE incidence in our country.

The increase from 2016 to 2020 in the prevalence of comorbidities among men and women with IE could partially obey population aging, as previously described in Spain and other countries [6,17,23–25]. Besides this increment in the comorbidity, the IHM did not show a significant increase over the study period, and this suggests that the management and pharmacological treatment of IE patients in Spain may be improving [6].

We detected that women underwent heart valve surgery and pacemaker implantation less often than men, whereas they received invasive lung ventilation more often than men, even after PSM. These facts are relevant since pacemaker implantation was associated with lower IHM among both sexes. We cannot dismiss the possibility of reverse causation in this association, as better clinical conditions may have prompted the implantation of the devices in patients prone to better outcomes. When surgery is indicated, failure to perform the operation was associated with the worst prognosis in one study [27,28]. Nevertheless, to make things more complex, other studies had reported worse outcomes for women when they were operated on because of IE [29].

Even after PSM, Streptococcus bacteremia was more incident among men, whereas Gram-negative bacilli bacteremia was more incident among women, in accordance with previous reports [8]. We might hypothesize that men have worse oral hygiene habits than women [30] and, consequently, a higher incidence of Streptococcus viridans bacteremias. Gram-negative bacilli bacteremias might derive from urinary tract infections, which are more common among women. Streptococcus bacteremia was associated with a lower IHM. This is coincidental from the previously published literature, especially when compared with Staphylococcus IE [6,27,31]. A higher incidence on native valves, a better profile of antimicrobial susceptibility, a lower capacity of valve destruction and abscess formation, and less common peripheral embolization could explain this better outcome for Streptococcus IE.

The odds of dying during hospitalization for IE were higher among women after PSM, which means that this finding is apparently not explained by the remaining variables analyzed. Conflicting results have been reported by previous work that studied the effect of sex on survival after the diagnosis of IE [3,7,10,32]. Varela-Barca et al. [10] communicated a 41% higher IHM among women with IE as compared with men in our country (OR, 1.41; 95% CI 1.21–1.65). Whereas a poorer overall baseline condition among women has been proposed to be responsible for this finding, it has been speculated that women develop heart disease later in life after the hormonal protective effects exerted by estrogens vanish [10,32].

We might theorize about a distinct biological basis or differences in the clinical profile to explain the worse outcomes seen among women, but we are more concerned about a possible gender bias in the clinical management of the condition beyond the measured factors. Physicians' perception of frailty may differ for female vs. male patients, and this perception might lead to the adoption of comfort measures earlier for female than for male patients, hence driving an unfair limitation on the therapeutic efforts among women [33–35]. In fact, in Spain, the higher mortality among women has been linked to different criteria to proceed with heart valve surgery depending on patients' gender [36]. Furthermore, IE could also be considered more often as a differential diagnosis in men than in women, thus allowing the diagnosis at an earlier stage, which would improve the prognosis. Future investigations should clarify these hypotheses.

In our population, the prevalence of congenital malformation of the heart was low compared to other recent investigations (2–4%) [37]. Van Melle et al. showed that 11% of the cases of IE in their cohort had a congenital malformation of the heart. We might argue that the data used in their registry probably overestimate the true prevalence of congenital malformation of the heart in people with IE since there is probably a selection bias (that registry offered the patients the possibility of being included in the registry after the diagnosis of IE, and perhaps those people aware of their chronic heart condition showed a higher predisposition to be included in the registry) [37]. However, the outcomes reported by Van Melle were better in this subpopulation for congenital malformation of the heart, with results that are in line with our findings [37].

A remarkable result of our investigation is the lower LOHS compared to other studies [6,10,26]. The reported LOHS for IE ranges between 7 and 43 days, with a substantial variation between studies from different countries, depending on the characteristics of the populations analyzed, data sources, and methods used [6,10,26,38,39]. A recent manuscript from Finland reports a median LOHS of 20.0 days in men and 18.0 days in women, which is quite similar to our results [38]. In the US, using data from the Nationwide Readmission Database for those patients who survived hospitalization for IE, the median length of stay was 10 (IQR, 6–17) days: much shorter than our results (18 days) [39]. Our data are from very recent years, and these figures probably reflect earlier diagnoses, more aggressive clinical management of the patients, and better results from surgery. However, future studies are needed to explain the differences in the LOHS reported.

The large sample size of this study, which includes data from 10,459 recent episodes of IE and the widespread coverage of the Spanish population by the RAE-CMBD (>95% of all hospital admissions), gives robustness to our results. However, some limitations should be pointed out. First, our data source was the RAE-CMBD, an administrative database that depends on the information that physicians include in the discharge report and on manual coding on behalf of administrative staff. Second, to our knowledge, the ICD-10 codes for IE in the RAE-CMBD have not been validated so far. However, the results from previous studies conducted in other countries using the International Classification of Disease, Ninth Revision, (ICD-9 and ICD-10) codes in hospital discharge databases suggested good accuracy for the detection of IE cases [24,25,40–43]. Third, it is unlikely that PSM could fully eliminate residual confounding. Fourth, we excluded 20 patients from the sample (<0.2%) due to missing data, though we believe that a selection bias that could impact the results is improbable. Fifth, the RAE-CMBD only collects information on the diagnosis and procedures for each patient during the hospitalization, but not the dates for each of these diagnoses nor the duration of the symptoms before hospitalization; therefore, it is not possible to calculate the time from the beginning of the symptoms to the diagnosis of IE. Sixth, it is common practice to admit every single case of IE to the hospital when it is the suspected diagnosis at admission. However, most of the cases were probably not suspected at admission but were diagnosed during the hospitalization period. For the latter category, fever, new-onset heart failure, or a general deterioration in the clinical status may have indicated the hospital admission. We cannot rule out some heterogeneity in the clinical presentation of the disease according to sex, but unfortunately, the initial reason for hospital admission was not collected in the database used. Furthermore, in our opinion, the sex differences found in the hospital department where patients were admitted may be justified by the differences in the symptoms of IE when they were admitted to the hospital, the comorbid conditions, and by the higher age of the women. The RAE-CMBD database is also limited by the lack of data on microbiological resistance patterns and the lack of information for identifying the foci of the pathogens isolated or if the IE is device-related. Future studies with more detailed clinical data should include these variables to assess sex differences in IE. Seventh, even if five years may be a short period of time to show a well-defined trend, we used data from 2016 onward because during that year, the RAE-CMBD moved from the ICD 9 to the ICD 10, and the effect of this change in the coding method could affect our results. Finally, the results of this study do not necessarily reflect the actual data from other countries.

5. Conclusions

Hospital admission for IE in adults in Spanish hospitals during the period 2016–2020 was more frequent among men than among women. The in-hospital mortality among those women admitted for IE was significantly higher than that among men. We observed a lower rate of invasive cardiac procedures among women admitted for IE. These and other factors should be better characterized to minimize the differences in mortality between the sexes for people admitted for IE.

Supplementary Materials: The following supporting information can be downloaded at: https://www.mdpi.com/article/10.3390/jcm11226847/s1, Table S1: Diagnosis, procedures, and pathogens analyzed with their corresponding ICD10 codes. Table S2: Hospital departments where patients with infective endocarditis were admitted according to sex. Hospital Discharge Records of the Spanish National Health System (RAE-CMBD) from 2016 to 20.

Author Contributions: Conceptualization, J.M.D.M.-Y., R.J.-G. and A.L.-d.-A.; methodology J.J.Z.-L. and C.N.; validation, D.C.-A.; data curation, V.H.-B.; Formal analysis, V.H.-B and J.D.M.-D.; Funding: A.L.-d.-A. and R.J.-G.; Writing—original draft, J.M.D.M.-Y., R.J.-G. and A.L.-d.-A.; Writing—review & editing, J.J.Z.-L., D.C.-A., C.N. and J.D.M.-D. All authors have read and agreed to the published version of the manuscript.

Funding: This study is a part of the research funded by: Convenio V-PRICIT de la Comunidad de Madrid y la Universidad Complutense de Madrid ("Programa de Excelencia para el Profesorado Universitario" INV.AY.20.2021.1E126). And by: Universidad Complutense de Madrid. Grupo de Investigación en Epidemiología de las Enfermedades Crónicas de Alta Prevalencia en España (970970).

Institutional Review Board Statement: Not applicable.

Informed Consent Statement: Not applicable.

Data Availability Statement: According to the contract signed with the Spanish Ministry of Health and Social Services, which provided access to the databases from the Spanish National Hospital Database (RAE-CMBD, *Registro de Actividad de Atención Especializada. Conjunto Mínimo Básico de Datos,* Registry of Specialized Health Care Activities. Minimum Basic Data Set), we cannot share the databases with any other investigator, and we have to destroy the databases once the investigation has concluded. Consequently, we cannot upload the databases to any public repository. However, any investigator can apply for access to the databases by filling out the questionnaire available at http://www.msssi.gob.es/estadEstudios/estadisticas/estadisticas/estMinisterio/SolicitudCMBDdocs/Formulario_Peticion_Datos_CMBD.pdf. All other relevant data are included in the paper. (accessed on 21 September 2022).

Conflicts of Interest: The authors declare no conflict of interest.

References

1. Ahtela, E.; Oksi, J.; Porela, P.; Ekström, T.; Rautava, P.; Kytö, V. Trends in occurrence and 30-day mortality of infective endocarditis in adults: Population-based registry study in Finland. *BMJ Open* **2019**, *9*, e026811. [CrossRef] [PubMed]
2. Sunder, S.; Grammatico-Guillon, L.; Lemaignen, A.; Lacasse, M.; Gaborit, C.; Boutoille, D.; Tattevin, P.; Denes, E.; Guimard, T.; Dupont, M.; et al. Incidence, characteristics, and mortality of infective endocarditis in France in 2011. *PLoS ONE* **2019**, *14*, e0223857. [CrossRef] [PubMed]
3. Polishchuk, I.; Stavi, V.; Awesat, J.; Ben Baruch Golan, Y.; Bartal, C.; Sagy, I.; Jotkowitz, A.; Barski, L. Sex differences in infective endocarditis. *Am. J. Med. Sci.* **2021**, *361*, 83–89. [CrossRef] [PubMed]
4. Mauvais-Jarvis, F.; Merz, N.B.; Barnes, P.J.; Brinton, R.D.; Carrero, J.J.; DeMeo, D.L.; De Vries, G.J.; Epperson, C.N.; Govindan, R.; Klein, S.L.; et al. Sex and gender: Modifiers of Health, Disease, and Medicine. *Lancet* **2020**, *396*, 565–582. [CrossRef]
5. Bansal, A.; Cremer, P.C.; Jaber, W.A.; Rampersad, P.; Menon, V. Sex differences in the utilization and outcomes of cardiac valve replacement surgery for infective endocarditis: Insights from the National Inpatient Sample. *J. Am. Heart Assoc.* **2021**, *10*, e020095. [CrossRef]

6. Olmos, C.; Vilacosta, I.; Fernández-Pérez, C.; Bernal, J.L.; Ferrera, C.; García-Arribas, D.; Pérez-García, C.N.; San Román, J.A.; Maroto, L.; Macaya, C.; et al. The evolving nature of infective endocarditis in Spain: A population-based study (2003 to 2014). *J. Am. Coll. Cardiol.* **2017**, *70*, 2795–2804. [CrossRef]
7. Chew, D.S.; Rennert-May, E.; Lu, S.; Parkins, M.; Miller, R.J.H.; Somavaji, R. Sex differences in health resource utilization, costs and mortality during hospitalization for infective endocarditis in the United States. *Am. Heart J. Plus.* **2021**, *3*, 100014. [CrossRef]
8. Sevilla, T.; Revilla, A.; López, J.; Vilacosta, I.; Sarriá, C.; Gómez, I.; García, H.; San Román, J.A. Influence of sex on left-sided infective endocarditis. *Rev. Esp. Cardiol.* **2010**, *63*, 1497–1500. [CrossRef]
9. Hernán, M.A.; Robins, J.M. Using big data to emulate a target trial when a randomized trial is not available. *Am. J. Epidemiol.* **2016**, *183*, 758–764. [CrossRef]
10. Varela Barca, L.; Vidal-Bonnet, L.; Fariñas, M.C.; Muñoz, P.; Valerio Minero, M.; de Alarcón, A.; Gutiérrez Carretero, E.; Gutiérrez Cuadra, M.; Moreno Camacho, A.; Kortajarena Urkola, X.; et al. Analysis of sex differences in the clinical presentation, management and prognosis of infective endocarditis in Spain. *Heart* **2021**, *107*, 1717–1724. [CrossRef]
11. Ministerio de Sanidad, Servicios Sociales e Igualdad. Real Decreto 69/2015, de 6 de Febrero, por el que se Regula el Registro de Actividad de Atención Sanitaria Especializada. (Spanish National Hospital Discharge Database) BOE 2015; 35: 10789-809. Available online: https://www.mscbs.gob.es/estadEstudios/estadisticas/docs/BOE_RD_69_2015_RAE_CMBD.pdf (accessed on 31 May 2022).
12. Sundararajan, V.; Henderson, T.; Perry, C.; Muggivan, A.; Quan, H.; Ghali, W.A. New ICD-10 version of the Charlson comorbidity index predicted in-hospital mortality. *J. Clin. Epidemiol.* **2004**, *57*, 1288–1294. [CrossRef] [PubMed]
13. Quan, H.; Sundararajan, V.; Halfon, P.; Fong, A.; Burnand, B.; Luthi, J.C.; Saunders, L.D.; Beck, C.A.; Feasby, T.E.; Ghali, W.A. Coding algorithms for defining comorbidities in ICD-9-CM and ICD-10 administrative data. *Med. Care* **2005**, *43*, 1130–1139. [CrossRef]
14. Instituto Nacional de Estadística Population Estimates. Available online: https://www.ine.es/dyngs/INEbase/es/operacion.htm?c=Estadistica_C&cid=1254736176951&menu=ultiDatos&idp=1254735572981 (accessed on 31 May 2022).
15. Austin, P.C. Comparing paired vs non-paired statistical methods of analyses when making inferences about absolute risk reductions in propensity-score matched samples. *Stat. Med.* **2011**, *30*, 1292–1301. [CrossRef] [PubMed]
16. Ministerio de Sanidad, Consumo y Bienestar Social. Solicitud de Extracción de Datos—Extraction Request (Spanish National Hospital Discharge Database). Available online: https://www.mscbs.gob.es/estadEstudios/estadisticas/estadisticas/estMinisterio/SolicitudCMBDdocs/2018_Formulario_Peticion_Datos_RAE_CMBD.pdf (accessed on 31 May 2022).
17. Sousa, C.; Nogueira, P.J.; Pinto, F.J. Gender based analysis of a population series of patients hospitalized with infective endocarditis in Portugal. How do women and men compare? *Int. J. Cardiovasc. Sci.* **2021**, *34*, 347–355. [CrossRef]
18. Talha, K.M.; Baddour, L.M.; Thornhill, M.H.; Arshad, V.; Tariq, W.; Tleyjeh, I.M.; Scott, C.G.; Hyun, M.C.; Bailey, K.R.; Anavekar, N.S.; et al. Escalating incidence of infective endocarditis in Europe in the 21st century. *Open Heart* **2021**, *8*, e001846. [CrossRef]
19. Talha, K.M.; Dayer, M.J.; Thornhill, M.H.; Tariq, W.; Arshad, V.; Tleyjeh, I.M.; Bailey, K.R.; Palraj, R.; Anavekar, N.S.; Rizwan Sohail, M.; et al. Temporal trends of infective endocarditis in North America from 2000 to 2017-A Systematic Review. *Open Forum. Infect. Dis.* **2021**, *8*, ofab479. [CrossRef] [PubMed]
20. Veloso, T.R.; Chaouch, A.; Roger, T.; Giddey, M.; Vouillamoz, J.; Majcherczyk, P.; Que, Y.A.; Rousson, V.; Moreillon, P.; Entenza, J.M. Use of a human-like low-grade bacteremia model of experimental endocarditis to study the role of Staphylococcus aureus adhesins and platelet aggregation in early endocarditis. *Infect. Immun.* **2013**, *81*, 697–703. [CrossRef] [PubMed]
21. Daniel, W.G.; Mügge, A.; Martin, R.P.; Lindert, O.; Hausmann, D.; Nonnast-Daniel, B.; Laas, J.; Lichtlen, P.R. Improvement in the diagnosis of abscesses associated with endocarditis by transesophageal echocardiography. *N. Engl. J. Med.* **1991**, *324*, 795–800. [CrossRef]
22. Shah, A.S.V.; McAllister, D.A.; Gallacher, P.; Astengo, F.; Rodríguez Pérez, J.A.; Hall, J.; Lee, K.K.; Bing, R.; Anand, A.; Nathwani, D.; et al. Incidence, Microbiology, and Outcomes in Patients Hospitalized With Infective Endocarditis. *Circulation* **2020**, *141*, 2067–2077. [CrossRef]
23. Jensen, A.D.; Bundgaard, H.; Butt, J.H.; Bruun, N.E.; Voldstedlund, M.; Torp-Pedersen, C.; Gislason, G.; Iversen, K.; Chamat, S.; Dahl, A.; et al. Temporal changes in the incidence of infective endocarditis in Denmark 1997–2017: A nationwide study. *Int. J. Cardiol.* **2021**, *326*, 145–152. [CrossRef]
24. Li, H.L.; Tromp, J.; Teramoto, K.; Tse, Y.K.; Yu, S.Y.; Lam, L.Y.; Li, K.Y.; Wu, M.Z.; Ren, Q.W.; Wong, P.F.; et al. Temporal trends and patterns of infective endocarditis in a Chinese population: A territory-wide study in Hong Kong (2002–2019). *Lancet Reg. Health West Pac.* **2022**, *22*, 100417. [CrossRef] [PubMed]
25. Toyoda, N.; Chikwe, J.; Itagaki, S.; Gelijns, A.C.; Adams, D.H.; Egorova, N.N. Trends in Infective Endocarditis in California and New York State, 1998–2013. *JAMA* **2017**, *317*, 1652–1660. [CrossRef] [PubMed]
26. Ortega-Loubon, C.; Muñoz-Moreno, M.F.; Andrés-García, I.; Álvarez, F.J.; Gómez-Sánchez, E.; Bustamante-Munguira, J.; Lorenzo-López, M.; Tamayo-Velasco, Á.; Jorge-Monjas, P.; Resino, S.; et al. Nosocomial Vs. Community-Acquired Infective Endocarditis in Spain: Location, Trends, Clinical Presentation, Etiology, and Survival in the 21st Century. *J. Clin. Med.* **2019**, *8*, 1755. [CrossRef] [PubMed]
27. Habib, G.; Erba, P.A.; Iung, B.; Donal, E.; Cosyns, B.; Laroche, C.; Popescu, B.A.; Prendergast, B.; Tornos, P.; Sadeghpour, A.; et al. Clinical presentation, aetiology and outcome of infective endocarditis. Results of the ESC-EORP EURO-ENDO (European infective endocarditis) registry: A prospective cohort study. *Eur. Heart J.* **2019**, *40*, 3222–3232. [CrossRef]

28. Habib, G. Infective endocarditis in Portugal: Changing epidemiology but still a deadly disease. *Rev. Port. Cardiol.* **2021**, *40*, 219–220. [CrossRef]
29. Curlier, E.; Hoen, B.; Alla, F.; Selton-Suty, C.; Schubel, L.; Doco-Lecompte, T.; Minary, L.; Erpelding, M.L.; Duval, X.; Chirouze, C.; et al. Relationships between sex, early valve surgery and mortality in patients with left-sided infective endocarditis analysed in a population-based cohort study. *Heart* **2014**, *100*, 1173–1178. [CrossRef]
30. Lipsky, M.S.; Su, S.; Crespo, C.J.; Hung, M. Men and oral health: A review of sex and gender differences. *Am. J. Mens. Health* **2021**, *15*, 15579883211016361. [CrossRef]
31. Mabilangan, C.; Cole, H.; Hiebert, B.; Keynan, Y.; Arora, R.C.; Shah, P. Short- and long-term outcomes of medically treated isolated left-sided endocarditis: A retrospective study with 5-year longitudinal follow-up. *Can. J. Cardiol.* **2020**, *36*, 1534–1540. [CrossRef]
32. Aksoy, O.; Meyer, L.T.; Cabell, C.H.; Kourany, W.M.; Pappas, P.A.; Sexton, D.J. Gender differences in infective endocarditis: Pre- and co-morbid conditions lead to different management and outcomes in female patients. *Scand. J. Infect. Dis.* **2007**, *39*, 101–107. [CrossRef]
33. Weber, C.; Gassa, A.; Rokohl, A.; Sabashnikov, A.; Deppe, A.C.; Eghbalzadeh, K.; Merkle, J.; Hamacher, S.; Liakopoulos, O.J.; Wahlers, T. Severity of presentation, not sex, increases risk of surgery for infective endocarditis. *Ann. Thorac. Surg.* **2019**, *107*, 1111–1117. [CrossRef]
34. Gordon, E.H.; Hubbard, R.E. Differences in frailty in older men and women. *Med. J. Aust.* **2020**, *212*, 183–188. [CrossRef] [PubMed]
35. Pal, L.M.; Manning, L. Palliative care for frail older people. *Clin. Med.* **2014**, *14*, 292–295. [CrossRef] [PubMed]
36. Sambola, A.; Fernández-Hidalgo, N.; Almirante, B.; Roca, I.; González-Alujas, T.; Serra, B.; Pahissa, A.; García-Dorado, D.; Tornos, P. Sex differences in native-valve infective endocarditis in a single tertiary-care hospital. *Am. J. Cardiol.* **2010**, *106*, 92–98. [CrossRef] [PubMed]
37. van Melle, J.P.; Roos-Hesselink, J.W.; Bansal, M.; Kamp, O.; Meshaal, M.; Pudich, J.; Luksic, V.R.; Rodriguez-Alvarez, R.; Sadeghpour, A.; Hanzevacki, J.S.; et al. Infective endocarditis in adult patients with congenital heart disease. *Int. J. Cardiol.* **2022**. [CrossRef] [PubMed]
38. Ahtela, E.; Oksi, J.; Vahlberg, T.; Sipilä, J.; Rautava, P.; Kytö, V. Short- and long-term outcomes of infective endocarditis admission in adults: A population-based registry study in Finland. *PLoS ONE* **2021**, *16*, e0254553. [CrossRef] [PubMed]
39. Morita, Y.; Haruna, T.; Haruna, Y.; Nakane, E.; Yamaji, Y.; Hayashi, H.; Hanyu, M.; Inoko, M. Thirty-Day Readmission After Infective Endocarditis: Analysis from a Nationwide Readmission Database. *J. Am. Heart Assoc.* **2019**, *8*, e011598. [CrossRef] [PubMed]
40. Tan, C.; Hansen, M.; Cohen, G.; Boyle, K.; Daneman, N.; Adhikari, N.K. Accuracy of administrative data for identification of patients with infective endocarditis. *Int. J. Cardiol.* **2016**, *224*, 162–164. [CrossRef] [PubMed]
41. Chiang, H.Y.; Liang, L.Y.; Lin, C.C.; Chen, Y.J.; Wu, M.Y.; Chen, S.H.; Wu, P.H.; Kuo, C.C.; Chi, C.Y. Electronic medical record-based deep data cleaning and phenotyping improve the diagnostic validity and mortality assessment of infective endocarditis: Medical big data initiative of CMUH. *Biomedicine* **2021**, *11*, 59–67. [CrossRef]
42. Fedeli, U.; Schievano, E.; Buonfrate, D.; Pellizzer, G.; Spolaore, P. Increasing incidence and mortality of infective endocarditis: A population-based study through a record-linkage system. *BMC Infect. Dis.* **2011**, *11*, 48. [CrossRef]
43. Schneeweiss, S.; Robicsek, A.; Scranton, R.; Zuckerman, D.; Solomon, D.H. Veteran's affairs hospital discharge databases coded serious bacterial infections accurately. *J. Clin. Epidemiol.* **2007**, *60*, 397–409. [CrossRef]

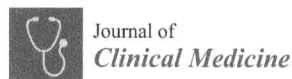

Article

Lipoprotein(a), Cardiovascular Events and Sex Differences: A Single Cardiological Unit Experience

Beatrice Dal Pino [1], Francesca Gorini [2], Melania Gaggini [2], Patrizia Landi [2], Alessandro Pingitore [2] and Cristina Vassalle [1,*]

[1] Fondazione Gabriele Monasterio CNR-Regione Toscana, 56124 Pisa, Italy
[2] Institute of Clinical Physiology, National Research Council, 56124 Pisa, Italy
* Correspondence: cristina.vassalle@ifc.cnr.it

Abstract: Lipoprotein(a)-Lp(a), which retains proatherogenic and prothrombotic properties, may be modified by hormonal and metabolic factors. However, few studies have focused on differences related to sex and cardiometabolic risk factors in the relationship between Lp(a) and cardiovascular disease, especially in terms of prognosis. This study aimed at evaluating the predictive value of Lp(a) (cut-off 30 mg/dL) for hard events (HEs: mortality and non-fatal myocardial infarction) according to sex and cardiometabolic risk factors in 2110 patients (1501 males, mean age: 68 ± 9 years) undergoing coronary angiography for known or suspected coronary artery disease. There were 211 events over a median follow-up period of 33 months. Lp(a) > 30 mg/dL did not confer a worse prognosis on the overall population. However, Kaplan–Meier subgroup analysis evidenced a worse prognosis in type 2 diabetes (T2D) females with elevated Lp(a) (log-rank test: $p = 0.03$) vs. T2D males and no-T2D patients, but not in other high-risk cardiovascular states (e.g., smoking, hypertension, reduced left ventricular ejection fraction or obesity). After Cox multivariate adjustment, Lp(a) remained an independent determinant for HEs in the T2D female subgroup, conferring an HR of 2.9 (95% CI 1.1–7.7, $p < 0.05$). Lp(a) is therefore a strong independent predictor of HR in T2D women, but not in T2D men, or in noT2D patients.

Keywords: Lp(a); biomarkers; mortality; non-fatal myocardial infarction; coronary artery disease; prognosis; sex-related differences; residual risk; type 2 diabetes

1. Introduction

Lipoprotein(a) (Lp(a)) is a low-density lipoprotein containing a molecule of apolipoprotein(a) and apolipoprotein B-100, with a structure similar to LDL cholesterol as well as plasminogen [1].

This molecule is associated with the pathogenesis and development of atherosclerotic damage, in view of its conformation, which gives Lp(a) proatherogenic and prothrombotic properties [1]. Accordingly, results from epidemiological and genetic studies have suggested the role of high Lp(a) as a biomarker of residual atherosclerotic risk and cardiovascular disease (CVD) [2–4]. Subsequent studies reinforced the importance of Lp(a), which should be assessed in all patients with premature coronary artery disease (CAD) in the absence of major coronary risk factors [5].

The 2019 ESC/EAS guidelines on dyslipidemia indicate that Lp(a) should be measured at least once in every person's lifetime, in order to identify individuals with very high inherited Lp(a) levels who are at very high risk for CVD [6]. In particular, the risk may significantly increase when Lp(a) is above 50 mg/dL [7], although other studies showed that values of Lp(a) >30 mg/dL are sufficient to increase the risk of cardiovascular events or all-cause mortality [8–10]. The function and atherogenicity of Lp(a) may be modulated by glycation, and is increased in diabetic patients [11,12]. Moreover, some studies suggest that estrogen may reduce Lp(a), which therefore increases in postmenopausal women and decreases in individuals on hormone replacement therapy (HRT) [13–15].

Citation: Dal Pino, B.; Gorini, F.; Gaggini, M.; Landi, P.; Pingitore, A.; Vassalle, C. Lipoprotein(a), Cardiovascular Events and Sex Differences: A Single Cardiological Unit Experience. *J. Clin. Med.* 2023, 12, 764. https://doi.org/10.3390/jcm12030764

Academic Editor: Alessandro Delitala

Received: 6 December 2022
Revised: 13 January 2023
Accepted: 15 January 2023
Published: 18 January 2023

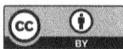

Copyright: © 2023 by the authors. Licensee MDPI, Basel, Switzerland. This article is an open access article distributed under the terms and conditions of the Creative Commons Attribution (CC BY) license (https://creativecommons.org/licenses/by/4.0/).

At present, few studies have explored sex differences in the relationship between serum Lp(a) and CVD, especially in terms of prognosis and secondary prevention, while the under-representation of women in most studies may indicate a gap in the evidence [16,17].

Therefore, the aim of this study was to assess the association between Lp(a) concentration and hard events (HEs: mortality and non-fatal myocardial infarction) in a large population of patients undergoing coronary angiography for known or suspected coronary artery disease (CAD) and in subgroups in relation to sex and in the presence of cardiometabolic risk factors, in particular type 2 diabetes (T2D).

2. Materials and Methods

2.1. Study and Population Characteristics

We conducted a longitudinal retrospective clinical cohort study to evaluate sex-related differences in cardiometabolic risk factors and survival in patients older than 50 years and admitted to the Cardiology Department of the Institute of Clinical Physiology, National Research Council, in Pisa, (Italy), who underwent coronary angiography for known or suspected CAD and were followed up for 10 years (2110 patients, 1501 males, mean age: 68 ± 9 years). All data were acquired in the setting of institutional assistance within clinical care purposes in a retrospective manner from our institution's patient dataset (image database), containing clinical characteristics, previous history, CAD risk factors, comorbidities, laboratory and instrumental results, pharmacological therapies and post-discharge follow-up outcomes, and analyzed anonymously as an aggregated group, not individually [18]. Exclusion criteria were applied as follows: unavailability of Lp(a) results, severe systemic diseases including neoplasia, acute or chronic inflammatory disease, immunological disease, HRT (for women) and patient refusal or inability to supply written informed consent.

Data on smoking (no smokers, smoking history), arterial hypertension (systolic blood pressure > 140 mmHg and/or diastolic pressure > 90 mmHg or use of antihypertensive agents), T2D (fasting plasma glucose > 126 mg/dL or use of antidiabetic treatment), obesity (defined as body mass index > 30 kg/m^2) and dyslipidemia (total cholesterol $\geq$ 200 mg/dL, triglyceride $\geq$ 150 mg/dL or current use of lipid-lowering therapy) were coded in a dichotomized manner. Previous medical therapy included angiotensin-converting-enzyme inhibitors, beta-blockers, lipid-lowering agents, antidiabetic agents, diuretics and aspirin.

The primary outcome was the occurrence of HEs. Follow-up was assessed by phone calls, personal communication with the patient's physician or outpatient follow-up visits. Patients were followed from admission until the end point (mortality, the information on which was obtained from medical records or death certificates) or for a maximum of 10 years from the time of enrollment. The definition of cardiac death required the following documentation: significant arrhythmias, cardiac arrest, death attributable to congestive heart failure or myocardial infarction in the absence of any other precipitating factors. The diagnosis of myocardial infarction was based on documentation of persistent electrocardiographic ST segment changes, or the development of new Q waves, in association with elevation of laboratory biomarkers.

2.2. Statistical Analysis

Data are presented as number and percentages for categorical variables and as means and standard deviations or median where appropriate for continuous variables. Statistical analysis included χ^2 tests for categorical variables. Estimates of survival probabilities were calculated using the Kaplan–Meier method and compared with the log-rank test. Variables were included in the multivariate Cox model based on significance in the univariate analyses to evaluate the effect of variables on survival time, reporting the hazard ratio (HR) with a 95% confidence interval of probability (95% CI). p values were two-sided with a significance threshold of 0.05. All statistical analyses were performed using Statview statistical package, version 5.0.1 (SAS Institute, Abacus Concept, Inc., Berkeley, CA, USA).

3. Results

Table 1 summarizes the study sample characteristics stratified by sex. Male patients were more likely to have a higher incidence of smoking history and were characterized by a higher proportion of subjects with reduced left ventricular ejection fraction (LVEF) (<50%), while female patients were likely to have a higher incidence of hypertension, CAD familiarity and obesity.

Table 1. Characteristics of the studied population.

Variable	Females n = 609	Males n = 1501	p Value
Age (50th percentile: 70 years for females, 67 years for males)	330 (54)	769 (51)	ns
Type 2 Diabetes	139 (23)	378 (25)	ns
Hypertension	379 (62)	850 (57)	<0.05
Dyslipidemia	465 (76)	1180 (79)	ns
Familiarity with CAD	317 (52)	677 (45)	<0.01
Smoking History	143 (23)	750 (50)	<0.001
Obesity (<30 kg/m^2)	172 (28)	323 (21)	<0.001
LVEF (<50%)	130 (21)	455 (30)	<0.001
Lp(a) (>30 mg/dL)	296 (49)	671 (45)	ns

Data are reported as number (%) in the female and male subgroups. Abbreviations: CAD: coronary artery disease; Lp(a): lipoprotein(a); LVEF: left ventricular ejection fraction; ns, not statistically significant.

The distribution of Lp(a) in the cohort of patients was skewed to the right (Figure 1). The median level of lipoprotein was 27 mg/dL (29 and 26 mg/dL in female and male patients, respectively).

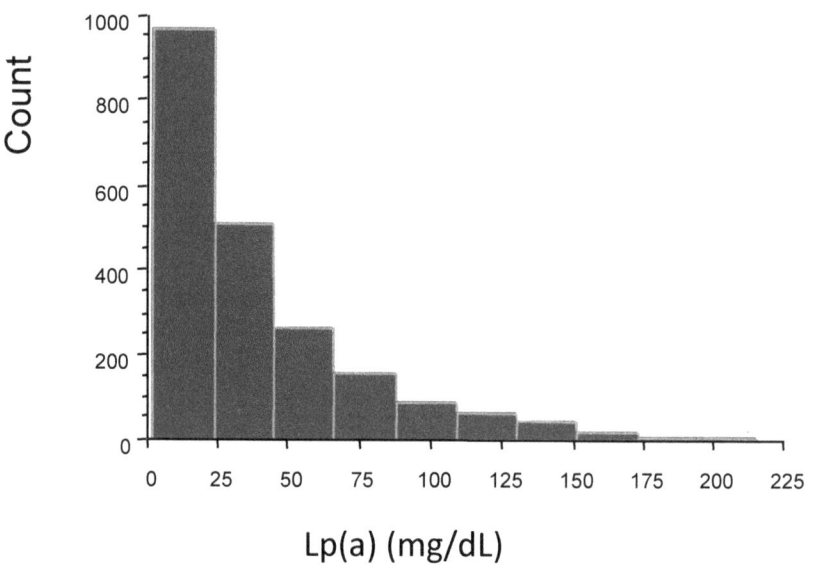

Figure 1. Lp(a) distribution in the overall population.

In both sexes, the percentage of subjects with increased Lp(a) (cut-off of 30 mg/dL) differed depending on the presence of dyslipidemia (40 vs. 51%, $p < 0.05$ and 35 vs. 47%,

$p < 0.001$ in females and males, respectively) and family history of CAD only in males (41 vs. 49%, $p < 0.01$) (Table 2).

Table 2. Number and percentage of subjects with Lp(a) > 30 mg/dL in female and male patients for each variable subgroup.

	Females $n = 609$		Males $n = 1501$	
Variable	Number of Subjects with Lp(a) > 30 mg/dL (%)	p Value	Number of Subjects with Lp(a) > 30 mg/dL (%)	p Value
Age (<50th percentile)	143 (51)	ns	337 (46)	ns
Age (≥50th percentile)	153 (46)		334 (43)	
no-T2D	235 (50)	ns	514 (46)	ns
T2D	61 (44)		157 (42)	
no-Hypertension	118 (51)	ns	294 (45)	ns
Hypertension	178 (47)		377 (44)	
no-Dyslipidemia	58 (40)	<0.05	111 (35)	<0.001
Dyslipidemia	238 (51)		560 (47)	
no-CAD Familiarity	138 (47)	ns	340 (41)	<0.01
CAD Familiarity	158 (50)		331 (49)	
no-Smoking History	222 (48)	ns	330 (44)	ns
Smoking History	74 (52)		341 (45)	
no-Obesity	210 (48)	ns	524 (45)	ns
Obesity	86 (50)		147 (45)	
LVEF (<50%)	67 (51)	ns	191 (42)	ns
LVEF (≥50%)	229 (48)		480 (46)	

Data are reported as the ratio between the number of individuals with Lp(a) > 30 mg/dL and the total number of subjects in each subgroup (%). Abbreviations: CAD: coronary artery disease; Lp(a): lipoprotein(a); LVEF: left ventricular ejection fraction; T2D: type 2 diabetes; ns, not statistically significant.

Overall, 211 HEs (161 deaths and 50 non-fatal myocardial infarctions) were recorded during a mean follow-up of 33 months. As determined by Kaplan–Meier analysis, elevated Lp(a) levels (>30 mg/dL) did not lead to a worse long-term prognosis (log-rank test p value 0.68). However, subgroups analysis showed a worse prognosis in T2D females with elevated Lp(a) (log-rank test p value 0.03) (Figure 2C) compared to T2D/no-T2D males and no-T2D female patients (Figure 2A,B,D).

In female patients with T2D, Cox regression analyses revealed a significant association of Lp(a) with outcomes; in particular, high Lp(a) levels (>30 mg/dL) were associated with HEs with an HR of 2.9 (95% CI 1.1–7.7, $p < 0.05$) after multivariate adjustment (Table 3).

In our cohort, high-sensitivity C-reactive protein (hsCRP), fibrinogen and the erythrocyte sedimentation rate (ESR) were available in a subset of patients, showing the following correlations with logLp(a) values: logLp(a) vs. logCRP (correlation not significant in 588 female patients, $r = 0.11$ $p < 0.001$ in 1451 males); logLp(a) vs. logESR ($r = 0.16$, $p < 0.001$ in 595 female patients, $r = 0.18$ $p < 0.001$ in 1465 males); logLp(a) vs. logfibrinogen (correlation not significant in 571 female patients, $r = 0.13$, $p < 0.001$ in 1410 males).

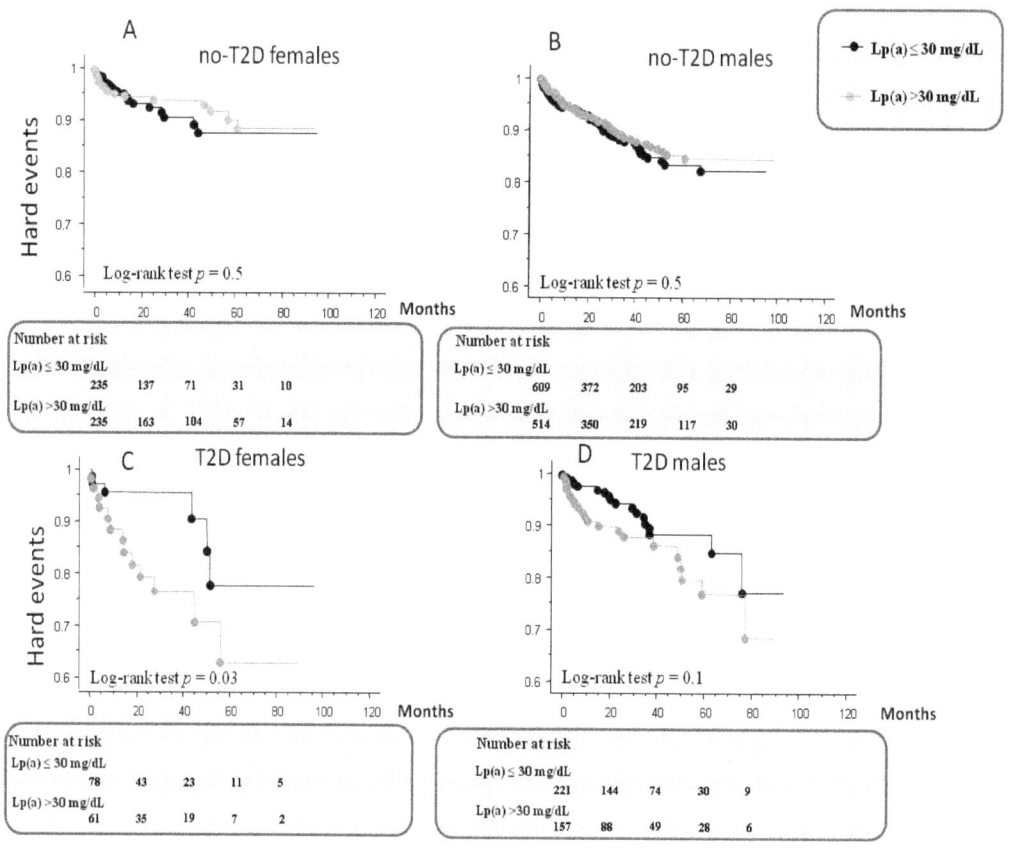

Figure 2. Kaplan–Meier survival curves according to Lp(a) levels in female and male patients with and without T2D (**A–D**), with hard events (mortality and non-fatal myocardial infarction) as end points.

Table 3. Univariate and multivariate COX analysis for HEs in T2D female patients.

Predictors	Univariate Analysis		Multivariate Analysis	
	HR (95%CI)	p Value	HR (95%CI)	p Value
Age (50th percentile)	2.5 (1–7.1)	<0.05	2.7 (1–7.7)	0.05
Hypertension	1.4 (0.5–3.8)	ns	-	-
Dyslipidemia	1.8 (0.4–8.0)	ns	-	-
Familiarity with CAD	0.5 (0.2–1.2)	ns	.	-
Smoking History	1.2 (0.4–3.9)	ns	-	-
Obesity (<30 kg/m^2)	0.7 (0.3–1.7)	ns	-	-
Left Ventricular Ejection Fraction (<50%)	1.6 (0.7–4.3)	ns	-	-
Lp(a) (>30 mg/dL)	2.7 (1–7.2)	<0.05	2.9 (1.1–7.7)	<0.05

Abbreviations: HR: hazard ratio; 95%CI: 95% confidence interval of probability; ns, not statistically significant.

4. Discussion

The main result of this study is the independent association of Lp(a) levels with HEs in a cohort of T2D women undergoing coronary angiography for known or suspected

CAD. Conversely, no relationship between events and Lp(a) levels in diabetic men or in non-diabetic subjects belonging to both sexes was observed.

Genetically predicted and measured Lp(a) values reveal a strong and consistent relationship with CAD risk and outcomes, identifying Lp(a) as an important element of residual cardiovascular risk [4,19]. In our overall population, Lp(a) > 30 mg/dL did not confer a worse prognosis, in contrast to several previous findings that identified Lp(a) as a prognostic independent risk factor for cardiovascular events, although it is important to remember that there is marked heterogeneity across studies evaluating the prognostic significance of Lp(a) [20]. This discrepancy may be due to different reasons. Importantly, the relationship between Lp(a) and CAD may vary depending on the patient's baseline risk based on demographic characteristics (e.g., age, sex) and the presence/absence of coexisting CAD risk factors, such as inflammation and/or a procoagulant status [21–24].

Specifically, in the Multi-Ethnic Study of Atherosclerosis (MESA) Apolipoprotein ancillary dataset, isolated Lp(a) elevation was not associated with increased CVD risk, whereas the combination of elevated Lp(a) ($\geq$50 mg/dL) and hsCRP ($\geq$2 mg/L) was independently associated with CVD risk (HR, 1.62; 95% CI, 1.25–2.10) and all-cause mortality (HR, 1.39; 95% CI, 1.12–1.72) [21,22]. Conversely, the relationship between Lp(a) and cardiovascular events may be attenuated in patients with lower low-density lipoprotein cholesterol values [20]. The data we obtained in a subgroup of patients evidenced correlations between logLp(a) values and CRP, fibrinogen and the erythrocyte sedimentation rate (ESR), confirming the relationship between Lp(a) and these pathways, which was especially evident in male patients. Thus, it is important to evaluate the independent and combined association of Lp(a) and hsCRP or other biomarkers with cardiovascular outcome in specific population subgroups. Moreover, using different methods to quantify Lp(a) may influence the final results [25–27].

The choice of cut-off may also be a key factor, because when Lp(a) is evaluated as a categorical variable, the thresholds for the categories may differ between studies. However, we observed that Lp(a) was not significantly associated with HEs as assessed considering the per unit increase in LogLp(a) (HR of 1.28, 95% CI: 1–1.8, $p = 0.16$), and using the categorical threshold of 50 mg/dL (HR 1.05, 95% CI: 0.8–1.4, $p = 0.7$) in the univariate analysis in the overall population.

In the context of T2D, Lp(a) is associated with T2D risk and CAD disease severity, as well as with microvascular and kidney complications and adverse events in patients with diabetes and elevated Lp(a) [28]. Lp(a) may increase the risk of the onset and development of T2D and the cardiometabolic burden via pro-atherogenic and pro-inflammatory effects, and induce a prothrombotic status through a variety of mechanisms (e.g., inhibition of the fibrinolytic system and enhancement of tissue-factor-mediated pathways). Conversely, a hyperglycemic status may promote the glycation of lipoproteins, while reduced insulin production can further exacerbate the increase in Lp(a) in T2D, as insulin inhibits hepatic apo(a) and apoB production through suppressed transcription [28].

Although sex differences in Lp(a)-related risk are still unclear, there is evidence that estrogen reduces Lp(a), as well as that Lp(a) rises in postmenopausal women, but its levels are reduced by HRT [29,30]. Accordingly, some data indicated that the relationship between elevated Lp(a) levels and increased CVD risk may be modulated by HRT, as the CV predictive role of Lp(a) in women not taking HRT was instead markedly attenuated in those taking HRT [31]. Women in the Nurses' Health Study with Lp(a) levels > 30 mg/dL had an increased risk of CAD events, which appeared to be modulated by thrombosis and inflammation [32]. Always in the Nurses' Health Study, T2D women with increased Lp(a) levels had a higher risk of developing CAD [33]. Previous findings also suggest that Lp(a) has a stronger association with coronary artery calcification in T2D females with respect to males with and without T2D or no-T2D women [30].

Taken together, these data may indicate that Lp(a) deserves to be evaluated as a potential risk predictor in high-risk T2D women. This finding may be of particular interest, as a woman's CV risk still has unknown specific characteristics and remains largely underestimated. Thus, research on and identification of reliable additive biomarkers for optimized CV assessment and improvement in CV management in women are expected and welcome. Moreover, conventional therapeutic strategies (such as statins) have resulted in a substantially ineffective reduction in Lp(a), and in some cases may even increase its concentration [34]. Other drugs that lower Lp(a) levels (e.g., niacin or cholesteryl ester transfer protein inhibitors) do not show significant beneficial effects on cardiovascular outcomes. However, some tools currently reduce Lp(a) while also lowering CV risk (e.g., PCSK9 inhibitors and lipoprotein apheresis). For PCSK9 inhibitors, the magnitude of clinical benefit is related to baseline Lp(a) value and associated with the degree of Lp(a) decrease. Therefore, the identification of patients that may benefit most from such therapies as well as the extent of Lp(a) reduction required to benefit the CV system represents a very important challenge in targeting this biomarker as a component of residual cardiovascular risk.

Other treatment options are currently available (e.g., gene silencing via RNA interference with use of antisense oligonucleotides or small interfering RNA molecules) that appear to reduce Lp(a) levels by more than 70%, and could be further evaluated for their reliability in reducing overall CV events in female patients with high-risk T2D [35].

Strengths and Limitations

The study may present limitations related to its retrospective nature, and the single-center experience, although the number of patients enrolled is large (even for the female counterpart), and the focus on sex differences is an aspect often neglected in research studies and clinical practice. The sample size is not necessarily balanced between sexes, as it is well known that CAD is more common in men than in women (men usually have a 2-fold higher incidence of CAD and related mortality than women) [36]. A further limitation is the lack of availability of information on menopausal status in female patients, although we included patients over 50 (only 28 women between 50 and 55 years), which is the average age at which menopause occurs among women from industrialized countries; thus, the large majority of female patients in our cohort were postmenopausal [37]. However, these data highlight that there may be potential sex-related mechanisms underlying the relationship between Lp(a), T2D and CAD, since Lp(a) would appear to predict additive risk in the case of women with T2D.

5. Conclusions

The concentration of Lp(a) is mainly determined by genetics (>90%), more than any other lipoprotein. In patients with suspected or known CAD, Lp(a) might represent an additive significant risk predictor in high-risk T2D women, but not in male patients with or without T2D or in non-diabetic women. Further studies are warranted to confirm our preliminary results and thus contribute to a better assessment of the risk profile of this specific population.

Author Contributions: Conceptualization, C.V.; writing—original draft preparation, C.V.; review and editing, B.D.P., F.G., M.G., P.L., A.P. and C.V. All authors have read and agreed to the published version of the manuscript.

Funding: This research received no external funding.

Institutional Review Board Statement: The study was conducted in accordance with the Declaration of Helsinki. All data were acquired in the context of institutional assistance within clinical care purposes in a retrospectively collected modality from our institution's patient dataset (image database), and analyzed anonymously as an aggregated group and not individually.

Informed Consent Statement: Informed consent was obtained from all subjects involved in the study.

Data Availability Statement: Data may be provided by the authors upon (reasonable) request.

Acknowledgments: The authors wish to thank Fabrizio Minichilli for his support in the statistical analysis.

Conflicts of Interest: The authors declare no conflict of interest.

Abbreviation

Lp(a)	lipoprotein(a)
CAD	coronary artery disease
T2D	type 2 diabetes
CVD	cardiovascular disease
HEs	hard events
HRT	hormone replacement therapy
LVEF	left ventricular ejection fraction
hsCRP	high-sensitivity C-reactive protein
ESR	erythrocyte sedimentation rate
HR	hazard ratio
95% CI	95% confidence interval of probability

References

1. Saeed, A.; Kinoush, S.; Virani, S.S. Lipoprotein (a): Recent Updates on a Unique Lipoprotein. *Curr. Atheroscler. Rep.* **2021**, *23*, 41. [CrossRef] [PubMed]
2. Yan, Z.; Liu, Y.; Li, W.; Zhao, X.; Lin, W.; Zhang, J.; Yu, S.; Ma, J.; Wang, J.; Yu, P.; et al. Liver fibrosis scores and prognosis in patients with cardiovascular diseases: A system-atic review and meta-analysis. *Eur J Clin Investig.* **2022**, *52*, 13855. [CrossRef] [PubMed]
3. Melita, H.; Manolis, A.A.; Manolis, T.A.; Manolis, A.S. Lipoprotein(a) and Cardiovascular Disease: A Missing Link for Premature Atherosclerotic Heart Disease and/or Residual Risk. *J. Cardiovasc. Pharmacol.* **2022**, *79*, 18–35. [CrossRef]
4. Rikhi, R.; Hammoud, A.; Ashburn, N.; Snavely, A.C.; Michos, E.D.; Chevli, P.; Tsai, M.Y.; Herrington, D.; Shapiro, M.D. Relationship of low-density lipoprotein-cholesterol and lipoprotein(a) to cardiovascular risk: The Multi-Ethnic Study of Atherosclerosis (MESA). *Atherosclerosis* **2022**, *363*, 102–108. [CrossRef]
5. Dal Pino, B.; Sbrana, F.; Coceani, M.; Bigazzi, F.; Sampietro, T. Lipoprotein(a) in familial hypercholesterolemia: Tips from family history. *Rev. Port. Cardiol.* **2021**, *40*, 225–227. [CrossRef] [PubMed]
6. Mach, F.; Baigent, C.; Catapano, A.L.; Koskinas, K.C.; Casula, M.; Badimon, L.; Chapman, M.J.; De Backer, G.G.; Delgado, V.; Ference, B.A. 2019 ESC/EAS Guidelines for the management of dyslipidaemias: Lipid modification to reduce cardiovascular risk: The Task Force for the management of dyslipidaemias of the European Society of Cardiology (ESC) and European Atherosclerosis Society. *Eur. Heart J.* **2020**, *1*, 111–188. [CrossRef] [PubMed]
7. Nordestgaard, B.G.; Chapman, M.J.; Ray, K.; Borén, J.; Andreotti, F.; Watts, G.F.; Ginsberg, H.; Amarenco, P.; Catapano, A.; Descamps, O.S.; et al. Lipoprotein(a) as a cardiovascular risk factor: Current status. *Eur. Heart J.* **2010**, *31*, 2844–2853. [CrossRef] [PubMed]
8. Jin, J.L.; Cao, Y.X.; Zhang, H.W.; Sun, D.; Hua, Q.; Li, Y.F.; Guo, Y.L.; Wu, N.Q.; Zhu, C.G.; Gao, Y.; et al. Lipoprotein(a) and cardiovascular outcomes in patients with coronary artery disease and prediabetes or diabetes. *Diabetes Care* **2019**, *42*, 1312–1318. [CrossRef]
9. Gao, S.; Ma, W.; Huang, S.; Lin, X.; Yu, M. Effect of Lipoprotein (a) Levels on Long-term Cardiovascular Outcomes in Patients with Myocardial Infarction with Nonobstructive Coronary Arteries. *Am. J. Cardiol.* **2021**, *152*, 34–42. [CrossRef]
10. Wang, Z.; Zhai, X.; Xue, M.; Cheng, W.; Hu, H. Prognostic value of lipoprotein (a) level in patients with coronary artery disease: A meta-analysis. *Lipids Health Dis.* **2019**, *18*, 150. [CrossRef]
11. Doucet, C.; Huby, T.; Ruiz, J.; Chapman, M.J.; Thillet, J. Non-enzymatic glycation of lipoprotein(a) in vitro and in vivo. *Atherosclerosis* **1995**, *118*, 135–143. [CrossRef] [PubMed]
12. Mahmoodi, M.R.; Najafipour, H. Association of C-peptide and lipoprotein(a) as two predictors with cardiometabolic biomarkers in patients with type 2 diabetes in KERCADR population-based study. *PLoS ONE* **2022**, *17*, e268927. [CrossRef] [PubMed]
13. Enkhmaa, B.; Berglund, L. Non-genetic influences on lipoprotein(a) concentrations. *Atherosclerosis* **2022**, *349*, 53–62. [CrossRef] [PubMed]
14. Liu, S.L.; Wu, N.Q.; Guo, Y.L.; Zhu, C.G.; Gao, Y.; Sun, J.; Xu, R.X.; Liu, G.; Dong, Q.; Li, J.J. Lipoprotein(a) and coronary artery disease in Chinese postmenopausal female patients: A large cross-sectional cohort study. *Postgrad. Med. J.* **2019**, *95*, 534–540. [CrossRef]
15. Anagnostis, P.; Galanis, P.; Chatzistergiou, V.; Stevenson, J.C.; Godsland, I.F.; Lambrinoudaki, I.; Theodorou, M.; Goulis, D.G. The effect of hormone replacement therapy and tibolone on lipoprotein (a) concentrations in postmenopausal women: A systematic review and meta-analysis. *Maturitas* **2017**, *99*, 27–36. [CrossRef]
16. Cook, N.R.; Mora, S.; Ridker, P.M. Lipoprotein(a) and Cardiovascular Risk Prediction Among Women. *J. Am. Coll. Cardiol.* **2018**, *72*, 287–296. [CrossRef]
17. Waldeyer, C.; Makarova, N.; Zeller, T.; Schnabel, R.B.; Brunner, F.J.; Jørgensen, T.; Linneberg, A.; Niiranen, T.; Salomaa, V.; Jousilahti, P.; et al. Lipoprotein(a) and the risk of cardiovascular disease in the European population: Results from the BiomarCaRE consortium. *Eur. Heart J.* **2017**, *38*, 2490–2498. [CrossRef]

18. Vassalle, C.; Maffei, S.; Bianchi, S.; Landi, P.; Carpeggiani, C. Prognostic role of heart rate in patients referred for coronary angiography: Age and sex differences. *Climacteric* **2014**, *17*, 260–267. [CrossRef]
19. Arsenault, B.J.; Kamstrup, P.R. Lipoprotein(a) and cardiovascular and valvular diseases: A genetic epidemiological perspective. *Atherosclerosis* **2022**, *349*, 7–16. [CrossRef]
20. O'Donoghue, M.L.; Morrow, D.A.; Tsimikas, S.; Sloan, S.; Ren, A.F.; Hoffman, E.B.; Desai, N.R.; Solomon, S.D.; Domanski, M.; Arai, K.; et al. Lipoprotein(a) for risk assessment in patients with established coronary artery disease. *J. Am. Coll. Cardiol.* **2014**, *63*, 520–527. [CrossRef]
21. Zhang, W.; Speiser, J.L.; Ye, F.; Tsai, M.Y.; Cainzos-Achirica, M.; Nasir, K.; Herrington, D.M.; Shapiro, M.D. High-Sensitivity C-Reactive Protein Modifies the Cardiovascular Risk of Lipoprotein(a): Multi-Ethnic Study of Atherosclerosis. *J. Am. Coll. Cardiol.* **2021**, *78*, 1083–1094. [CrossRef]
22. Ong, K.L.; McClelland, R.L.; Allison, M.A.; Cushman, M.; Garg, P.K.; Tsai, M.Y.; Rye, K.A.; Tabet, F. Lipoprotein (a) and coronary artery calcification: Prospective study assessing interactions with other risk factors. *Metabolism* **2021**, *116*, 154706. [CrossRef]
23. Jin, J.L.; Zhang, H.W.; Liu, H.H.; Zhu, C.G.; Guo, Y.L.; Wu, N.Q.; Xu, R.X.; Dong, Q.; Li, J.J. Lipoprotein(a) and Cardiovascular Outcomes in Patients With Coronary Artery Disease and Different Metabolic Phenotypes. *Front. Cardiovasc. Med.* **2022**, *9*, 1–9. [CrossRef] [PubMed]
24. Yuan, D.; Wang, P.; Jia, S.; Zhang, C.; Zhu, P.; Jiang, L.; Liu, R.; Xu, J.; Tang, X.; Song, Y.; et al. Lipoprotein(a), high-sensitivity C-reactive protein, and cardiovascular risk in patients undergoing percutaneous coronary intervention. *Atherosclerosis* **2022**, *363*, 109–116. [CrossRef] [PubMed]
25. Vasquez, N.; Joshi, P.H. Lp(a): Addressing a Target for Cardiovascular Disease Prevention. *Curr. Cardiol. Rep.* **2019**, *21*, 102. [CrossRef] [PubMed]
26. Forbes, C.A.; Quek, R.G.W.; Deshpande, S.; Worthy, G.; Wolff, R.; Stirk, L.; Kleijnen, J.; Gandra, S.R.; Djedjos, S.; Wong, N.D. The relationship between Lp(a) and CVD outcomes: A systematic review. *Lipids Health Dis.* **2016**, *15*, 95. [CrossRef]
27. Marcovina, S.M.; Albers, J.J. Lipoprotein (a) measurements for clinical application. *J. Lipid Res.* **2016**, *57*, 526–537. [CrossRef]
28. Lamina, C.; Ward, N.C. Lipoprotein (a) and diabetes mellitus. *Atherosclerosis* **2022**, *349*, 63–71. [CrossRef]
29. Kim, C.J.; Ryu, W.S.; Kwak, J.W.; Park, C.T.; Ryoo, U.H. Changes in Lp(a) lipoprotein and lipid levels after cessation of female sex hormone production and estrogen replacement therapy. *Arch. Intern. Med.* **1996**, *156*, 500–504. [CrossRef]
30. Qasim, A.N.; Martin, S.S.; Mehta, N.N.; Wolfe, M.L.; Park, J.; Schwartz, S.; Schutta, M.; Iqbal, N.; Reilly, M.P. Lipoprotein(a) is strongly associated with coronary artery calcification in type-2 diabetic women. *Int. J. Cardiol.* **2011**, *150*, 17–21. [CrossRef]
31. Danik, J.S.; Rifai, N.; Buring, J.E.; Ridker, P.M. Lipoprotein(a), Hormone Replacement Therapy, and Risk of Future Cardiovascular Events. *J. Am. Coll. Cardiol.* **2008**, *52*, 124–131. [CrossRef] [PubMed]
32. Shai, I.; Rimm, E.B.; Hankinson, S.E.; Cannuscio, C.; Curhan, G.; Manson, J.A.E.; Rifai, N.; Stampfer, M.J.; Ma, J. Lipoprotein (a) and coronary heart disease among women: Beyond a cholesterol carrier? *Eur. Heart J.* **2005**, *26*, 1633–1639. [CrossRef] [PubMed]
33. Shai, I.; Schulze, M.B.; Manson, J.E.; Stampfer, M.J.; Rifai, N.; Hu, F.B. A prospective study of lipoprotein(a) and risk of coronary heart disease among women with type 2 diabetes. *Diabetologia* **2005**, *48*, 1469–1476. [CrossRef] [PubMed]
34. Schwartz, G.G.; Ballantyne, C.M. Existing and emerging strategies to lower Lipoprotein(a). *Atherosclerosis* **2022**, *349*, 110–122. [CrossRef]
35. Gareri, C.; Polimeni, A.; Giordano, S.; Tammè, L.; Curcio, A.; Indolfi, C. Antisense Oligonucleotides and Small Interfering RNA for the Treatment of Dyslipidemias. *J. Clin. Med.* **2022**, *11*, 3884.
36. Gao, Z.; Chen, Z.; Sun, A.; Deng, X. Gender differences in cardiovascular disease. *Med. Nov. Technol. Devices* **2019**, *4*, 100025. [CrossRef]
37. Gold, E.B. The Timing of the Age at Which Natural Menopause Occurs. *Obstet. Gynecol. Clin. N. Am.* **2011**, *38*, 425–440. [CrossRef]

Disclaimer/Publisher's Note: The statements, opinions and data contained in all publications are solely those of the individual author(s) and contributor(s) and not of MDPI and/or the editor(s). MDPI and/or the editor(s) disclaim responsibility for any injury to people or property resulting from any ideas, methods, instructions or products referred to in the content.

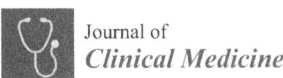

Article

Sex-Related Differences in Outpatient Healthcare of Acute Coronary Syndrome: Evidence from an Italian Real-World Investigation

Raffaella Ronco [1,2], Federico Rea [1,2,*], Amelia Filippelli [1,3], Aldo Pietro Maggioni [4] and Giovanni Corrao [1,2]

1. National Centre for Healthcare Research and Pharmacoepidemiology, University of Milano-Bicocca, 20126 Milan, Italy; raffaella.ronco@unimib.it (R.R.); afilippelli@unisa.it (A.F.); giovanni.corrao@unimib.it (G.C.)
2. Unit of Biostatistics, Epidemiology and Public Health, Department of Statistics and Quantitative Methods, University of Milano-Bicocca, 20126 Milan, Italy
3. Department of Medicine, Surgery, and Dentistry, University of Salerno, 84081 Baronissi, Italy
4. ANMCO Research Center, 50121 Florence, Italy; maggioni@heartcarefoundation.it
*   Correspondence: federico.rea@unimib.it; Tel.: +39-026-448-5859

Abstract: At the time of first acute coronary syndrome (ACS) hospital admission, women are generally older and have more comorbidities than men, which may explain differences in their short-term prognosis. However, few studies have focused on differences in the out-of-hospital management of men and women. This study investigated (i) the risk of clinical outcomes, (ii) the use of out-of-hospital healthcare and (iii) the effects of clinical recommendations on outcomes in men vs. women. A total of 90,779 residents of the Lombardy Region (Italy) were hospitalized for ACS from 2011 to 2015. Exposure to prescribed drugs, diagnostic procedures, laboratory tests, and cardiac rehabilitation in the first year after ACS hospitalization were recorded. To evaluate whether sex can modify the relationship between clinical recommendations and outcomes, adjusted Cox models were separately fitted for men and women. Women were exposed to fewer treatments, required fewer outpatient services than men and had a lower risk of long-term clinical events. The stratified analysis showed an association between adherence to clinical recommendations and a lower risk of clinical outcomes in both sexes. Since improved adherence to clinical recommendations seems to be beneficial for both sexes, tight out-of-hospital healthcare control should be recommended to achieve favourable clinical benefits.

Keywords: acute coronary syndrome; sex-differences; healthcare; public health; real-world

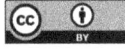

1. Introduction

Acute coronary syndrome (ACS) includes multiple manifestations of myocardial ischemia, including ST-segment elevation myocardial infarction (STEMI), non-ST-segment elevation myocardial infarction (NSTEMI) and unstable angina (UA). In Italy, twenty-eight-day case cardiac fatalities decreased by almost two-thirds during the 1990s [1], likely due to impressive improvements in medical treatments. This led to an increased number of patients who survived an ACS episode. Therefore, the clinical management of ACS patients after hospital discharge became a major challenge to improving long-term prognosis [2]. Although evidence-based guidelines have been developed for the secondary prevention of cardiovascular events and death [3,4], the risk of adverse outcomes in these patients is still high [5]. This is partially due to suboptimal adherence to current clinical practice guidelines [6,7].

Several studies have reported that women have worse short-term outcomes after ACS treatment. This is likely because they experience their first ACS episode at an older age when their clinical profile is already compromised by other comorbidities [8–12].

However, few studies have investigated differences in the out-of-hospital management of ACS between men and women, and those that have evaluated drug treatment and long-term prognosis observed conflicting findings [13–15].

Based on these premises, a large real-world study of a cohort of patients admitted to the hospital for their first episode of ACS was performed to evaluate sex-related differences in both out-of-hospital healthcare and short- and long-term clinical outcomes. A further aim was to assess whether sex modified the relationship between post-discharge healthcare and clinical outcomes.

2. Materials and Methods

2.1. Setting

Data used for this study were retrieved from the healthcare utilization databases of Lombardy, a region of Italy that accounts for about 16% of its population (about 10 million individuals). All Italian citizens have equal access to health care services as part of the National Health Service (NHS).

Automated healthcare utilization databases allow the Lombardy Region to collect various information, including (i) demographic and administrative data on NHS beneficiaries, (ii) private and public hospital discharge records coded according to the International Classification of Diseases, 9th Revision Clinical Modification (ICD-CM-9) classification system; (iii) outpatient drug prescriptions coded with the Anatomical Therapeutic Chemical (ATC) classification system; and (iv) data on outpatient services, including specialist visits and diagnostic examinations reimbursable by the NHS.

Records are linked between databases through a single identification code. To preserve privacy, each identification code is automatically converted into an anonymous code. Patient identification by the Regional Health Authority is only allowed upon request by judicial authorities.

Studies on the healthcare utilization databases of Lombardy in the field of cardiovascular diseases have been carried out [16–18]. Supplementary Table S1 lists the codes that were used to identify hospitalizations, prescriptions and information of interest to the current paper.

2.2. Cohort Selection

The target population consisted of residents of Lombardy aged 40–90 years. As shown in Figure 1, to assess (i) in-hospital all-cause mortality, (ii) out-of-hospital clinical outcomes, and (iii) healthcare provision to cohort members, three cohorts were identified and evaluated as described below.

First, patients who were hospitalized via the emergency room with an ACS diagnosis from 2011–2015 were identified, and the dates of admission and discharge from their first hospitalization during this period were recorded as "index admission" and "index discharge", respectively. Patients who were beneficiaries of the NHS for less than five years prior to the index hospital admission, or who had a previous hospitalization for ACS during the same period, were excluded from the study cohort, as information from previous years was used to characterize cohort members. The remaining patients were included in the "first cohort" and were studied to evaluate in-hospital all-cause mortality.

Aiming to evaluate clinical outcomes after hospital discharge, subjects who survived the index hospitalization were selected for the "second cohort". This latter group calculated person-years of follow-up from the index discharge until an end outcome (see below) or censoring event (death, emigration, or end of follow-up, i.e., 30 June 2018) occurred.

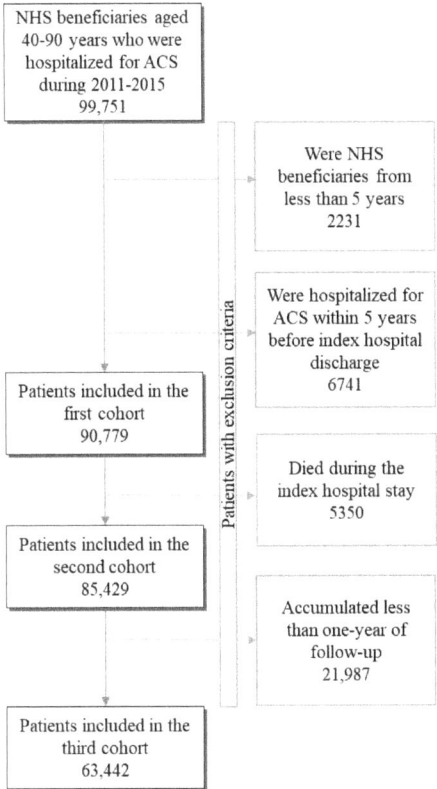

Figure 1. Flowchart of selection of the cohorts.

Finally, aiming to guarantee at least one year of observations to track outpatient services and treatments, patients who experienced a relevant clinical outcome (death or readmission for any cardiovascular causes) in the first year after hospital discharge were excluded from the "third cohort". Patients of the third cohort were followed up until clinical outcomes or censoring as defined for the second cohort were met.

2.3. Cohort Baseline Characteristics

Baseline characteristics included those measured at the index admission, including sex, age, ACS type and comorbidities as drawn from in-hospital diagnoses and drugs dispensed within five years of the index admission: hypertension, dyslipidaemia, cerebrovascular disease, diabetes, chronic renal failure, chronic obstructive pulmonary disease (COPD), depression and cancer. Patient clinical status was assessed by the Multisource Comorbidity Score (MCS) [19], a comorbidity index that has been shown to predict mortality and other clinical outcomes in the Italian population better than other commonly used comorbidity scores. Four comorbidity profile categories were established: good (MCS: 0–4), intermediate (5–9), poor (10–14), and very poor (≥ 15).

2.4. Clinical Outcomes

In-hospital mortality of the first cohort was recorded. Of those who survived the index hospitalization and the first year of follow-up (i.e., patients included in the second and third cohorts), (i) hospital readmission for ACS, (ii) readmission for any cardiovascular cause, and (iii) all-cause mortality were evaluated as long-term clinical outcomes.

2.5. Adherence to Recommendations

To evaluate the use of out-of-hospital healthcare services in the first year following index hospital discharge, the following information was recorded: (i) prescribed drugs, (ii) access to outpatient clinical controls, and (iii) cardiac rehabilitation programs. Adherence to each of these healthcare categories was studied separately.

With respect to medications of interest, the prescription of renin–angiotensin system blockade agents (angiotensin-converting enzyme inhibitors or angiotensin receptor blockers), beta-blockers, statins and dual antiplatelet treatment (DAPT) was recorded. Two drug therapy outcomes were recorded: (i) starting drug treatment (i.e., at least one prescription) and (ii) adherence to drug treatment. To assess the latter, the period covered by the prescription was calculated according to the defined daily dose (DDD) metric. However, since beta-blockers are likely prescribed at doses lower than those established for treating hypertension following myocardial infarction [20], the corresponding dosage was carefully chosen by a working group of experts (Supplementary Table S2). For overlapping prescriptions, the individual was assumed to have completed the former one before starting the second. Adherence to drug therapy was assessed as the cumulative number of days during which the medication was available divided by the number of days of follow-up (365 days), a quantity defined as the "proportion of days covered" (PDC) [21]. Cohort members were considered adherent to each drug treatment if they had a PDC >75%, and to overall drug recommendations if they were adherent to at least 3 out of 4 therapies.

As far as outpatient services are concerned, cardiology visits, echo-electrocardiograms, and lipid profile tests were considered. Cohort members were classified as adherent to services if at least one outpatient service was prescribed during the first year after the ACS episode. Subjects were considered adherent to the overall recommendation if they underwent at least 2 of the 3 services.

Finally, participation in an outpatient cardiac rehabilitation program was recorded and patients were considered adherent if they used the program at least once.

2.6. Data Analysis

The chi-square test, or its version for the trend, was used to compare the demographic and clinical characteristics of men and women of the first cohort. As the sample size affects whether the results are significant, and about 100 thousand patients were included in our study (Figure 1), the standardized mean differences were also computed to better interpret the results [22]. A between-group mean standardized difference of <0.1 was considered negligible.

Aiming to evaluate associations between sex and intra-hospital mortality, logistic regression models were used to estimate the odds ratio (OR) and 95% confidence interval (CI). Regression was controlled for baseline age, MCS and comorbidities at the index date.

Since men and women had different clinical profiles and clinical characteristics, propensity score matching was used for the second and third cohorts. Propensity scores were derived through a logistic regression model that included age, type of ACS and comorbidities at baseline as covariates. Men and women were 1:1 matched using the nearest neighbour matching algorithm [23].

Of the matched and unmatched patients of the second cohort, the probability of experiencing a specific outcome (ACS, cardiovascular event or death) from the day after the index discharge until the end of follow-up was estimated using the cause-specific cumulative incidence function [24], which takes into account the competing nature of the considered outcomes (e.g., hospital readmission for ACS or other cardiovascular causes likely affects the subsequent probability of death). With this approach, a subject belonging to the second cohort was assumed to experience only one outcome (the one which comes first), and overall incidence at a given time was calculated as the sum of the individual cumulative incidence functions for each outcome.

In order to highlight significant differences in the out-of-hospital healthcare of the men and women in the third cohort, adherence to recommendations was compared using the McNemar test and the standardized mean differences.

To assess whether out-of-hospital healthcare has a different effect on clinical outcomes between men and women, a stratification approach was adopted [25]. Adjusted proportional hazard regression models were fitted to the men and women of the third cohort to estimate associations between adherence to clinical recommendations and the clinical composite outcome (i.e., hospital readmission for any cardiovascular cause or death). Heterogeneity between sex was tested by Cochran's Q test [26].

All analyses were performed using Statistical Analysis System Software (version 9.4; SAS Institute, Cary, NC, USA). For all hypotheses tested, two-tailed p-values less than 0.05 were considered significant.

3. Results

3.1. Patients

Of the approximately 100 thousand NHS beneficiaries from the Lombardy region aged 40–90 years who were hospitalized for ACS from 2011 to 2015, 90,779 met the inclusion criteria for the first cohort, as shown in Figure 1.

There were 59,108 men (65%) and 31,671 women (35%), with mean ages of 67.6 and 75.1 years, respectively. STEMI was the most diagnosed type of ACS in both sexes (42% and 47% in women and men, respectively), followed by NSTEMI (36% and 33%, respectively) and unstable angina (21% and 20%, respectively). Women had more comorbidities (e.g., hypertension, COPD and depression) and a worse overall clinical profile based on the MCS (Table 1).

Table 1. Baseline characteristics of the 90,779 patients diagnosed with acute coronary syndrome in the Lombardy Region, Italy, 2011–2015.

	Whole Population (N = 90,779)	Women (N = 31,671)	Men (N = 59,108)	SD	p-Value *
Age (years)				0.66	<0.001
40–60	21,443 (23.6%)	3924 (12.4%)	17,519 (29.6%)		
61–70	20,798 (22.9%)	5368 (17.0%)	15,430 (26.1%)		
71–80	26,573 (29.3%)	10,063 (31.8%)	16,510 (27.9%)		
81–90	21,965 (24.2%)	12,316 (38.9%)	9649 (16.3%)		
ACS diagnosis				0.12	<0.001
STEMI	41,450 (45.7%)	13,366 (42.2%)	28,084 (47.5%)		
NSTEMI	30,812 (33.9%)	11,531 (36.4%)	19,281 (32.6%)		
Unstable angina	18,517 (20.4%)	6774 (21.4%)	11,743 (19.9%)		
Clinical profile †				0.31	<0.001
Good	22,808 (25.1%)	5503 (17.4%)	17,305 (29.3%)		
Intermediate	28,062 (30.9%)	9666 (30.5%)	18,396 (31.1%)		
Poor	29,323 (32.3%)	12,337 (39.0%)	16,986 (28.7%)		
Very poor	10,586 (11.7%)	4105 (13.2%)	6421 (10.9%)		
Comorbidities ‡					
Hypertension	66,561 (73.3%)	25,997 (82.1%)	40,564 (68.6%)	0.32	<0.001
Dyslipidaemia	34,649 (38.2%)	12,227 (38.6%)	22,422 (37.9%)	0.01	0.047
Cerebrovascular disease	7148 (7.9%)	2987 (9.4%)	4161 (7.0%)	0.09	<0.001
Diabetes	21,373 (23.5%)	7856 (24.8%)	13,517 (22.9%)	0.05	<0.001
Chronic renal failure	1042 (1.2%)	334 (1.1%)	708 (1.2%)	0.01	0.054
COPD	28,421 (31.3%)	11,104 (35.1%)	17,317 (29.3%)	0.12	<0.001
Depression	17,305 (19.1%)	9215 (29.1%)	8090 (13.7%)	0.38	<0.001

ACS: acute coronary syndrome; NSTEMI: non-ST elevation myocardial infarction; SD: Standardized difference; STEMI: ST elevation myocardial infarction ‡ Comorbidity and Multisource Comorbidity Score both measured according to hospital admission and drug prescriptions experienced five years before the date of index admission. † Multisource Comorbidity Score is a comorbidity index obtained from inpatient diagnostic information and outpatient drug prescriptions, validated using Italian data. Four categories of clinical profiles were considered: good (MCS: 0–4), intermediate (5–9), poor (10–14) or very poor ($\geq$15). * According to the chi-square test or its version for the trend.

3.2. Clinical Outcomes

A total of 2492 (8%) women and 2843 (5%) men died during the index hospitalization. Compared with men, the unadjusted odds of death were 1.69 (95% CI, 1.60 to 1.79) times greater among women. In-hospital deaths were equivalent between sexes after adjusting for baseline characteristics (OR: 1.02, 0.96 to 1.08) (Table 2).

Table 2. Odds ratio (OR) and 95% confidence intervals (CI) of the risk of intra-hospital mortality associated with sex. The first cohort was considered (see text).

	OR (95% CI)
Sex: Women vs. Men	1.02 (0.96–1.08)
Age (years)	
40–60	1.00 [Reference]
61–70	1.67 (1.44–1.92)
71–80	2.89 (2.53–3.30)
81–90	6.30 (5.23–7.19)
ACS diagnosis	
Unstable angina	1.00 [Reference]
NSTEMI	1.40 (1.28–1.53)
STEMI	2.16 (1.98–2.35)
Comorbidities ‡	
Hypertension	2.06 (1.85–2.30)
Dyslipidaemia	0.73 (0.69–0.78)
Cerebrovascular disease	1.28 (1.17–1.39)
Diabetes	1.15 (1.08–1.23)
Chronic renal failure	1.01 (0.81–1.25)
COPD	0.91 (0.86–0.97)
Depression	1.28 (1.20–1.36)
Clinical profile †	
Good	1.00 [Reference]
Intermediate	1.09 (0.97–1.21)
Poor	1.54 (1.38–1.72)
Very poor	2.57 (2.26–2.92)

ACS: acute coronary syndrome. ‡ Comorbidity and Multisource Comorbidity Score both measured according to hospital admission and drug prescriptions experienced five years before the date of index admission. † Multisource Comorbidity Score is a comorbidity index obtained from inpatient diagnostic information and outpatient drug prescriptions, validated using Italian data. Four categories of clinical profiles were considered: good (MCS: 0–4), intermediate (5–9), poor (10–14) or very poor ($\geq$15).

The 85,429 cohort members who survived the index hospitalization accumulated 273,228 person-years (86,189 in women and 187,039 in men) and generated 22,125 clinical outcomes (8780 in women and 13,345 in men). After matching, 20,079 couples were identified. The characteristics of cohort members included in the second cohort before and after matching are shown in Supplementary Table S3.

Before matching, women had more clinical outcomes than men (54% vs. 44%, $p < 0.001$), especially in the first year after the hospital discharge (30% vs. 23%, $p < 0.001$) (Supplementary Figure S1). However, after matching, men had a slightly higher risk of clinical outcomes at one year (28% vs. 30%, $p < 0.001$) and five years of follow-up (50% vs. 53%, $p < 0.001$). The cumulative incidence functions are shown in Figure 2.

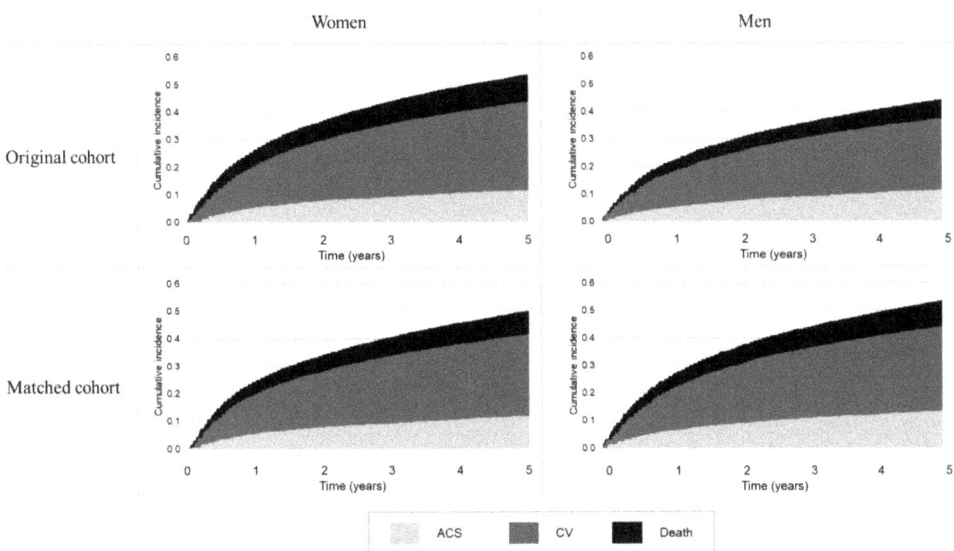

Figure 2. Cumulative incidences of health-related outcomes (ACS hospitalization, cardiovascular hospitalization, and all-cause mortality) among Propensity Score 1:1 matched and non-matched cohorts, according to sex.

3.3. Out-Of-Hospital Healthcare

Of the 63,442 patients who did not experience a clinical outcome in the first year after hospital discharge (i.e., patients included in the third cohort), 20,450 were women and 42,992 were men. The matching procedure identified 14,354 couples. Characteristics of the original and matched third cohort are shown in Supplementary Table S4.

In the original cohort, women were less treated than men in all out-of-hospital healthcare services according to the McNemar test (Table 3). Higher differences were observed for some drug therapies (statins and DAPT), cardiology visits, and cardiac rehabilitation (standardized difference ≥ 0.1).

Table 3. Exposure to healthcare management strategies in the first year after discharge from the index hospital admission for acute coronary syndrome. The third cohort was considered (see text).

	Original Cohort (N = 63,442)				Matched Cohort (N = 28,708)			
	Women (N = 20,450)	Men (N = 42,992)	SD	*p*-Value *	Women (N = 14,354)	Men (N = 14,354)	SD	*p*-Value *
Drug therapies Prescription								
Renin–angiotensin system blockers	15,285 (74.7%)	33,716 (78.4%)	0.09	<0.001	10,726 (74.7%)	11,346 (79.0%)	0.10	<0.001
Beta-blockers	16,372 (80.1%)	35,820 (83.3%)	0.08	<0.001	11,665 (81.3%)	11,696 (81.5%)	0.01	<0.001
Statins	15,988 (78.2%)	38,621 (89.8%)	0.32	<0.001	11,471 (79.9%)	12,578 (87.6%)	0.21	<0.001
Dual antiplatelet treatment	12,290 (60.1%)	31,995 (74.4%)	0.31	<0.001	8772 (61.1%)	10,257 (71.5%)	0.22	<0.001
Three out of four	14,596 (71.4%)	35,810 (83.3%)	0.29	<0.001	10,442 (72.8%)	11,600 (80.8%)	0.19	<0.001
Adherence §								
Renin–angiotensin system blockers	8772 (57.4%)	20,251 (60.1%)	0.05	<0.001	6165 (57.5%)	6829 (60.2%)	0.06	<0.001

Table 3. Cont.

	Original Cohort (N = 63,442)				Matched Cohort (N = 28,708)			
	Women (N = 20,450)	Men (N = 42,992)	SD	p-Value *	Women (N = 14,354)	Men (N = 14,354)	SD	p-Value *
Beta-blockers	8988 (54.9%)	21,005 (58.6%)	0.08	<0.001	6500 (55.7%)	6620 (56.6%)	0.02	<0.001
Statins	10,428 (65.2%)	29,711 (76.9%)	0.26	<0.001	7651 (66.7%)	9290 (73.9%)	0.16	<0.001
Dual antiplatelet treatment	6913 (56.3%)	20,527 (64.2%)	0.16	<0.001	5040 (57.5%)	6410 (62.5%)	0.10	<0.001
Three out of four	5966 (40.9%)	17,709 (49.5%)	0.17	<0.001	4396 (42.1%)	5507 (47.5%)	0.11	<0.001
Cardiac controls								
Cardiologic visits	14,461 (70.7%)	32,350 (75.3%)	0.10	<0.001	10,330 (72.0%)	10,597 (73.8%)	0.04	<0.001
ECO-Electrocardiograms	16,256 (79.5%)	35,668 (83.0%)	0.09	<0.001	11,588 (80.7%)	11,775 (82.0%)	0.03	<0.001
Test for lipid profile	16,524 (80.8%)	34,982 (81.4%)	0.01	<0.001	11,690 (81.4%)	11,708 (81.6%)	0.00	<0.001
Two out of three	16,230 (79.4%)	35,689 (83.0%)	0.09	<0.001	11,581 (80.7%)	11,779 (82.1%)	0.04	<0.001
Cardiac rehabilitation	413 (2.0%)	2092 (4.9%)	0.16	<0.001	327 (2.3%)	565 (3.9%)	0.10	<0.001

SD: Standardized difference. § Patients adherent to specific drug therapies among those who were prescribed at least one prescription of that treatment. * According to the McNemar test.

For example, 90% of men and 78% of women were prescribed statins, while the corresponding figures for DAPT were 74% vs. 60%, respectively. Among those prescribed drugs, men were more adherent to drug therapies (e.g., 77% vs. 65% among statin users). Only 5% and 2% of men and women went to cardiac rehabilitation.

Albeit the sex differences in all out-of-hospital healthcare services were confirmed in the matched cohort according to the McNemar test, some of these differences were reduced (e.g., cardiac controls) (Table 3).

3.4. Sex, Out-Of-Hospital Healthcare and Clinical Outcomes

The effects of out-of-hospital healthcare services on composite clinical outcomes are shown in Table 4.

Table 4. Hazard ratios (HR), and 95% confidence intervals (CI), of the risk of composite outcome (cardiovascular hospitalization or death) associated with exposure to out-of-hospital healthcare, stratified by sex. The third cohort was considered (see text).

	Men	Women	p-Value *
Out-of-hospital healthcare †			
Drug therapies	0.80 (0.75–0.85)	0.85 (0.79–0.92)	0.21
Cardiac controls	0.85 (0.79–0.91)	0.81 (0.76–0.87)	0.35
Cardiac rehabilitation	0.81 (0.67–0.97)	0.65 (0.48–0.87)	0.23

† Patients were considered exposed to dispensed drugs if they adhered to at least 3 out of 4 drug therapies; patients were considered exposed to cardiac controls if they underwent at least 2 out of 3 services. * Test for heterogeneity was considered.

Compared with non-adherent patients, those who adhered to drug therapies, outpatient services and cardiac rehabilitation programs had a lower risk of cardiovascular admission or death. There was no difference in the association between out-of-hospital healthcare services and clinical outcomes between men and women (all p-value > 0.05).

4. Discussion

The present study provides real-world evidence of sex-related differences in the health-related outcomes and out-of-hospital healthcare pathways of patients who were discharged after an episode of ACS.

At the time of their first ACS episode, women were older and had a worse clinical profile than men, findings confirmed by prior literature [27]. These characteristics may explain their higher risk of in-hospital mortality. Indeed, after adjusting for age and other baseline characteristics, there was no evidence that men and women had different in-hospital mortality risks. These results are consistent with those reported by the Italian National

Outcome Program [28], showing the absence of sex differences in short-term mortality post-acute myocardial infarction. Among those who survived the first hospitalization, several patients experienced a second episode of ACS or another related cardiovascular event, mainly in the first year after discharge. This observation highlights the importance of a timely and efficient therapeutic and surveillance program that may reduce the risk of subsequent morbidity/mortality and promptly identify subsequent cardiovascular events.

The novel findings of the present study, however, rely on observed sex differences in the out-of-hospital provision of healthcare services. Women were less commonly prescribed recommended drug treatments than men, especially DAPT (74% of men vs. 60% of women). Lower DAPT prescription rates among women were also observed in previous studies [29], and Moriel et al. suggested that this could be explained by a greater prevalence of renal failure in women with STEMI [30]. While several patients were prescribed other drug therapies (about 80% for renin–angiotensin system blockers, statins and beta-blockers), only approximately three out of five patients adhered to treatment. As supported by several prior studies [29,30], women who were prescribed drug therapies were generally less willing to adhere to them than men. Weaker differences were observed among outpatient controls and diagnostic tests. To the best of our knowledge, no prior studies have compared access to these services between sexes.

Finally, cardiac rehabilitation was utilized by nearly double the number of men compared with women, although these programs were poorly attended by both sexes (less than 5% of the whole cohort). Since the use of outpatient cardiac rehabilitation programs has consistently been shown to be associated with more favourable cardiovascular outcomes, including mortality [31–33], there is still significant potential for cardiac rehabilitation to improve the long-term prognosis of ACS patients.

The most remarkable differences between men and women in receiving medical care are reported by studies in the United States, where services are paid for. Women usually have lower incomes than men and this may, at least in part, explain the large differences observed. However, in the Italian setting, this problem should not be so relevant, as women and men have an equal right to healthcare services.

As international guidelines do not include different out-of-hospital service recommendations between men and women [34], and there is no evidence that adherence to out-of-hospital healthcare improves long-term prognosis differently in men and women, emphasis should be placed on the greater use of healthcare resources by men compared with women.

The present study has several strengths. First, it was based on a very large and unselected population, made possible by the inclusion of nearly all citizens in Italy's free healthcare system. Second, healthcare utilization databases provide highly accurate data, as all services claimed by the health providers for reimbursement by the Regional Health Authority are checked, and incorrect reports may have legal consequences. Finally, patients were identified based on their first hospitalization for ACS, allowing the complete sequence of post-discharge healthcare services supplied by the NHS to be identified.

Some limitations should be considered when properly interpreting our findings. Exposure misclassification may affect our findings in several ways. First, adherence to dispensed drugs was evaluated according to the DDD metric. Although guidelines do not recommend different drug therapy dosages for men and women, there may be differences in the prescribed dosage. Second, bias associated with our inability to account for out-of-pocket clinical evaluations, such as private cardiologist visits, should be noted [35,36]. However, estimates would not be biased if the use of out-of-pocket clinical evaluations similarly affected cohort members regardless of sex. Another limitation is that an intention-to-treat approach was adopted when considering healthcare exposure during follow-up, which was presumed to be consistent with the exposure level observed during the first year after index discharge, which may not be the case. Finally, like other administrative databases, the Lombardy database does not include clinical data (e.g., blood pressure), physical characteristics (e.g., body mass index) and lifestyle information (e.g., smoking status). In addition, the cause of death and other in-hospital data were not recorded in our database. Thus, we cannot examine the association between sex and intermediate clinical outcomes, and we cannot rule out the possibility that these unmeasured factors may confound associations between sex and clinical adherence. To minimize the potential for residual confounding, the propensity score matching design was adopted. Of course, this does not entirely avoid the problem of confounding, and thus further evidence is thus needed to confirm our findings.

5. Conclusions

Women were older and had a more compromised clinical profile at the time of their first ACS admission than men, which explains their observed short-term higher risk of death and cardiovascular events. Women were less treated and less adherent to clinical recommendations than men, although advantages derived from improved adherence to guideline-driven recommendations were expected for women just as much as for men. Tight out-of-hospital healthcare surveillance of ACS patients must be considered the cornerstone of optimizing the clinical outcomes of these patients.

Supplementary Materials: The following supporting information can be downloaded at: https://www.mdpi.com/article/10.3390/jcm12082972/s1, Table S1: Clinical diagnoses, drugs and outpatient services codes used for the study purpose; Table S2: Weights used to adjust the drug coverage of beta-blockers prescriptions; Table S3: Characteristics of cohort 2 members before and after matching; Table S4: Characteristics of cohort 3 members before and after matching.

Author Contributions: Conceptualization, G.C.; methodology, R.R., F.R. and G.C.; software, R.R.; validation, A.F. and A.P.M.; formal analysis, R.R.; investigation, R.R.; resources, R.R.; data curation, R.R.; writing—original draft preparation, R.R.; writing—review and editing, F.R., A.F., A.P.M. and G.C.; visualization, R.R.; supervision, G.C.; project administration, G.C.; funding acquisition, G.C. All authors have read and agreed to the published version of the manuscript.

Funding: This research was funded by the Italian Ministry of the Education, University and Research ('Fondo d'Ateneo per la Ricerca' portion, year 2019) and from the Italian Ministry of Health ('Ricerca Finalizzata 2016', NET-2016-02363853). The funding sources had no role in the design of the study, the collection, analysis and interpretation of the data, or the decision to approve the publication of the finished manuscript.

Institutional Review Board Statement: Not applicable.

Informed Consent Statement: Not applicable.

Data Availability Statement: The data that support the findings of this study are available from the Lombardy Region, but restrictions apply to the availability of these data, which were used under license for the current study, and so are not publicly available. Data are however available from the Lombardy Region upon reasonable request.

Conflicts of Interest: Giovanni Corrao received research support from the European Community (EC), the Italian Medicines Agency (AIFA), and the Italian Ministry of Education, University and Research (MIUR). He took part in a variety of projects that were funded by pharmaceutical companies (i.e., Novartis, GSK, Roche, AMGEN and BMS). He also received honoraria from Roche as a member of its Advisory Board. Other authors declare that they have no conflict of interest to disclose.

References

1. Ferrario, M.M.; Fornari, C.; Bolognesi, L.; Gussoni, M.T.; Benedetti, M.; Sega, R.; Borchini, R.; Cesana, G. Recent time trends of myocardial infarction rates in northern Italy. Results from the MONICA and CAMUNI registries in Brianza: 1993–1994 versus 1997–1998. *Ital. Heart J.* **2003**, *4* (Suppl. 8), 651–657.
2. Barchielli, A.; Balzi, D.; Pasqua, A.; Buiatti, E. Incidence of acute myocardial infarction in Tuscany, 1997–2002: Data from the Acute Myocardial Infarction Registry of Tuscany (Tosc-AMI). *Epidemiol. Prev.* **2006**, *30*, 161–168. [PubMed]
3. Amsterdam, E.A.; Wenger, N.K.; Brindis, R.G.; Casey, D.E.; Ganiats, T.G.; Holmes, D.R.; Jaffe, A.S.; Jneid, H.; Kelly, R.F.; Kontos, M.C.; et al. AHA/ACC guideline for the management of patients with non-ST-elevation acute coronary syndromes: Executive summary: A report of the American College of Cardiology/American Heart Association Task Force on Practice Guidelines. *Circulation* **2014**, *130*, 2354–2394. [CrossRef] [PubMed]

4. Ibanez, B.; James, S.; Agewall, S.; Antunes, M.; Bucciarelli-Ducci, C.; Bueno, H.; Caforio, A.; Crea, F.; Goudevenos, J.; Halvorsen, S.; et al. ESC Guidelines for the management of acute myocardial infarction in patients presenting with ST-segment elevation: The Task Force for the management of acute myocardial infarction in patients presenting with ST-segment elevation of the European Society of Cardiology (ESC). *Eur. Heart J.* **2017**, *39*, 119–177.
5. Piironen, M.; Ukkola, O.; Huikuri, H.; Havulinna, A.S.; Koukkunen, H.; Mustonen, J.; Ketonen, M.; Lehto, S.; Airaksinen, J.; Kesaeniemi, Y.A.; et al. Trends in long-term prognosis after acute coronary syndrome. *Eur. J. Prev. Cardiol.* **2017**, *24*, 274–280. [CrossRef]
6. Bansilal, S.; Castellano, J.M.; Garrido, E.; Wei, H.G.; Freeman, A.; Spettell, C.; Garcia-Alonso, F.; Lizano, I.; Arnold, R.J.; Rajda, J.; et al. Assessing the impact of medication adherence on long-term cardiovascular outcomes. *J. Am. Coll. Cardiol.* **2016**, *68*, 789–801. [CrossRef]
7. Choudhry, N.K.; Glynn, R.J.; Avorn, J.; Lee, J.L.; Brennan, T.A.; Reisman, L.; Toscano, M.; Levin, R.; Matlin, O.S.; Antman, E.M.; et al. Untangling the relationship between medication adherence and post-myocardial infarction outcomes: Medication adherence and clinical outcomes. *Am. Heart J.* **2014**, *167*, 51–58.e5. [CrossRef]
8. Worrall-Carter, L.; McEvedy, S.; Wilson, A.; Rahman, M.A. Gender Differences in Presentation, Coronary Intervention, and Outcomes of 28,985 Acute Coronary Syndrome Patients in Victoria, Australia. *Women's Health Issues* **2016**, *26*, 14–20. [CrossRef]
9. Lee, C.Y.; Liu, K.T.; Lu, H.T.; Ali, R.M.; Fong, A.Y.Y.; Ahmad, W.A.W. Sex and gender differences in presentation, treatment and outcomes in acute coronary syndrome, a 10 year study from a multi-ethnic Asian population: The Malaysian National Cardiovascular Disease Database-Acute Coronary Syndrome (NCVD-ACS) registry. *PLoS ONE* **2021**, *16*, e0246474. [CrossRef]
10. Haaf, M.E.T.; Bax, M.; Berg, J.M.T.; Brouwer, J.; Hof, A.W.V.; van der Schaaf, R.J.; Stella, P.R.; Gin, R.M.T.J.; Tonino, P.A.; de Vries, A.G.; et al. Sex differences in characteristics and outcome in acute coronary syndrome patients in the Netherlands. *Neth. Heart J.* **2019**, *27*, 263–271. [CrossRef]
11. Hao, Y.; Liu, J.; Liu, J.; Yang, N.; Smith, S.C.S., Jr.; Huo, Y.; Fonarow, G.C.; Ge, J.; Taubert, K.A.; Morgan, L.; et al. Sex Differences in In-Hospital Management and Outcomes of Patients With Acute Coronary Syndrome. *Circulation* **2019**, *139*, 1776–1785. [CrossRef] [PubMed]
12. Malacrida, R.; Genoni, M.; Maggioni, A.P.; Spataro, V.; Parish, S.; Palmer, A.; Collins, R.; Moccetti, T. A comparison of the early outcome of acute myocardial infarction in women and men. The Third International Study of Infarct Survival Collaborative Group. *N. Engl. J. Med.* **1998**, *388*, 8–14. [CrossRef] [PubMed]
13. Lin, C.F.; Shen, L.J.; Hsiao, F.Y.; Gau, C.S.; Wu, F.L.L. Sex differences in the treatment and outcome of patients with acute coronary syndrome after percutaneous coronary intervention: A population-based study. *J. Women's Health* **2014**, *23*, 238–245. [CrossRef] [PubMed]
14. Alabas, O.A.; Gale, C.P.; Hall, M.; Rutherford, M.J.; Szummer, K.; Lawesson, S.S.; Alfredsson, J.; Lindahl, B.; Jernberg, T. Sex Differences in Treatments, Relative Survival, and Excess Mortality Following Acute Myocardial Infarction: National Cohort Study Using the SWEDEHEART Registry. *J. Am. Heart Assoc.* **2017**, *6*, e007123. [CrossRef]
15. Hyun, K.; Negrone, A.; Redfern, J.; Atkins, E.; Chow, C.; Kilian, J.; Rajaratnam, R.; Brieger, D. Gender Difference in Secondary Prevention of Cardiovascular Disease and Outcomes Following the Survival of Acute Coronary Syndrome. *Heart Lung Circ.* **2021**, *30*, 121–127. [CrossRef]
16. Trifirò, G.; Gini, R.; Barone-Adesi, F.; Beghi, E.; Cantarutti, A.; Capuano, A.; Carnovale, C.; Clavenna, A.; Dellagiovanna, M.; Ferrajolo, C.; et al. The Role of European Healthcare Databases for Post-Marketing Drug Effectiveness, Safety and Value Evaluation: Where Does Italy Stand? *Drug Saf.* **2019**, *42*, 347–363. [CrossRef]
17. Rea, F.; Ronco, R.; Pedretti, R.F.; Merlino, L.; Corrao, G. Better adherence with out-of-hospital healthcare improved long-term prognosis of acute coronary syndromes: Evidence from an Italian real-world investigation. *Int. J. Cardiol.* **2020**, *318*, 14–20. [CrossRef]
18. Rea, F.; Cantarutti, A.; Merlino, L.; Ungar, A.; Corrao, G.; Mancia, G. Antihypertensive Treatment in Elderly Frail Patients: Evidence From a Large Italian Database. *Hypertension* **2020**, *76*, 442–449. [CrossRef]
19. Corrao, G.; Rea, F.; Di Martino, M.; De Palma, R.; Scondotto, S.; Fusco, D.; Lallo, A.; Belotti, L.M.B.; Ferrante, M.; Addario, S.P.; et al. Developing and validating a novel multisource comorbidity score from administrative data: A large population-based cohort study from Italy. *BMJ Open* **2017**, *7*, e019503. [CrossRef]
20. Goldberger, J.J.; Bonow, R.O.; Cuffe, M.; Dyer, A.; Rosenberg, Y.; O'Rourke, R.; Shah, P.K.; Smith, S.C.S., Jr.; PACE-MI Investigators. beta-blocker use following myocardial infarction: Low prevalence of evidence-based dosing. *Am. Heart J.* **2010**, *160*, 435–442. [CrossRef]
21. Andrade, S.E.; Kahler, K.H.; Frech, F.; Chan, K.A. Methods for evaluation of medication adherence and persistence using automated databases. *Pharmacoepidemiol. Drug Saf.* **2006**, *15*, 565–574. [CrossRef] [PubMed]
22. Austin, P. Balance diagnostics for comparing the distribution of baseline covariates between treatment groups in propensity-score matched samples. *Stat Med.* **2009**, *28*, 3083–3107. [CrossRef] [PubMed]
23. Austin, P. A comparison of 12 algorithms for matching on the propensity score. *Stat. Med.* **2014**, *33*, 1057–1069. [CrossRef]
24. Fine, J.; Gray, R.J. A Proportional hazards model for the subdistribution of a competing risk. *J. Am. Stat. Ass.* **1999**, *94*, 496–509. [CrossRef]
25. Buckley, J.P.; Doherty, B.T.; Keil, A.P.; Engel, S.M. Statistical Approaches for Estimating Sex-Specific Effects in Endocrine Disruptors Research. *Environ. Health Perspect.* **2017**, *125*, 067013. [CrossRef]

26. Higgins, J.; Thompson, S.; Deeks, J.; Altman, D. Measuring inconsistency in meta-analyses. *BMJ* **2003**, *327*, 557–560. [CrossRef]
27. Kawamoto, K.; Davis, M.; Duvernoy, C. Acute Coronary Syndromes: Differences in Men and Women. *Curr. Atheroscler. Rep.* **2016**, *18*, 73. [CrossRef]
28. *Programma Nazionale Esiti, Report 2021*; Ministero della Salute, 2021. Available online: https://pne.agenas.it/main/doc/Report_PNE_2021.pdf (accessed on 17 April 2023).
29. Mallidi, J.; Lata, K. Role of Gender in Dual Antiplatelet Therapy After Acute Coronary Syndrome. *Curr. Atheroscler. Rep.* **2019**, *21*, 34. [CrossRef]
30. Moriel, M.; Tzivoni, D.; Behar, S.; Zahger, D.; Hod, H.; Hasdai, D.; Sandach, A.; Gottlieb, S. Contemporary treatment and adherence to guidelines in women and men with acute coronary syndromes. *Int. J. Cardiol.* **2008**, *131*, 97–104. [CrossRef]
31. Ji, H.; Fang, L.; Yuan, L.; Zhang, Q. Effects of Exercise-Based Cardiac Rehabilitation in Patients with Acute Coronary Syndrome: A Meta-Analysis. *Med. Sci. Monit.* **2019**, *25*, 5015–5027. [CrossRef]
32. Sunamura, M.; ter Hoeve, N.; Berg-Emons, R.J.G.V.D.; Boersma, E.; van Domburg, R.T.; Geleijnse, M.L. Cardiac rehabilitation in patients with acute coronary syndrome with primary percutaneous coronary intervention is associated with improved 10-year survival. *Eur. Heart J. Qual. Care Clin. Outcomes* **2018**, *4*, 168–172. [CrossRef] [PubMed]
33. Rodrigues, P.; Santos, M.; Sousa, M.J.; Brochado, B.; Anjo, D.; Barreira, A.; Preza-Fernandes, J.; Palma, P.; Viamonte, S.; Torres, S. Cardiac Rehabilitation after an Acute Coronary Syndrome: The Impact in Elderly Patients. *Cardiology* **2015**, *131*, 177–185. [CrossRef] [PubMed]
34. Collet, J.-P.; Thiele, H.; Barbato, E.; Barthélémy, O.; Bauersachs, J.; Bhatt, D.; Dendale, P.; Dorobantu, M.; Edvardsen, T.; Folliguet, T.; et al. 2020 ESC Guidelines for the management of acute coronary syndromes in patients presenting without persistent ST-segment elevation: The Task Force for the management of acute coronary syndromes in patients presenting without persistent ST-segment elevation. *Eur. Heart J.* **2021**, *42*, 1289–1367. [CrossRef] [PubMed]
35. Gamble, M.; McAllister, F.A.; Johnson, J.A.; Eurich, D.T. Quantifying the impact of drug exposure misclassification due to restrictive drug coverage in administrative databases: A simulation cohort study. *Value Health* **2012**, *15*, 191–197. [CrossRef] [PubMed]
36. Pauly, N.J.; Talbert, J.C.; Brown, J. Low-cost generic program use by Medicare beneficiaries: Implications for medication exposure misclassification in administrative claims data. *J. Manag. Care. Spec. Pharm.* **2016**, *22*, 741–751. [CrossRef]

Disclaimer/Publisher's Note: The statements, opinions and data contained in all publications are solely those of the individual author(s) and contributor(s) and not of MDPI and/or the editor(s). MDPI and/or the editor(s) disclaim responsibility for any injury to people or property resulting from any ideas, methods, instructions or products referred to in the content.

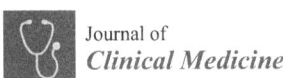

Journal of Clinical Medicine

Article

Sex Differences in Repolarization Markers: Telemonitoring for Chronic Heart Failure Patients

Federica Moscucci [1,*], Susanna Sciomer [2], Silvia Maffei [3], Antonella Meloni [4], Ilaria Lospinuso [2], Myriam Carnovale [2], Andrea Corrao [2], Ilaria Di Diego [2], Cristina Caltabiano [2], Martina Mezzadri [2], Anna Vittoria Mattioli [5], Sabina Gallina [6], Pietro Rossi [7], Damiano Magrì [8] and Gianfranco Piccirillo [2]

[1] Department of Internal Medicine and Medical Specialties, Policlinico Umberto I, Viale del Policlinico n. 155, 00161 Rome, Italy

[2] Dipartimento di Scienze Cliniche, Internistiche, Anestesiologiche, Cardiovascolari, "Sapienza" University of Rome, 00185 Rome, Italy; susanna.sciomer@uniroma1.it (S.S.); lospinuso.i@gmail.com (I.L.); myriam.carnovale@uniroma1.it (M.C.); andrea.corrao@uniroma1.it (A.C.); ilaria.didiego@uniroma1.it (I.D.D.); cristina.caltabiano@uniroma1.it (C.C.); martina.mezzadri@uniroma1.it (M.M.); gianfranco.piccirillo@uniroma1.it (G.P.)

[3] Endocrinologia Cardiovascolare Ginecologica ed Osteoporosi, Fondazione G. Monasterio CNR-Regione Toscana, 56124 Pisa, Italy; silvia.maffei@ftgm.it

[4] Department of Radiology, Fondazione G. Monasterio CNR-Regione Toscana, 56124 Pisa, Italy; antonella.meloni@ftgm.it

[5] Surgical, Medical and Dental Department of Morphological Sciences Related to Transplant, Oncology and Regenerative Medicine, University of Modena and Reggio Emilia, 42121 Modena, Italy; annavittoria.mattioli@unimore.it

[6] Department of Neuroscience, Imaging and Clinical Sciences, Institute of Advanced Biomedical Technologies, "G. D'Annunzio" University, 66100 Chieti, Italy; s.gallina@unich.it

[7] Arrhythmology Unit, Fatebenefratelli Hospital Isola Tiberina—Gemelli Isola, 00186 Rome, Italy; rossi.ptr@gmail.com

[8] Dipartimento di Medicina Clinica e Molecolare, S. Andrea Hospital, "Sapienza" University of Rome, 00185 Rome, Italy; damiano.magri@uniroma1.it

* Correspondence: federica.moscucci@uniroma1.it

Abstract: Aging and chronic heart failure (CHF) are responsible for the temporal inhomogeneity of the electrocardiogram (ECG) repolarization phase. Recently, some short period repolarization–dispersion parameters have been proposed as markers of acute decompensation and of mortality risk in CHF patients. Some important differences in repolarization between sexes are known, but their impact on ECG markers remains unstudied. The aim of this study was to evaluate possible differences between men and women in ECG repolarization markers for the telemonitoring of CHF patients. Method: 5 min ECG recordings were collected to assess the mean and standard deviation (SD) of the following variables: QT end (QTe), QT peak (QTp), and T peak to T end (Te) in 215 decompensated CHF (age range: from 49 to 103 years). Thirty-day mortality and high levels of NT-pro BNP (<75 percentile) were considered markers of decompensated CHF. Results: A total of 34 patients (16%) died during the 30-day follow-up, without differences between sexes. Women showed a more preserved ejection fraction and higher LDL and total cholesterol levels. Among female patients, implantable cardioverter devices, statins, and antiplatelet agents were less used. Data for Te mean showed increased values among deceased men and women compared to survival, but Te$_{SD}$ was shown to be the most reliable marker for CHF reacutization in both sexes. Conclusion: Te$_{SD}$ could be considered a risk factor for CHF worsening and complications for female and male patients, but different cut offs should be taken into account. (ClinicalTrials.gov number, NCT04127162.)

Keywords: myocardial repolarization; Tend; sex differences; chronic heart failure telemonitoring

Citation: Moscucci, F.; Sciomer, S.; Maffei, S.; Meloni, A.; Lospinuso, I.; Carnovale, M.; Corrao, A.; Di Diego, I.; Caltabiano, C.; Mezzadri, M.; et al. Sex Differences in Repolarization Markers: Telemonitoring for Chronic Heart Failure Patients. *J. Clin. Med.* **2023**, *12*, 4714. https://doi.org/10.3390/jcm12144714

Academic Editor: Andrea Fabbri

Received: 15 June 2023
Revised: 10 July 2023
Accepted: 14 July 2023
Published: 16 July 2023

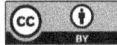

Copyright: © 2023 by the authors. Licensee MDPI, Basel, Switzerland. This article is an open access article distributed under the terms and conditions of the Creative Commons Attribution (CC BY) license (https://creativecommons.org/licenses/by/4.0/).

1. Introduction

Acutely decompensated chronic heart failure (CHF) is among the most frequent causes of hospitalization in Western countries [1], presenting a high mortality rate and a serious burden for patients' quality of life and for cost charges in the health systems. Mortality for CHF depends on sex, age, reacutization frequency, comorbidities, and severity of the CHF itself. According to recent evidence, proper early risk stratification and management could help reduce the burden of this chronic disorder [2]; thus, telemonitoring is promising and undelayable, using accurate prognostic markers for optimal risk stratification and early intervention for high-risk patients.

Aside from blood tests and echocardiography, electrocardiogram (ECG) is one of the essential tools in the investigation, management, and follow-up of heart failure among both in-patients and out-patients [3–6]. In particular, ECG is readily available, inexpensive, and could be a useful indicator of re-exacerbation in CHF patients [7]. However, gender-specific data of the prognostic value of ECG measurements are lacking.

As evidenced by many recent studies [8–14], heart failure in women shows extremely peculiar characteristics. In fact, a later age at the diagnosis [8] affects more women than men; less women receive implantable devices and resynchronization therapy [8,9]. These characteristics are strictly related to the protective role of estrogens during the fertility age; these hormones have been demonstrated to enhance the endothelial nitric oxide synthase (eNOS) role in the endothelium layer, ameliorating the flux-mediated vasodilatation, and preventing atherosclerotic and ischemic damage [10–12]. The physiopathology of the ischemic damage is strictly related to the endothelial dysfunction and micro-vessel damage [15–17], which, in women, lead to a CHF with a more preserved ejection fraction than in men [8]. For this reason, symptoms, clinical course, therapeutic response, and prognosis [13,18–20] (Table 1) are peculiar, and the repolarization ECG patterns [21,22] and specific markers of clinical curse and prognosis should also be evaluated [13,14,16,17].

Table 1. Peculiarities of chronic heart failure among women.

Specific Characteristics of Chronic Heart Failure in Women	
Pathophysiology	- Endotelial dysfunction, microvessel damage (diabetes, arterial hypertension, estrogens depletion after menopause, etc.)
Symptoms	- More severe weakness, reduced exercise tolerance, diaphoresis, more pronounced dyspnea, precordial palpitations
Diagnostic delay determining a later-in-life diagnosis	- High degree of polypathology, polypharmacy, and iatrogenic damage - Reduced access to the heart transplant - Exclusion from clinical trials
Difficult prognostic evaluation	- Scores/risk charts formulated on male models, and therefore not designed and studied for women - No score currently takes into account sex-specific risk factors.
High "revolving door" risk	- High costs for the health systems - Reduced patients' quality of life

Specific diagnostic and therapeutic interventions, together with an education program to enhance clinicians' and women's awareness, are desirable [23].

All in all, these patients, especially the oldest ones, frequently show an increased incidence of arrhythmias and electrical conduction disturbances (atrial fibrillation, premature beats, bundle branch block, etc.), so they are often excluded from trials [8], despite being the group with the more impaired quality of life and more severe lack of independence in everyday life activities.

Therefore, we studied the repolarization variables (thus, sinus rhythm was not necessary) in order to better understand sex differences in heart failure repolarization markers and to better estimate arrhythmic risk, and those variables were specifically customed for telemonitoring devices.

2. Methods and Materials

2.1. Participants and Protocol

A total of 215 consecutive symptomatic outpatients with acutely decompensated chronic heart failure (adCHF) were enrolled at admission to the Geriatric, Internal Medicine and Cardiovascular divisions of Policlinico Umberto I in Rome from January 2019 to October 2022, with an enrollment interruption of 14 months from March 2020 due to the SARS-CoV2 pandemic. Decompensated CHF were defined as patients with at least one symptom or sign compatible with a reacutization and a previous documented history of CHF, following European Society of Cardiology guidelines (2016 and 2021) [24,25]. At the time of hospitalization, all patients underwent full clinical history, physical examination, standard electrocardiogram (ECG) evaluation and transthoracic echocardiography, 5 min of II lead ECG (Miocardio EventTM, Rome, Italy) recording, and a blood sample for routine plasma tests (serum electrolytes, creatinine, urea, ultra-sensible troponin T, C-reaction protein -CRP-, and NT-pro Brain Natriuretic Peptide -NT-pro-BNP, etc.). Among the twenty-four hours before the planned hospital discharge, the patients repeated the 5 min ECG recording and the NT-pro BNP plasma level dosage. To assess the creatinine clearance, the Cockcroft–Gault formula was used.

2.2. Off-Line Data Analysis

A custom-designed card (National Instruments USB-6008; National Instruments, Austin, TX) was used to acquire and digitalize the ECG signals; the sampling frequency was 500 Hz. A single physician (G.P.) rechecked the ECG recordings in a single-blind manner. The same software was used to calculate the study ECG intervals, as described in detail in previous papers—LabView program (National Instruments, Austin, TX, USA). In particular, the following intervals from the respective time series in ECG recordings were analyzed: R-R mean (RR), Q-R mean (QR), Q-R-S mean (QRS), Q-T mean (QT), S-T mean (ST), and T peak to T end mean (Te) intervals (Figure 1).

To identify the repolarization intervals, we used a software originally proposed by Berger [26] and validated in other subsequent studies [4–7]. Moreover, we have analyzed the standard deviation (QTe_{SD}, QTp_{SD}, Te_{SD}) values for each of these repolarization phase intervals. Software for data analysis was designed and produced by our research group with the LabView program (National Instruments, Austin, TX, USA).

2.3. Statistical Analysis

All variables with normal distribution were expressed as means ± standard deviation, whereas non-normally distributed variables were expressed as median and inter-quartile range (i.r.) and categorical variables as frequencies and percentages (%). Subjects were grouped in 30-day deceased/survivors and positive to Januzzi NT-proBNP cut off/negative. Moreover, mortality, adCHF were analysed in male and female patients separately. One-way ANOVA and Bonferroni tests were used to compare data for the normally distributed variables; Kruskal–Wallis tests were used to compare non-normally distributed variables (as evaluated by the Kolmogorov–Smirnov test); and categorical variables were analyzed with the χ^2 test. Uni- and multivariable forward (A. Wald) stepwise logistic regression analysis were used to determine the association between mortality or worsening of CHF and other selected clinical and repolarization variables included in the study. In particular, it was considered dependent on variable 30-day mortality and, as covariates, on the following parameters: QTend (QTe) mean, QTpeak (QTp) mean, Tend standard deviation (Te)$_{SD}$ mean, QTend standard deviation (QTe$_{SD}$), QTpeak standard deviation (QTp$_{SD}$), Tend standard deviation (Te$_{SD}$). The same method was applied to NT-pro BNP Januzzi cut off with the same ECG variables as covariates. Stepwise multiple regression analysis was used to determine possible relationships between the studied variables. Receiver operating characteristic (ROC) curves were used to determine the sensitivity and specificity of the studied parameters predicting mortality and adCHF as well as areas under curves (AUCs), and 95% confidence intervals (CI) were calculated to compare the diagnostic accuracy in all patients but separately with males and females. All data were evaluated by use of database SPSS-PC+ (SPSS-PC+ Inc., Chicago, IL, USA).

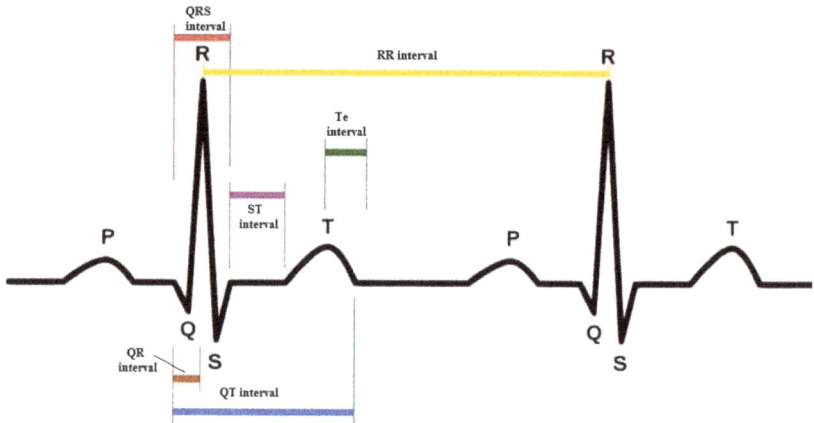

Figure 1. Intervals observed and analyzed during the 5 min ECG recordings.

3. Results

Considering the initial 239 eligible patients with symptoms of decompensated CHF, 24 patients were excluded because of poor-quality ECGs. Consequently, 215 CHF patients (M/F: 107/108) were finally studied (Table 2).

A total of thirty-four patients died (overall mortality rate, 16%, M/F:17/17), fifteen (7%, M/F: 6/9) died of bronchopneumonia and respiratory failure, fourteen of terminal heart failure (7%, M/F: 9/14), two of fatal myocardial infarction (1%, M/F: 1/1), and three of sudden cardiac death (1%, M/F: 1/2) (of the latter, two of sustained ventricular tachycardia and ventricular fibrillation, and one of acute "cor pulmonale" secondary to a massive embolism). Difference were found regarding causes of death among the two sexes (Table 2).

The general characteristics of the males and females were quite similar (Table 2) except for some data. In particular, women reported significantly higher levels of blood pressures ($p < 0.05$), HDL-cholesterol ($p < 0.05$), and LDL-cholesterol than the male group (Table 2). On the contrary, male patients showed a significant increase in the left ventricular mass index ($p < 0.001$), end-diastolic diameter ($p < 0.001$), and creatinine clearance ($p < 0.05$). Women had a more preserved ejection fraction ($p < 0.05$), while men showed a more frequent history of myocardial ischemia ($p < 0.001$), more premature ventricular complexes ($p < 0.05$), and left ($p < 0.05$) or right ($p < 0.05$) bundle branch blocks. Moreover, men have been implanted with a pacemaker or ICD ($p < 0.05$) more frequently than women (Table 2). Finally, women used statins ($p < 0.005$) and antiplatelet drugs ($p < 0.05$) significantly less often (Table 2).

Table 2. General Characteristics of the Study Subjects.

	All Subjects N:215	Male Subjects N:107	Female Subjects N:108	p
Age, years	84 ± 8	81 ± 10	85 ± 9	**0.003**
BMI, kg/m^2	24.3 ± 3.0	26.3 ± 5.0	25.3 ± 4.7	0.131
Heart Rate, beats/m	76 ± 15	73 ± 14	76 ± 12	0.214
Systolic Blood Pressure, mm Hg	127 ± 18	122 ± 19	129 ± 19	**0.010**
Diastolic Blood Pressure, mm Hg	70 ± 11	68 ± 10	72 ± 11	**0.005**
Left Ventricular Ejection Fraction, %	44 ± 9	40 ± 11	44 ± 10	**0.009**
Left Ventricular Mass Index, g/m^2	143 ± 29	145 ± 36	127 ± 31	**<0.001**
Left Ventricular End-Diastolic Diameter, mm	53 ± 6	56 ± 7	50 ± 7	**<0.001**
Posterior Wall Thickness, mm	12 ± 1	11 ± 2	11 ± 1	0.994
Interventricular Septum Thickness, mm	12 ± 2	12 ± 1	12 ± 1	0.629
Left Atrial Transversal Diameter, mm	47 ± 7	48 ± 6	46 ± 7	0.103
Tricuspid Annular Plane Systolic Excursion, mm	21 ± 5	20 ± 4	20 ± 4	0.956
Tricuspid Regurgitation Peak Gradient, mmHg	44 ± 15	44 ± 15	44 ± 12	0.836
Heart Failure with Reduced Ejection Fraction, n(%)	98(46)	58(54)	40(37)	**0.011**
Heart Failure with Mildy Reduced Ejection Fraction, n(%)	32(15)	13(12)	19(18)	0.262
Heart Failure with Preserved Ejection Fraction, n(%)	85(40)	36(34)	49(45)	0.079
NT-pro BNP, pg/mL	2895[7350]	2951[8235]	2865[6489]	0.886
C-reactive protein (mg/dl)	3.7[8.7]	3.4[8.4]	4.4[9.0]	0.127
High sensitivity cardiac troponin/(pg/L)	42[59]	43[60]	41[59]	0.365
Creatinine clearance (mL/m)	44 ± 25	53 ± 29	44 ± 31	**0.039**
Fasting glucose (mmol/L)	6.46 ± 1.93	6.48 ± 2.25	7.12 ± 2.46	0.057
HbA$_{1c}$ (%)	6.01 ± 1.20	5.87 ± 1.20	6.40 ± 1.49	**0.010**
Total Cholesterol (mmol/L)	3.70 ± 1.00	3.55 ± 1.01	3.85 ± 1.05	0.119
HDL-cholesterol (mmol/L)	1.13 ± 0.42	1.02 ± 0.33	1.15 ± 0.40	**0.048**
LDL –cholesterol (mmol/L)	1.99 ± 0.81	1.85 ± 0.81	2.16 ± 0.84	**0.041**
Triglycerides (mmol/L)	1.67 ± 1.49	1.80 ± 1.34	1.56 ± 0.91	0.254
Hypertension, n (%)	166(77)	80(75)	86(80)	0.395
Hypercholesterolemia, n (%)	98(46)	55(51)	43(40)	0.088
Diabetes, n (%)	90(42)	44(41)	46(43)	0.827
Renal Insufficiency, n (%)	105(49)	57(53)	48(44)	0.195
Known Myocardial Ischemia History, n (%)	75(35)	51(48)	24(22)	**<0.001**
Premature Supraventricular Complexes, n (%)	20(9)	14(13)	6(6)	0.057
Premature Ventricular Complexes, n (%)	48(22)	30(28)	18(17)	**0.045**
Permanent Atrial fibrillation, n (%)	76(35)	37(35)	39(36)	0.814
Left Bundle Branch Block, n (%)	44(21)	28(26)	16(15)	**0.039**
Right Bundle Branch Block, n (%)	33(15)	24(22)	9(8)	**0.004**
Pacemaker-ICD, n (%)	48(22)	32(30)	16(15)	**0.008**
Deceased Subjects, n (%)	34(16)	17(16)	17(16)	0.976
β-blockers, n (%)	144(67)	73(68)	71(66)	0.699
Furosemide, n (%)	166(77)	84(79)	82(76)	0.652
ACE/Sartans	87(41)	44(41)	43(40)	0.845
Aldosterone antagonists, n (%)	31(14)	14(13)	17(16)	0.579
Potassium, n (%)	15(7)	5(5)	10(9)	0.187
Nitrates, n (%)	28(13)	14(13)	14(13)	0.979
Digoxin, n (%)	10(4)	6(6)	4(4)	0.507
Statins, n (%)	64(30)	42(39)	22(20)	**0.002**
Antiplatelet drugs, n (%)	83(39)	51(48)	32(30)	**0.007**
Oral Anticoagulants, n (%)	61(28)	27(25)	34(32)	0.310
Diltiazem or Verapamil, n (%)	7(3)	2(2)	5(5)	0.254
Dihydropyridine Calcium channel blockers, n (%)	28(13)	13(12)	15(14)	0.705
Propafenone, n (%)	2(0.9)	0(0)	2(1.9)	0.157
Amiodarone, n (%)	19(9)	11(10)	8(7)	0.458
Valsartan/Sacubitril, n (%)	4(1.9)	2(2)	2(2)	0.993

Data are expressed as mean ± SD, or median [interquartile range], or number of patients (%).

Regarding the ECG variables, male subjects reported a significant increase in QR (49 ± 21 versus 44 ± 16 ms, $p < 0.05$), QRS (112 ± 35 versus 99 ± 32 ms, $p < 0.05$), QT (479 ± 91 versus 444 ± 75 ms, $p < 0.05$), and ST (366 ± 81 versus 345 ± 61 ms, $p < 0.001$) intervals than female patients. The other examined ECG parameters did not show significant sex differences. Considering all study subjects without sex division, the deceased patients reported a significant increase in Te (121 ± 77 versus 102 ± 26 ms, $p < 0.001$) and Te$_{SD}$ (9i.r6 versus 7i.r.5 ms, $p < 0.05$) in comparison to survival subjects (Figure 2A,C).

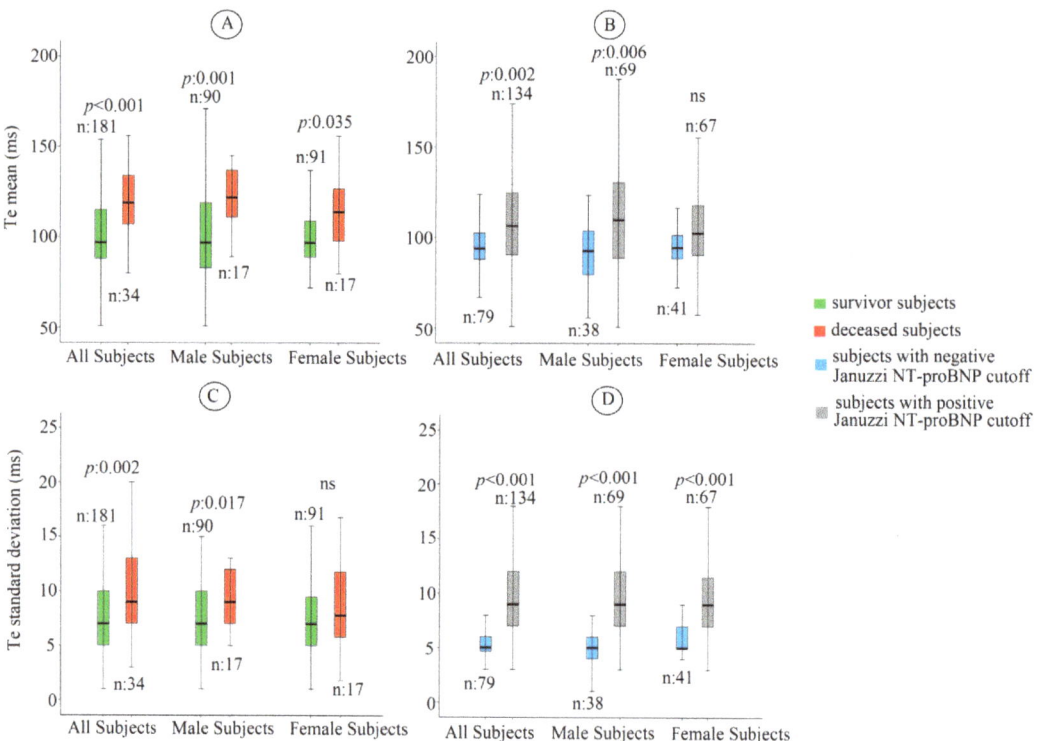

Figure 2. Te mean and Tend SD for survived patients and deceased ones (**A**,**C**) and for subjects with increased and normal levels of NT-proBNP (**B**,**D**).

Regarding the Te and Te$_{SD}$, males reported a similar trend (Te: 126 ± 23 versus 102 ± 28 ms, $p < 0.05$; TeSD: 9i.r.6 versus 7i.r.5 ms, $p < 0.05$) (Figure 2A,C). On the contrary, deceased women confirmed only the significant increase in Te (117 ± 29 versus 103 ± 26 ms, $p < 0.05$) (Figure 2A), but Te$_{SD}$ (9 i.r. 6 versus 7 i.r 5 ms, p: 0.062) did not reach the statistical significance (Figure 2C). Finally, we observed a significant increase in Te and Te$_{SD}$ in men (Te: 111 ± 30 versus 95 ± 23 ms, $p < 0.05$; Te$_{SD}$: 9 interquartile ratio—i.r.—5 versus 5 i.r.2 ms, $p < 0.001$) with higher levels of NT-proBNP (Figure 2B,D). On the contrary, the female patients with higher NT-proBNP levels only showed an increased Te$_{SD}$ (Te: 108 ± 28 versus 100 ± 23 ms, p: 0.114; Te$_{SD}$: 9i.r5 versus 5 i.q.2 ms, $p < 0.001$). Male CHF patients with higher NT-proBNP (Jannuzzi cut-off) showed a significant increase in QR$_{SD}$ (6i.r.7 versus 3i.r.5 ms, $p < 0.05$), QRS$_{SD}$ (8i.r.7 versus 5i.r.5 ms, $p < 0.05$), QT (497 ± 98 versus 448 ± 69, $p < 0.05$), QT$_{SD}$ (11i.r.5 versus 7i.r.6 ms, $p < 0.05$), ST (381 ± 91 ms, $p < 0.05$), and ST$_{SD}$ (9i.r. versus 7i.r. ms, $p < 0.05$). On the other hand, the female CHF patients confirmed a significant increase only for QT$_{SD}$ (10i.r.4 versus 7i.r.6, $p < 0.05$) and ST$_{SD}$ (9i.r.4 versus 7i.r.5 ms, $p < 0.05$).

All studied variables obtained from the last part of the repolarization reported a significant specificity-sensitivity curve for mortality (Figure 3A,C,E) and for high levels of NT-proBNP (Figure 3B,D,F).

The NT-proBNP levels were significantly related to Te$_{SD}$ (Figure 4A–C) in both men and women.

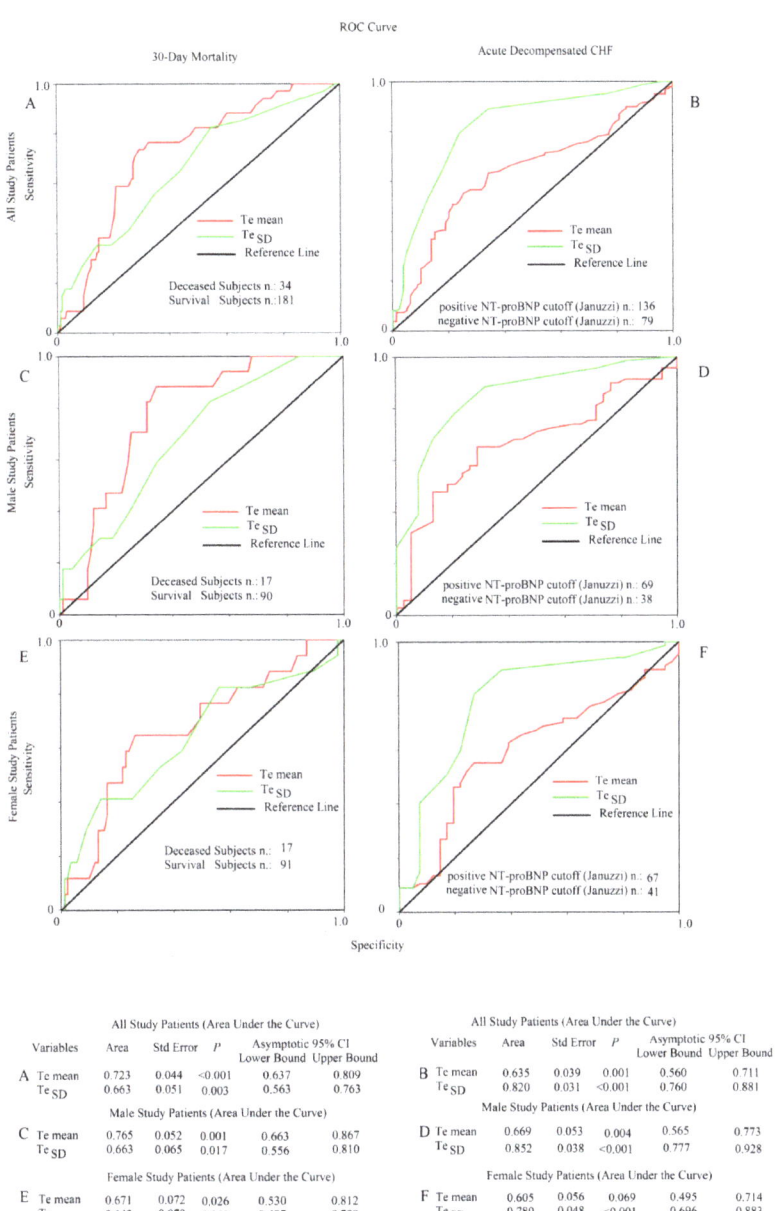

Figure 3. Receiving operating curves for Te mean and Te standard deviation for mortality based on NT-proBNP levels. (**A**) Mortality among all patients for Te mean and Te Standard Deviation (SD) markers. (**B**) Heart failure decompensation related to NT-proBNP levels among all patients for Te mean and Te SD markers. (**C**) Mortality among male patients related to to Te mean and TeSD. (**D**) Heart failure decompensation among male patients related to Te mean and TeSD markers. (**E**) Mortality among female patient related to Te mean and Te SD markers. (**F**) Heart failure decompensation among female patients related to Te mean and TeSD markers.

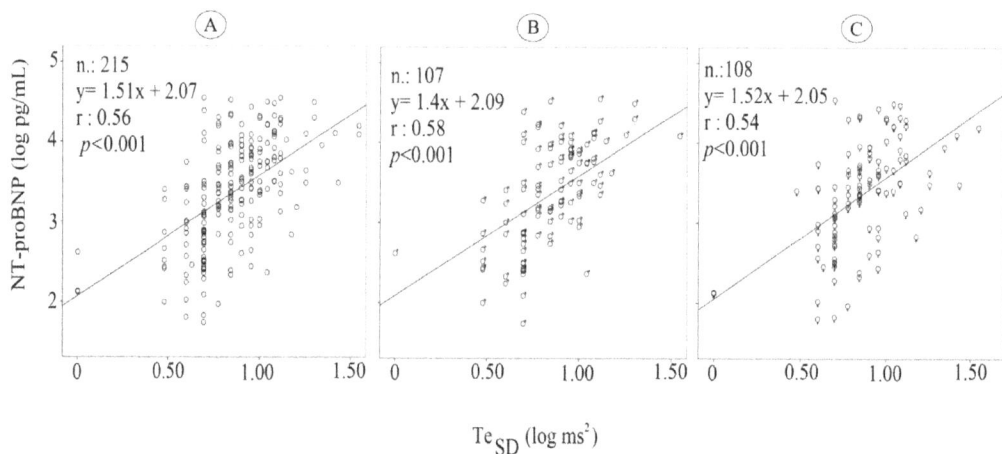

Figure 4. NT-proBNP and Te$_{SD}$ correlations in all patients (**A**), among men (**B**), and among women (**C**).

4. Discussion

The main results of our study demonstrated that male and female patients with CHF have different conditions and parameters to be considered in clinical practice [8,12,13]. As already highlighted in previous studies [8,19], women suffering from heart failure have a substantially more preserved ejection fraction than men (Table 2); this aspect is easily explained considering the CHF physiopathology, characterized by the greater prevalence of hypertensive heart disease, diabetic disorders, and microvessel impairment, rather than the well-known ischemic heart disease affecting the large epicardial coronary vessels among men. For these reasons, some authors have recently felt the need to reevaluate the guidelines and reinterpret the data from the clinical trials in the light of the known clinical and therapeutic differences that HFpEF shows [27]. This demonstrates how the scientific community has understood the importance of evaluating the various clinical phenotypes of heart failure in a more precise and selective manner in order to give increasingly appropriate and equitable responses to the clinical, therapeutic, and quality of life needs of patients, men, and women.

Moreover, from the data collected in our study, women presented higher values of total cholesterol, LDL, and blood pressure. Women frequently reach a late diagnosis [8] with a more severe clinical decompensation [19,28]. In addition, undertreatment largely depends on the erroneous belief that women, even with high cholesterol levels or hypertensive disorders, are protected during their fertile life by estrogens, which, as known, have a protective activity on endothelium and cardiomyocytes. However, the concept of "lipid-load" is increasingly affirming, deserving the clinical community's attention for a more appropriate use of anti-lipid agents even among young patients [29]. The same underestimation and undertreatment attitude often occur for hypertensive disorders [30]. Conversely, men had a higher left ventricular myocardial index, a sign of more severe hypertensive heart disease, and a better creatinine clearance. Women were significantly older, which was coherent with the epidemiological data in the literature [8].

In order to ensure correct monitoring, even remotely, of patients suffering from heart failure, numerous studies have been produced for the creation of devices and models for risk stratification of exacerbations and acute heart failure [31–34]. The effort to prevent reacutization must be undertaken using some routinely collected clinical data, such as those derived from ECG repolarization intervals and clinical biomarkers (NT-proBNP).

The Tend mean and the T end standard deviation have been shown to be effective in predicting the mortality of patients hospitalized for acute heart failure in various associated pathological conditions [3–5,7,35]. Moreover, they seem to be useful for intercepting those patients who deserve higher attention for progressive hemodynamic lability [3–5,7,34]. In our study, an accurate evaluation was carried out for disaggregated data by sex, which was guaranteed to highlight how the Tend SD, and not the Tend mean, is a reliable parameter in the female population for predicting mortality and reacutization in CHF patients.

These data will therefore be carefully considered in the creation of risk models as specific sex markers for specific cardiovascular preventions [36]. The use of electrocardiographic variables that take into consideration the ventricular repolarization marker for early risk stratification of adCHF patients is a promising field of clinical research [3–5]. In fact, together with the evaluation of NT-proBNP and the use of eHealth, artificial intelligence, and machine learning tools, it could be possible to produce predictive models with these inexpensive, easily available parameters for patient monitoring.

5. Study Limitations

An actual limitation of the study is the absence of patients treated with SGLT2 inhibitors. The sample was, in fact, largely studied before the recent indications provided by the European Society of Cardiology guidelines [25] on the use in class I evidence A of these drugs in subjects with HF and diabetes, hence the impact on repolarization, frequency of reacutizations, and clinical outcomes. Further enrollment in this registry will help fill this gap. Moreover, an interventional study could definitively assess the power and utility of such evidence.

Author Contributions: F.M.: conceptualization. methodology, data curation, writing original draft, validation, I.L., M.C., A.C., I.D.D., C.C. and M.M.: data collection, supervision, enrollment, final validation, S.S., S.M., A.M., A.V.M., S.G. and P.R.: conceptualization, project administration, software, resources, validation, D.M.: methodology, validation, writing—review and editing, G.P.: conceptualization, data curation, formal analysis, project administration, writing original draft. All authors have read and agreed to the published version of the manuscript.

Funding: This research has not received any financial support by private or public institutions.

Institutional Review Board Statement: Policlinico Umberto I Ethical Committee was informed of and approved the study. The ClinicalTrials.gov number is NCT04127162.

Informed Consent Statement: All patients at the moment of the test signed an informed consent, aware that their clinical information could be analyzed anonymously at any time for research purpose.

Data Availability Statement: All data, materials, and codes used in this study are available upon request from the corresponding author.

Conflicts of Interest: Authors deny personal or financial conflicts of interest regarding this paper.

References

1. Gallego-Colon, E.; Bonaventura, A.; Vecchié, A.; Cannatà, A.; Fitzpatrick, C.M. Cardiology on the cutting edge: Updates from the European Society of Cardiology (ESC) Congress 2020. *BMC Cardiovasc. Disord.* **2020**, *20*, 448. [CrossRef]
2. Sabovčik, F.; Ntalianis, E.; Cauwenberghs, N.; Kuznetsova, T. Improving predictive performance in incident heart failure using machine learning and multi-center data. *Front. Cardiovasc. Med.* **2022**, *9*, 1011071. [CrossRef]
3. Piccirillo, G.; Moscucci, F.; Corrao, A.; Carnovale, M.; Di Diego, I.; Lospinuso, I.; Caltabiano, C.; Mezzadri, M.; Rossi, P.; Magrì, D. Noninvasive Hemodynamic Monitoring in Advanced Heart Failure Patients: New Approach for Target Treatments. *Biomedicines* **2022**, *10*, 2407. [CrossRef] [PubMed]
4. Piccirillo, G.; Moscucci, F.; Mariani, M.V.; Di Iorio, C.; Fabietti, M.; Mastropietri, F.; Crapanzano, D.; Bertani, G.; Sabatino, T.; Zaccagnini, G.; et al. Hospital mortality in decompensated heart failure. A pilot study. *J. Electrocardiol.* **2020**, *61*, 147–152. [CrossRef] [PubMed]
5. Piccirillo, G.; Moscucci, F.; Bertani, G.; Lospinuso, I.; Sabatino, T.; Zaccagnini, G.; Crapanzano, D.; Di Diego, I.; Corrao, A.; Rossi, P.; et al. Short-period temporal repolarization dispersion in subjects with atrial fibrillation and decompensated heart failure. *Pacing Clin. Electrophysiol.* **2021**, *44*, 327–333. [CrossRef] [PubMed]
6. Baumert, M.; Porta, M.; Vos, M.A.; Malik, M.; Couderc, J.P.; Laguna, P.; Piccirillo, G.; Smith, G.L.; Tereshchenko, L.G.; Volders, P.G.A. QT interval variability in body surface ECG: Measurement, physiological basis, and clinical value: Position statement and consensus guidance endorsed by the European Heart Rhythm Association jointly with the ESC Working Group on Cardiac Cellular Electrophysiology. *Europace* **2016**, *19*, 925–944.

7. Piccirillo, G.; Moscucci, F.; Bertani, G.; Lospinuso, I.; Mastropietri, F.; Fabietti, M.; Sabatino, T.; Zaccagnini, G.; Crapanzano, D.; Di Diego, I.; et al. Short-Period Temporal Dispersion Repolarization Markers Predict 30-Days Mortality in Decompensated Heart Failure. *J. Clin. Med.* **2020**, *9*, 1879. [CrossRef]
8. Crousillat, D.R.; Ibrahim, N.E. Sex differences in the management of advanced heart failure. *Curr. Treat. Options Cardiovasc. Med.* **2018**, *20*, 88. [CrossRef] [PubMed]
9. Han, Z.; Chen, Z.; Lan, R.; Di, W.; Li, X.; Yu, H.; Ji, W.; Zhang, X.; Xu, B.; Xu, W. Sex-specific mortality differences in heart failure patients with ischemia receiving cardiac resynchronization therapy. *PLoS ONE* **2017**, *12*, e0180513. [CrossRef] [PubMed]
10. Shuaishuai, D.; Jingyi, L.; Zhiqiang, Z.; Guanwei, F. Sex differences and related estrogenic effects in heart failure with preserved ejection fraction. *Heart Fail. Rev.* **2022**, *28*, 937–948. [CrossRef] [PubMed]
11. Cesaroni, G.; Mureddu, G.F.; Agabiti, N.; Mayer, F.; Stafoggia, M.; Forastiere, F.; Latini, R.; Masson, S.; Davoli, M.; Boccanelli, A.; et al. Sex differences in factors associated with heart failure and diastolic left ventricular dysfunction: A cross-sectional population-based study. *BMC Public Health* **2021**, *21*, 415. [CrossRef] [PubMed]
12. Geraghty, L.; Figtree, G.A.; Schutte, A.E.; Patel, S.; Woodward, M.; Arnott, C. Cardiovascular Disease in Women: From Pathophysiology to Novel and Emerging Risk Factors. *Heart Lung Circ.* **2021**, *30*, 9–17. [CrossRef] [PubMed]
13. Scicchitano, P.; Paolillo, C.; De Palo, M.; Potenza, A.; Abruzzese, S.; Basile, M.; Cannito, A.; Tangorra, M.; Guida, P.; Caldarola, P.; et al. Sex Differences in the Evaluation of Congestion Markers in Patients with Acute Heart Failure. *J. Cardiovasc. Dev. Dis.* **2022**, *9*, 67. [CrossRef] [PubMed]
14. Prajapati, C.; Koivumäki, J.; Pekkanen-Mattila, M.; Aalto-Setälä, K. Sex differences in heart: From basics to clinics. *Eur. J. Med. Res.* **2022**, *27*, 241. [CrossRef]
15. Yerly, A.; van der Vorst, E.P.C.; Baumgartner, I.; Bernhard, S.M.; Schindewolf, M.; Döring, Y. Sex-specific and hormone-related differences in vascular remodelling in atherosclerosis. *Eur. J. Clin. Investig.* **2023**, *53*, e13885. [CrossRef]
16. de Miguel-Balsa, E. Risk stratification and health inequalities in women with acute coronary syndrome: Time to move on. *Lancet* **2022**, *400*, 710–711. [CrossRef]
17. Wenzl, F.A.; Kraler, S.; Ambler, G.; Weston, C.; Herzog, S.A.; Räber, L.; Muller, O.; Camici, G.G.; Roffi, M.; Rickli, H.; et al. Sex-specific evaluation and redevelopment of the GRACE score in non-ST-segment elevation acute coronary syndromes in populations from the UK and Switzerland: A multinational analysis with external cohort validation. *Lancet* **2022**, *400*, 744–756. [CrossRef]
18. De Bellis, A.; De Angelis, G.; Fabris, E.; Cannatà, A.; Merlo, M.; Sinagra, G. Gender-related differences in heart failure: Beyond the "one-size-fits-all" paradigm. *Heart Fail. Rev.* **2020**, *25*, 245–255. [CrossRef]
19. Sciomer, S.; Moscucci, F.; Salvioni, E.; Marchese, G.; Bussotti, M.; Corrà, U.; Piepoli, M.F. Role of gender, age and BMI in prognosis of heart failure. *Eur. J. Prev. Cardiol.* **2020**, *27* (Suppl. S2), 46–51. [CrossRef]
20. Regitz-Zagrosek, V. Sex and Gender Differences in Heart Failure. *Int. J. Heart Fail.* **2020**, *2*, 157–181. [CrossRef]
21. Bazzett, H. An analysis of the time-relations of electrocardiograms. *Heart* **1920**, *7*, 353–370. [CrossRef]
22. Surawicz, B.; Parikh, S.R. Differences between ventricular repolarization in men and women: Description, mechanism and implications. *Ann. Noninvasive Electrocardiol.* **2003**, *8*, 333–340. [CrossRef] [PubMed]
23. Moscucci, F.; Lavalle, C.; Politi, C.; Campanale, M.; Baggio, G.; Sciomer, S. Acute Coronary Syndrome in Women: A new and specific approach is needed. *Eur. J. Prev. Cardiol.* **2022**, *29*, e305–e308. [CrossRef]
24. Ponikowski, P.; Voors, A.A.; Anker, S.D.; Bueno, H.; Cleland, J.G.F.; Coats, A.J.S.; Falk, V.; González-Juanatey, J.R.; Harjola, V.P. 2016 ESC Guidelines for the diagnosis and treatment of acute and chronic heart failure: The Task Force for the diagnosis and treatment of acute and chronic heart failure of the European Society of Cardiology (ESC) Developed with the special contribution of the Heart Failure Association (HFA) of the ESC. *Eur. Heart J.* **2016**, *37*, 2129–2200.
25. McDonagh, T.A.; Metra, M.; Adamo, M.; Gardner, R.S.; Baumbach, A.; Böhm, M.; Burri, H.; Butler, J.; Čelutkienė, J.; Chioncel, O.; et al. 2021 ESC Guidelines for the diagnosis and treatment of acute and chronic heart failure: Developed by the Task Force for the diagnosis and treatment of acute and chronic heart failure of the European Society of Cardiology (ESC). With the special contribution of the Heart Failure Association (HFA) of the ESC. *Eur. J. Heart Fail.* **2021**, *24*, 4–131.
26. Berger, R.D.; Kasper, E.K.; Baughman, K.L.; Marban, E.; Calkins, H.; Tomaselli, G.F. Beat-to-beat QT interval variability: Novel evidence for repolarization lability in ischemic and nonischemic dilated cardiomyopathy. *Circulation* **1997**, *96*, 1557–1565. [CrossRef]
27. Desai, A.S.; Lam, C.S.P.; McMurray, J.J.V.; Redfield, M.M. How to Manage Heart Failure with Preserved Ejection Fraction: Practical Guidance for Clinicians. *JACC Heart Fail.* **2023**, *11*, 619–636. [CrossRef] [PubMed]
28. Nanna, M.G.; Wang, T.Y.; Xiang, Q.; Goldberg, A.C.; Robinson, J.G.; Roger, V.L.; Virani, S.S.; Wilson, P.W.F.; Louie, M.J.; Koren, A.; et al. Sex Differences in the Use of Statins in Community Practice. *Circ. Cardiovasc. Qual. Outcomes* **2019**, *12*, e005562. [CrossRef]
29. Setny, M.; Jankowski, P.; Krzykwa, A.; Kamiński, K.A.; Gąsior, Z.; Haberka, M.; Czarnecka, D.; Pająk, A.; Kozieł, P.; Szóstak-Janiak, K.; et al. Management of Dyslipidemia in Women and Men with Coronary Heart Disease: Results from POLASPIRE Study. *J. Clin. Med.* **2021**, *10*, 2594. [CrossRef]
30. Choi, H.Y.; Kim, E. Factors Influencing the Control of Hypertension According to the Gender of Older Adults. *Healthcare* **2021**, *11*, 1595. [CrossRef]

31. Imamura, T.; Kinugawa, K. Clinical insight of remote dielectric sensing-guided congestive heart failure management in outpatient clinic. *J. Cardiol. Cases* **2022**, *26*, 426–428. [CrossRef] [PubMed]
32. Olesen, A.S.O.; Miger, K.; Fabricius-Bjerre, A.; Sandvang, K.D.; Kjesbu, I.E.; Sajadieh, A.; Høst, N.; Køber, N.; Wamberg, J.; Pedersen, L.; et al. Remote dielectric sensing to detect acute heart failure in patients with dyspnoea: A prospective observational study in the emergency department. *Eur. Heart J. Open* **2022**, *2*, oeac073. [CrossRef] [PubMed]
33. Faragli, A.; Abawi, D.; Quinn, C.; Cvetkovic, M.; Schlabs, T.; Tahirovic, E.; Düngen, H.D.; Pieske, B.; Kelle, S.; Edelmann, F.; et al. The role of non-invasive devices for the telemonitoring of heart failure patients. *Heart Fail. Rev.* **2021**, *26*, 1063–1080. [CrossRef] [PubMed]
34. Piccirillo, G.; Moscucci, F.; Mezzadri, M.; Caltabiano, C.; Di Diego, I.; Carnovale, M.; Corrao, A.; Stefano, S.; Scinicariello, C.; Giuffrè, M.; et al. Electrocardiographic and other Noninvasive Hemodynamic Markers in Decompensated CHF Patients. *J. Cardiovasc. Dev. Dis.* **2023**, *10*, 125. [CrossRef]
35. Piccirillo, G.; Moscucci, F.; Fabietti, M.; Di Iorio, C.; Mastropietri, F.; Sabatino, T.; Crapanzano, D.; Bertani, G.; Zaccagnini, G.; Lospinuso, I.; et al. Age, gender and drug therapy influences on Tpeak-tend interval and on electrical risk score. *J. Electrocardiol.* **2020**, *59*, 88–92. [CrossRef]
36. Mattioli, A.V.; Moscucci, F.; Sciomer, S.; Maffei, S.; Nasi, M.; Pinti, M.; Bucciarelli, V.; Dei Cas, A.; Parati, G.; Ciccone, M.; et al. Cardiovascular prevention in women: An update by the Italian Society of Cardiology working group on 'Prevention, hypertension and peripheral disease'. *J. Cardiovasc. Med.* **2023**, *24* (Suppl. S2), e147–e155. [CrossRef]

Disclaimer/Publisher's Note: The statements, opinions and data contained in all publications are solely those of the individual author(s) and contributor(s) and not of MDPI and/or the editor(s). MDPI and/or the editor(s) disclaim responsibility for any injury to people or property resulting from any ideas, methods, instructions or products referred to in the content.

MDPI
St. Alban-Anlage 66
4052 Basel
Switzerland
www.mdpi.com

Journal of Clinical Medicine Editorial Office
E-mail: jcm@mdpi.com
www.mdpi.com/journal/jcm

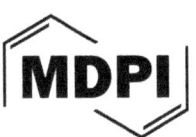

Disclaimer/Publisher's Note: The statements, opinions and data contained in all publications are solely those of the individual author(s) and contributor(s) and not of MDPI and/or the editor(s). MDPI and/or the editor(s) disclaim responsibility for any injury to people or property resulting from any ideas, methods, instructions or products referred to in the content.

www.ingramcontent.com/pod-product-compliance
Lightning Source LLC
LaVergne TN
LVHW070558100526
838202LV00012B/504